OXFORD MEDICAL PUBLICATIONS

Epidemiological methods in life course research

Epidemiological methods in life course research

Edited by

Andrew Pickles

School of Epidemiology and Social Statistics
University of Manchester
Manchester, UK

Barbara Maughan

MRC Social, Genetic and Developmental Psychiatry Centre
King's College London
Institute of Psychiatry
London, UK

Michael Wadsworth

MRC National Survey of Health and Development
Department of Epidemiology and Public Health
University College London
London, UK

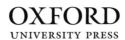

OXFORD
UNIVERSITY PRESS

OXFORD

UNIVERSITY PRESS

Great Clarendon Street, Oxford OX2 6DP

Oxford University Press is a department of the University of Oxford.
It furthers the University's objective of excellence in research, scholarship,
and education by publishing worldwide in

Oxford New York

Auckland Cape Town Dar es Salaam Hong Kong Karachi
Kuala Lumpur Madrid Melbourne Mexico City Nairobi
New Delhi Shanghai Taipei Toronto

With offices in

Argentina Austria Brazil Chile Czech Republic France Greece
Guatemala Hungary Italy Japan Poland Portugal Singapore
South Korea Switzerland Thailand Turkey Ukraine Vietnam

Oxford is a registered trade mark of Oxford University Press
in the UK and in certain other countries

Published in the United States
by Oxford University Press Inc., New York

British Library Cataloguing in Publication Data

Data available

Library of Congress Cataloging-in-Publication Data
Epidemiological methods in life course research / edited by Andrew Pickles,
Barbara Maughan, Michael Wadsworth.
  p. ; cm. -- (Life course approach to adult health series)
 Includes bibliographical references and index.
 ISBN 978-0-19-852848-7 (alk. paper)

1. Epidemiology -- Longitudinal studies. 2. Life cycle, Human -- Health aspects.
3. Lifestyles -- Health aspects. 4. Life change events -- Health aspects.
I. Pickles, Andrew. II. Maughan, Barbara, 1946- III. Wadsworth, Michael E. J.
(Michael Edwin John) IV. Series.
 [DNLM: 1. Epidemiologic Methods. 2. Data Interpretation, Statistical.
3. Models, Statistical. 4. Risk Assessment. WA 950 E627 2007]
 RA652.E64515 2007
 614.4--dc22

                                                                    2007009405

Typeset by Cepha Imaging Private Ltd., Bangalore, India
Printed in Great Britain
on acid-free paper by
Ashford Colour Press Ltd, Gosport, Hants

ISBN 978-0-19-8528-487

10 9 8 7 6 5 4 3 2 1

To Sara, Amy and Madeleine for
providing necessary distraction

Contents

Contributors

Adrian Angold
Associate Professor
Developmental Epidemiology
Department of Psychiatry and
Behavioral Sciences
Duke University Medical
School, USA

Paul Clarke
Senior Lecturer
Department of Epidemiology and
Population Health, London School of
Hygiene and Tropical Medicine
University of London, UK

Tim Cole
Professor
Centre for Paediatric Epidemiology
and Biostatistics
Institute of Child Health
University College London, UK

Jane Costello
Professor
Developmental Epidemiology
Department of Psychiatry and
Behavioral Sciences
Duke University Medical School, USA

Rebecca Hardy
MRC Senior Scientist and
Senior Lecturer
MRC National Survey of
Health and Development
Department of Epidemiology and
Public Health
Royal Free and University College
London Medical School
University of London, UK

Clyde Hertzman
Fellow, Canadian Institute for Advanced
Research
Professor and Director of the
Human Early Learning Partnership
University of British Columbia, Canada

Barbara Maughan
Reader in Developmental Psychopathology
MRC Social, Genetic and Developmental
Psychiatry Centre
King's College London
Institute of Psychiatry, UK

Andrew Pickles
Professor
Biostatistics, Informatics and Health
Economics
School of Community Medicine
University of Manchester, UK

Bianca De Stavola
Reader in Biostatistics
Department of Epidemiology and
Population Health
London School of Hygiene and Tropical
Medicine
University of London, UK

Camilla Stoltenberg
Associate Professor
The Norwegian University of Science and
Technology
Director of the Division of Epidemiology
Norwegian Institute of Public Health,
Norway

Michael Wadsworth
Professor
MRC National Survey of Health and
Development,
Department of Epidemiology and Public
Health
University College London
London, UK

Preface

Andrew Pickles, Michael Wadsworth
and Barbara Maughan

Although we tend to think of life course epidemiology as a recent development, in practice, pointers to life course effects began to emerge from some of the earliest epidemiological studies of individual differences in health. Widdowson, for example, asked why children having identical diets in two orphanages gained height at different rates, and found the adverse effect on height growth of a negative emotional environment.[1] Dubos *et al.* showed that 'when newborn animals are nursed by mothers fed diets that are slightly inadequate, their size remains subnormal throughout their lifespan, even though the young are fed an adequate diet after weaning. A similar depression of growth can be produced by subclinical infections shortly after birth'.[2] Reid presented evidence suggesting that the beginnings of adult-onset bronchitis might lie in childhood,[3] while Illsley and Kincaid noted in the findings from the first British national perinatal mortality study the 'strong implication that physical growth and development are related to later obstetric performance'.[4] In an article entitled *Biological Freudianism*, Dubos *et al.* concluded that 'socially and individually, the response of human beings to the conditions of the present is always conditioned by the biological remembrance of things past'.[2]

What distinguishes these researchers as forerunners of what is now called life course epidemiology is their pursuit of answers across different kinds of data sources and investigative methods, including ecological studies that looked at risk in age cohorts as children and adults, natural experiments, migration studies and follow-up studies. Like their predecessors, today's life course epidemiologists, whose scope, concepts and findings are brought together by Kuh and Ben-Shlomo in the first volume of this series,[5] use a wide range of investigative methods, have ingeniously sought new opportunities for quasi-experimental design and have patiently developed new sources of life course data. Our intention in this volume is to describe the methods now used and being developed to study individual differences in reaction to adverse exposures across the life course, and the mechanisms by which risk factors may influence present but, in particular, future health, that is the essential temporal and developmental aspect of life course epidemiology. A second, and equally strong theme is that of the permeability of health domains: the pervasive effects of stress on both psychological and physical health, the widespread occurrence of co-morbidity and the frequent co-occurrence of risk factors of varied kinds and environments that are toxic for a wide range of health outcomes. A third and increasingly important theme is the incorporation of genetics into aetiological models and analysis—and in particular in a form that progresses beyond the unproductive antithesis of nature versus nurture to investigate gene–environment interplay. The demands presented by these last two themes result in an additional distinctive feature of much of life course epidemiology, namely its highly interdisciplinary character—an appreciation that an understanding of disease aetiology will not come from any one discipline alone, and a recognition of the need to be familiar with the concepts and putative aetiological mechanisms of disciplines beyond one's own.

As a consequence, we have neither disease-specific chapters nor chapters concerning single disciplines, such as methods for genome-wide screening for disease loci. Instead, for the most part, each chapter focuses on a cross-cutting theme elaborating issues such as measurement, design and analysis likely to be important in interdisciplinary studies of almost any disease.

The book falls into two main parts, the first broadly concerned with design and measurement, the second with methods of analysis. Chapter 1 provides an overview of models of the development of risk throughout the life course, and how data sources to test these models are being developed. Chapter 2 deals with traditional and some new designs and measurement considerations for studies that focus on individual differences and processes. In contrast, Chapter 3 focuses on design and measurement in studies that examine mechanisms beyond the individual, where social interaction and context are key. Chapter 4 examines the promise of the very large (primarily cohort) studies, with designs that have been driven by the search for genetic effects, that are currently receiving heavy investment in a number of countries. Chapter 5 examines the conceptual background, potential scope and design of intervention studies of interest from a life course perspective.

The second part of the book deals with analytical issues. A common question for much life course analysis is how to analyse the effects of a time-varying exposure. Chapter 6 explains some of the complexities of this comparatively simple problem, and describes and illustrates simple and reliable solutions. Chapter 7 surveys alternative treatments for the ubiquitous problem of missing data. Life course research questions frequently involve a profile of health outcomes (either over time, or over a set of outcomes), that have both shared and distinctive predictors. The research questions are also often developmental, with a concern to identify pathways that might involve precursor stages, mediating variables and chains of effect. A central theme of Chapter 8 thus concerns analysis of a multivariate outcome and of sets of linked equations. However, the traditional concern of epidemiology to take account of the effects of confounders remains, and although life course data allow some new possibilities for tackling this problem, they also bring additional complexities of their own. Thus this chapter is also concerned to outline the range of approaches, both new and older, some more conceptual others more technical, that tackle different versions of the problem of estimating causal, as distinct from mere associational, effects. These include structural equation modelling and marginal structural modelling. Chapter 9 surveys the range of approaches that can be used for the analysis of event data, from the various forms of survival analysis, to trajectory analysis that yields a typology of developmentally distinct patterns of onset.

Finally, in the light of the arguments put forward in this volume, in an Afterword we briefly review the methodological challenges and difficulties of life course epidemiology, describing both the progress achieved thus far, and the work that remains to be done.

Preparation of this volume has been very much a joint enterprise. First and foremost, our thanks are due to our contributors, who responded so willingly to the request to share their expertise in life course research. In addition, we are grateful to the Series Editors for their encouragement and constructive guidance; to colleagues at the University of Manchester, the Institute of Psychiatry and the MRC National Survey of Health and Development for discussions that have shaped our thinking on life course issues over many years; to Angela Butterworth, Helen Liepman and Georgia Pinteau of OUP, for their expert help in smoothing our way through the production process; and to Sally Cartwright and Wendy Lamb, who assisted in several unenviable tasks with such care and good humour.

References

1. Widdowson EM (1951). Mental contentment and physical growth. *Lancet* i, 1316–1318.
2. Dubos R, Savage D, Schaedler R (1966). Biological Freudianism: lasting effects of early environmental influences. *Pediatrics* 38, 789–800.
3. Reid DD (1968). The beginnings of bronchitis. *Proceedings of the Royal Society of Medicine* 62, 311–316.
4. Illsley R, Kincaid JC (1963). Social correlations of perinatal mortality. In: Butler NR, Bonham DG, ed. *Perinatal mortality*. E & S Livingstone, Edinburgh, pp. 270–286.
5. Kuh D, Ben Shlomo Y, ed. (2004). *A life course approach to chronic disease epidemiology*, 2nd edn. Oxford University Press, Oxford.

Chapter 1

Introduction: development and progression of life course ideas in epidemiology

Michael Wadsworth, Barbara Maughan
and Andrew Pickles

Abstract

Increasing demand for life course data and life course findings requires developments in methods of modelling life course trajectories and analysis of life course data. In this chapter, we illustrate the progression of ideas in epidemiological life course studies, and the main strands of thinking about how risk develops and is modified. Innovative methods for obtaining life course data are described, and the reasons for development of new sources of life course data are outlined.

1.1 **Introduction**

For centuries there has been a fascination with the processes of human development and the extent to which early life influences adulthood. It is, however, only of relatively recent times that the subject has been systematically addressed. The social sciences and psychology have taken a broad approach to lifespan influence and development, ranging from Freud to Terman and Oden[1] to Elder.[2] The life sciences concerned with human mental health and development also have a long history of systematic research into life course effects,[3-7] as do those concerned with human physical health.[8-11]

Over the last 25 years, epidemiological thinking about life course processes has developed considerably. Studies of physical health have progressed from ecological comparative investigations of health and mortality in specific geographic areas at different historical times,[12,13] to identification of pathways over long periods of life,[11,14] and to hypotheses that suggest biological processes that may explain how the effects of environmental exposures and individual characteristics appear to affect biological function and disease risk.[15] In mental health, these kinds of studies have, in addition, shown direction and reversibility of effect, particularly in childhood[16] and in later life.[17]

These new insights have been facilitated by, and have also prompted, new approaches to data acquisition. New sources of data have been found for opportunistic use, for example follow-up of individuals who experienced serious difficulties likely to impact on health,[18,19] and the follow-up of populations identified from routine health or demographic records.[20,21] Life course studies that accrue new data have also greatly improved. The objective is no longer solely to identify illness and risk of illness, but also to measure function in order to study pathways to functional change with age.[7,11] For example, clinically validated scales have been developed that allow reliable identification of minor mental health problems, and screening for more severe ones, in large-scale studies.[22–24] Scales to measure memory and other aspects of cognitive function have been developed for use in studies of cognitive ageing,[25] and measures of well-being are being developed.[26] Improved measures of the social environment have been devised to capture, for example, the extent of social integration and support at the individual level[27] and in international comparisons.[28] More easily useable, valid and reliable biological measures have also been developed, for example of cardiovascular function,[29] and the collection of source material for making DNA can now be undertaken at home visits by data collectors with little training, or by self-administration.

During the same period, life course analysis methods used by epidemiologists have progressed from basic regression-based methods to those concerned specifically with the requirements of long-term epidemiological studies. Identification of life course pathways has been helped by development of methods such as latent class analysis,[30] and by multilevel modelling, sensitivity methods and Cox modelling.[31,32] Missing cases and missing values, that tend to become an increasing problem as long-term studies continue, are no longer simply omitted from analyses. Instead, as discussed in Chapter 7, cases are weighted, values multiply imputed or partial records included using increasingly sophisticated analysis methods that allow for varying degrees of selective loss.[32–34]

New demands for life course epidemiological studies of health, and new approaches to study design, are being driven essentially by three sources of influence. First is the increasing pressure to understand the processes of development of disease risk and of physical and mental ageing as the demographic structure changes, and as the care of chronic illness and disability, and the drive to prevent them early in the disease risk process, become dominant health activities. Second is the general acceptance that early life physical and mental development play a part in relation to most if not all outcomes of epidemiological concern, and need to be taken into account in life course approaches. Third is the new accessibility of genetic information about individuals.

The aim of much new life course epidemiological research is to replicate findings and re-test them in other social, geographical and historical contexts, and to investigate the roles that gene–environment interplay and gene–gene interactions play in life course pathways to disease risk and disease. Most of the existing data sources that have genome and good phenome characterization are on the margins of statistical viability because of their sample size.[35,36] Consequently, studies of this kind now need to pool existing life course data resources, and in the long run also to use the new and much larger sample size data resources in study samples currently in childhood or adolescence or in studies that are just beginning.[37]

The concern of this book is to show how life course epidemiology is handling the implications of the new demands through development of methods of measurement, and of data management and analysis. This first chapter sets the scene by outlining the development of life course thinking using examples from research on physical and mental health, and summaries of work on the measurement of the development of risk and resilience, and of how research has coped with the reality of less than perfect measures.

The second section of the book is concerned with study design in terms of measurement, dealing first with methods of studying individual differences, next with measurement of the effects of the social environment, and then with the new large-scale study designs, with genetically informed designs, and with the methods used in life course intervention epidemiology.

The third section reviews both conventional methods used in analysis of life course epidemiological data and the innovative methods required when using data covering many years of life.

1.2 Three summary examples of the development of life course ideas

1.2.1 A biological example

The biological example concerns cardiovascular health. Since this problem usually becomes evidently symptomatic in later middle life or the later years, and is manifest earlier in men than in women, the original British epidemiological prospective research into cause used samples of men and began in middle life, as did some important successor studies;[38,39] in the USA, the Framingham study was at that time a notable exception.[40] Risk was sought in obesity, current habits of diet, exercise and smoking, and in personality and temperament. Later, two ideas suggested the possible earlier beginnings of risk of cardiovascular disease, each concerned with exposure to a changing environment. Forsdahl[12] wondered whether children born in times of scarcity who did not grow well were then in effect programmed to handle poor diets. If they lived their adult lives in times of plenty, they would be more inclined than others to become obese adults and at risk earlier than others of raised cholesterol levels. Barker[13] observed in demographic statistical data that geographical areas of high premature heart disease mortality also had high infant mortality, and wondered whether the two phenomena were related. Migration studies showed that those born in low risk geographical areas tended to carry that level of risk, even after migrating to higher risk areas,[41] although that was not true of all kinds of risk.[42] Then came long-term follow-up studies that showed indicators of poor growth in early life (usually using low weight at birth) to be associated with raised risk of adult heart disease.[10,43] The biological programming hypothesis developed from that work stated that the lifetime resource of biological functional capacity was established in pre-natal and early post-natal life, and that subsequent challenges to that resource conditioned disease onset.[10] Subsequent work then asked what affected growth in early life, and what made the individual vulnerable initially to poor growth and to later challenge.[21] Consequent modification of the programming hypothesis was achieved by showing that the pathway from poor growth and poor socio-economic circumstances in early life to the disease outcome was influenced by other forms of risk, particularly that involving chronic exposure to stressful psychological and socio-economic circumstances in childhood and also in adult life.[44–46] Now new life course hypotheses about the development of heart disease risk have been developed that propose biologically plausible links between growth, the socio-economic environment and in particular exposure to chronic stress, using the hypothalamic–pituitary–adrenal (HPA) axis.[15] This is one of the first working examples of programmed progression. It helped to progress understanding of an apparent discontinuity between early life effects and later outcomes, and to explain individual variation in risk impact. Similarly Whincup et al.[47] point out the imprecision of earlier blood pressure measures in explaining intra-individual variation. New current work that is concerned with genetic sources of risk and their interaction with environmental exposures will continue that work.[37]

1.2.2 A psychological example

In contrast to much chronic physical disease, many severe psychiatric disorders—such as autism and hyperactivity—onset early in childhood; rates of others—such as depression— rise sharply in adolescence. We take depression as our 'psychological' example here. Like most psychiatric disorders, depression is now considered to be multifactorially determined: heritable influences are important, cognitive/psychological vulnerabilities are often evident, and many episodes are immediately precipitated by exposure to adverse life events or stress. From Freud onwards, however, theorists have also posited that early experience is a key determinant of vulnerability. Over time, empirical studies have tested and refined models deriving from this approach. In part, these efforts have focused on identifying the *source* of early risk: notions that parental loss might be the key element, for example, have gradually given way to an awareness that inadequacies in parental care are likely to constitute one core feature. Secondly, investigators have attempted to clarify the *mechanisms* whereby early adversity contributes to later risk. Brown and his colleagues,[48] for example, have proposed two pathways, one 'internal', operating via psychological vulnerabilities laid down in childhood, the second 'external', whereby adverse childhood social conditions operate via environmental or behavioural pathways to increase risks of later exposure to adult stress. Where childhood exposures are severe—as, for example, in the case of physical or sexual abuse— evidence now suggests that biological systems, including HPA function, may also be affected. Though depression *per se* is rare in childhood, it is now clear that depressed adults have often shown other emotional and/or behavioural difficulties earlier in development,[49] and prospective studies suggest that childhood risks may be especially salient for early onset of depression, beginning in the early to mid teens.[50] As with many physical disorders, the experience of a first episode of depression may also influence later risk: evidence suggests, for example, that associations with 'triggering' life events are stronger in first episodes than for recurrences, suggesting either a 'kindling' effect, whereby sensitivity to stressors is reduced as time goes on, or an increased stress sensitivity such that with repeated episodes, much more minor stressors are sufficient to trigger effects.[51]

1.2.3 A social example

Studies of antisocial behaviour and crime provide a third example of the insights emerging from a life course approach. Here, age trends typically follow a different pattern from that for chronic disease: in most Western societies, for example, rates of antisocial behaviour are relatively low in childhood, rise steeply in the teens, then fall again in the 20s and 30s. Cross-sectional studies in adolescence (the peak period for 'participation' in antisocial behaviour) have highlighted a plethora of potential risks. Criminologists were also, however, among the first to undertake long-term longitudinal studies, tracking outcomes for antisocial children later in life. These longitudinal data highlighted an apparent paradox. Looking backwards from adulthood, continuities in antisocial behaviour were strong: almost all severely antisocial adults have been antisocial in childhood. Looking forwards from childhood, in contrast, only about a third of antisocial children went on to have major criminal histories later in their lives,[52] although childhood exposure to parental separation has been show to be associated with a range of internalizing and externalizing outcomes.[53] Over time, attempts to reconcile these observations led to evidence that the overall 'pool' of antisocial individuals is made up of distinct subgroups, each with quite different developmental histories and sources of risk.[54] Childhood onset difficulties, for example, are often associated with both individual and environmental risks: neuropsychological deficits and adverse temperamental features appear to interact with adverse rearing environments to contribute to risk for 'life course persistent' antisocial behaviour. Adolescent onset difficulties, in contrast, seem predominantly socially determined, with peer influences and the adolescent 'maturity gap' playing key roles. As these issues have been clarified, so new life course questions have emerged. At the time of writing, two such questions are attracting particular attention. First, what accounts for the well-nigh universal desistance from crime observed in most individuals at some stage in adult life? Do childhood risk factors still predict behavioural trajectories later in development, or, as some investigators[55] have argued, do new adult experiences constitute the crucial 'turning points' that redirect trajectories later in life? Secondly, what accounts for the high rates of *heterotypic continuity* to risk for other mental health problems—including phenomena as seemingly diverse as depression and schizophreniform disorders—now known to be later sequelae of childhood and adolescent conduct problems?[49]

1.3 The progression of ideas in epidemiological life course analysis

These three examples show how initially observation, both clinical and epidemiological, began the progression of development of life course hypotheses. Explanations were then sought at the individual level for the nature and development of risk, why risk varied with age, what were the 'drivers' and transmitters of risk, and what were the modifiers of risk. The main arguments concerned with the development of risk are now summarized.

1.3.1 Critical and sensitive periods

Explanation for why risk was greater at particular ages in life asked whether it was because these were life stages uniquely sensitive to the processes hypothesized to be the sources of risk, and if so whether that was the result of intrinsic processes (e.g. because cellular development has a unique developmental period), extrinsic influences (e.g. exposure to poverty), or an interaction between them.

The concept of developmental stages is fundamental in both biology and psychology. It refers, in terms of age, to windows of opportunity during which a particular form of development normally occurs. Those windows are referred to as critical or sensitive periods: those terms are sometimes used interchangeably: critical in this context implies irreversibility.

Life course epidemiological studies of physical health in Britain initially suggested that factors that affected developmental progress *in utero*, particularly concurrent maternal health and the supply of nutrient to the fetus, were in effect also programming the future of the fetus in terms of functional capacity throughout the whole of life. This is known as the *biological programming hypothesis*.[13] The implication of determinism that the hypothesis originally carried was modified by the recognition that the environmental and social context of the critical or sensitive period was usually a defining aspect of the nature of the effect, and an indicator of how its effect was likely to continue. For example, poor maternal nutrition and exercise and maternal smoking that had adversely affected cardiovascular fetal development during a critical period of pre-natal development would also be likely to influence post-natal growth in adverse ways. Rutter *et al.*[16] further differentiated two kinds of developmental programming, experience-expectant and experience-adaptive. In experience-expectant developmental programming, 'normal somatic development *requires* particular experiences during the relevant sensitive phase of development if the somatic structure is to be laid down'.[56] Visual development is given as an example in which appropriate visual stimulation during early infancy is necessary for normal visual development. In contrast, in experience-adaptive developmental programming, 'somatic development, both structural and functional, is shaped by the specifics of experiences during a relatively sensitive phase of development in such a way that there is optimal adaptation to the specifics of that environment'.[57,58] This is exemplified by the effect of early life subnutrition that programmes the individual to function with low nutrition and thus for risk if richer diets are subsequently encountered.

Boyce and Keating (2004) describe sensitive and critical periods in neurological development in this way:[59]

> All the basic pathways involved in human emotion, volition, movement, and thought are already in place at birth, awaiting the experiential input that will propel latent pathways into the neural substrates of individual personalities, predispositions, talents and failings. Over the course of the next several postnatal months, this rich neural network is progressively 'pruned', selectively eliminating neurones (through apotosis, or programmed cell death) and synapses from the less utilised pathways and circuits. It appears that this process of neural elimination is as essential to the emergence of normal intelligence, behaviour, and mental functioning, as is the stage of neuronal proliferation that precedes it in fetal life.

Thus, a process of interaction between the developing organism and the environment, described by Boyce and Keating in the quotation above as 'experiential input', continues to affect the developmental course well after birth.[59] In some processes, such as height growth, that process continues until the late teenage years.

However, for some functions, one characteristic of early development continues to be detectable in the form of *tracking*. Tracking of some aspects of physical function (e.g. blood pressure, respiratory function) as well as cognitive function, refers to the likelihood of the individual remaining in the same sector of the measurement distribution at the population level throughout adulthood. Tracking implies that biological programming, in its original sense, is a valuable concept. However, it does not necessarily imply that a function cannot be modified, as shown by the rapidly increasing prevalence of medication that effectively modifies blood pressure.

Similarly the childhood social environment can also have a long-term effect, but the processes by which it does so are greatly varied. The processes are likely to include adverse continuing circumstances that retard physical and cognitive growth and development, such as poor nutrition, emotional insecurity and inconsistency, low intellectual stimulation, and parental smoking. In the long run, not all effects of adverse childhood circumstances are irreversible, and some forms of intervention to counteract adverse childhood circumstances seem very effective.[18,47,60] Effects of early life interventions are not necessarily measurable on a short time scale, and long-term life course studies have yet to show whether apparent reversal or mitigation of adverse childhood effects is sustained over many years of life.

Resilience is not yet a well-defined working concept in life course epidemiology. Resilience in the sense of resistance to vulnerability, has been shown to be associated, for example, with the quality of enduring relationships with partners and with high self-esteem. Childhood origins of such resilience have been found in habitual pro-social behaviour in the developmental period.[61] Examples of such resilience have been described by Rodgers,[62] Bifulco and Moran,[63] and Ryff et al.,[64] who showed that women vulnerable to adult depression because of emotionally disturbing experience in childhood were resilient to that risk if they were in a stable relationship in adult life. Resilience, in the sense of resistance to circumstances that are sources of health risk for many, has been shown in perceived high control of and reward from work circumstances,[65] but little is yet known about whether these perceptions originate in childhood. It has been suggested that chains of protection may develop from childhood 'that predispose towards the pursuit of health-protective developmental trajectories'.[59]

Pathways from early life to adult health have generally been modelled either in terms of a *latent effect* of an adverse impact in a critical or sensitive period, or in terms of a position on a *pathway* that begins at that time.[66] Latent effect models describe a source of vulnerability established during a critical period and eventually triggered into effect by an additional problem encountered later on in life, or by age. Pathway models, in contrast, describe the processes in terms of accumulating risk or cascades of risk, in which health risks or adverse social circumstances increase vulnerability to subsequent health risks and problems.

1.3.2 Development of risk

As these models imply, life course studies are also characterized by a focus on the development and elaboration of risk—whether biological, social, psychological or behavioural—throughout the life course. Effects associated with the biological processes of development, growth and ageing are considered in conjunction with the unfolding effects of life course variations in social circumstances, in psychosocial strengths, supports and vulnerabilities, and in the development of health-relevant behaviours, to build a comprehensive picture of age-related influences on health and disease. This emphasis on the development or *accumulation* of risk across the life course has proved important in two complementary ways. First, exposures at critical or sensitive developmental periods may be modified by later exposures: research in coronary heart disease, for example, has shown that associations with low birth weight are especially marked, and sometimes only apparent, in individuals who become obese later in life.[67] Similarly Rodgers showed that in women, vulnerability to depression was established through childhood experience of parental separation that was only triggered into depression by adult experience of separation from a partner.[62] Secondly, even in the absence of critical or sensitive period effects, risks may cumulate across development, with the number and/or duration of exposures gradually incrementing the overall burden of risk. Figure 1.1 (adapted from Kuh *et al.*[68]) provides a schematic illustration of some of the differing patterns of risk accumulation that have been described.

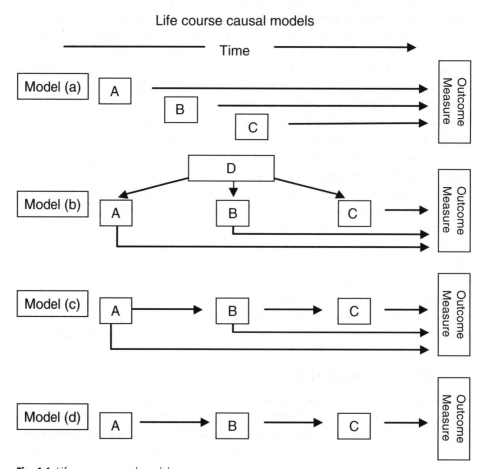

Fig. 1.1 Life course causal models.

Model (a), the simplest account, shows differing sources of risk emerging at different stages in the life course, each exerting independent, additive effects. Though some risk effects doubtless follow this pattern, empirical findings suggest that the more complex scenarios illustrated in later models are in practice far more typical. Model (b) illustrates a *clustering* of risks, whereby an exposure at one life stage gives rise to a range of more specific risk processes. Poor social circumstances in childhood, for example, may contribute to risk for later respiratory disease through a variety of different processes, some environmental (through poor early nutrition, or exposure to effects of passive smoking), some biological (through effects of intrauterine growth on lung development and risk of early infection) and some behavioural (through increased risk of later smoking or poor diet).

In Model (b), each of these pathways has distinct and separable effects on disease outcome. Models (c) and (d) illustrate more complex patterns, whereby early risk factors impact not only on final disease outcome but also on the likelihood of later risk exposures. To pursue our socio-economic status (SES) example: poor childhood SES may contribute directly to risk for lung disease through exposure to early adverse environmental conditions. Low SES may also, however, influence progress on other risk pathways—constraining educational attainments, for example, or affecting the development of poor health behaviours—which, later in the life course, may contribute independently to risk. *Pathways* models of this kind have attracted increasing attention in charting the elaboration of risk processes for a wide range of both physical and mental health outcomes. In relation to mental health difficulties, behavioural styles set up in childhood may function to 'select' individuals into stress-prone environments (physical, social or relational) later in life. Severe antisocial behaviour in childhood, for example, is known to have wide-ranging effects on later social functioning, spanning problems in employment, in making and maintaining close relationships and in increased risks of alcohol and drug use.[69] Though largely dependent on prior behaviours, these 'intermediate' outcomes could in themselves compromise social circumstances, reduce the availability of supports and give rise to stressors, so heightening risk for both physical and mental health problems later in life. Models (c) and (d) illustrate differing ideal-type processes whereby effects of this kind might be carried forward. Model (c) is the most complex, suggesting separable effects on both later risk exposures and on ultimate outcomes. Model (d) is a special case of this model—sometimes referred to in terms of *chains of risk* or *stepping stone* effects—whereby early risk factors are primarily or exclusively important in increasing exposure to later risks. If progression from risk A to risk B can be halted—if the chain can, as it were, be broken—the likelihood of disease outcome is eliminated or greatly reduced.

These models suggest dynamic processes of risk accumulation across the life course, varying among individuals. Sociological models of the life course (see, for example, Elder and Shanahan[2]) have proposed a variety of constructs that have proved helpful in conceptualizing dynamic processes of this kind. Following these formulations, diverse aspects of the life course can be characterized in terms of developmental *trajectories* (spanning relatively extended developmental periods), punctuated by *transitions* between individual states. Trajectories may be defined in terms of social statuses such as employment or marriage and parenthood, psychological states such as the experience of depressive episodes, or physiological states such as blood pressure or the development and decline in lung function. Transitions on an employment trajectory might include moving from school to work; promotions or periods of unemployment; and eventual moves to retirement. Transitions on trajectory of blood pressure might mark changes from low to somewhat elevated risk, and later into the pathogenic range.

As these examples suggest, individuals will vary in their relative positions on any specific trajectory. In some instances it may be appropriate to envisage a single underlying 'normative' trajectory, around which individuals deviate. Increasingly, however, researchers in the behavioural domain are using newly developed statistical tools (see, for example, Nagin and Land[70] and Chapter 9) to group individuals into *trajectory classes* based on repeated measures of their behaviour over time. In relation to childhood conduct problems, for example, studies typically identify three or four main trajectory classes, one (usually large) compromising children who are rarely if ever antisocial, a second (usually small) who show consistently high rates of aggression or rule-breaking at each measurement point, and others that show rising or falling rates of difficulty across developmental time.[71] Similar approaches are now being applied to aspects of physical development,[72] and to characterize population heterogeneity in vulnerability to affective disturbances.[73] The use of trajectory classes of this kind may add precision in the identification of risk processes, and models of differing trajectory class memberships could of course be applied to dynamic variations in risk exposures just as much as to health or behavioural outcomes.

Transitions in the course of developmental trajectories—changes from one state to another—may be of interest from a variety of perspectives. In some cases, their *timing* may be salient for later outcomes: though young people vary widely in their ages at and rates of pubertal development, for example, studies suggest that being markedly 'off-time' (either early or late) in relation to age-peers can increase vulnerability to psychological distress.[74] In other instances, the patterning of transitions, or their inter-relationships across trajectories, may be of concern: very early childbearing, for example, before the completion of education, and especially if embarked upon without regular support from a partner, is associated with adverse outcomes for both mother and child.[75] While many transitions are normative, and typically lead to incremental progress along an established trajectory, some changes are more major, and lead to a marked redirection in development. *Turning points* of this kind may occur in a variety of domains; to date, they have been examined most widely in relation to experiences which contribute to previously high-rate offenders' desistance from crime.[76]

As risk factors accumulate, so does the process of disease. In common with other branches of epidemiology, life course studies have been concerned with a variety of issues and distinctions here. First, the term *embodiment* is used to describe processes whereby extrinsic factors (whether associated with developments at critical periods, learning, insult or trauma, or repair) are inscribed in the body's functions or structures—how, as it were, risk or protective factors 'get under the skin'.[77] Though much research focuses on *risk factors*, understanding *risk mechanisms* of this kind may be critical not only to advance in theory, but also to the development of appropriate interventions, as Hertzman discusses in the Chapter 5. Secondly, life course researchers are often concerned to trace *induction periods* (the time between exposure and the onset of a disease process) and *latency periods* (the time between disease onset and detection).[78] In practice, distinctions of this kind are often difficult to determine: disease processes may begin before symptoms are apparent, and symptoms themselves may only be recognized when individuals make contact with a healthcare system. In some psychiatric disorders (especially in relation to psychoses), interest has also centred on identifying *prodromal* states in at-risk individuals, when social functioning begins to deteriorate and some symptoms are evident, but before the full disorder is manifest. Here too, however, ambiguities have arisen as longitudinal studies have traced apparently meaningful behavioural precursors much earlier in development.[79] Should these too be regarded as part of the prodrome (though they affect much larger groups than those who eventually develop psychoses), or are they more appropriately regarded as risk or vulnerability factors for disorder? What accounts for transitions from precursors to prodrome, and from prodrome to the development of full psychotic states? As some life course questions have been answered, so others continue to emerge, contributing to an iterative process of refinement of both hypotheses and substantive knowledge.

1.3.3 Modification of risk

Up to this point, the discussion has proceeded as though the impact of risk factors is the same for all individuals. In practice, of course, we know that this is far from the case: risk–outcome associations are probabilistic rather than deterministic and, even when exceptionally robust risk associations have been demonstrated (such as, for example, the link between smoking and lung cancer), or when individuals have faced exceptionally severe insults (such as exposure to major trauma), variability in outcomes is common. This in turn suggests that modification of risk—whether associated with variations in individual characteristics or prior risk exposure—is also common, and will often require explicit examination in life course research.

A wide variety of factors may be implicated in risk moderation of this kind. Especially in long-term longitudinal studies, effects of later-life risk exposures may depend heavily on variations in vulnerability or resilience set up earlier in development. In addition, individual characteristics are also likely to be key. The wide-ranging evidence for sex-based differences in biology,[80] for example, in conjunction with gender differences in many health-related roles and expectations, makes examination of sex differences in risk impact and processes a core element in much epidemiological enquiry; racial/ethnic variations, and differential effects depending on developmental timing of exposures, are also of central concern in life course research. In recent years, some of the most exciting developments have been in the area of gene–environment interplay, with demonstrations that the impact of risk exposures varies systematically with aspects of the individual's genotype.[79] In relation to cardiovascular disease, for example, replicated findings have now shown that associations between high dietary fat intake and abnormal high-density lipoprotein (HDL) cholesterol concentrations depend on individuals' genotype on the polymorphic hepatic lipase (HL) gene promoter,[81,82] while in the mental health arena risk for depression in the face of adverse life events has been shown to depend on variations in a functional polymorphism in the promoter region of the serotonin transporter gene.[83] Shanahan and Hofer[84] have proposed four 'ideal-type' models whereby genetic influences may vary according to environmental circumstances. First, as suggested by the examples cited above, environmental influences may trigger genetic susceptibilities. Secondly, social context factors may compensate for a genetic diathesis, in some instances reflecting a positive protective effect. Thirdly, environmental constraints may reduce the role of genetic influences; and fourthly, environmental contexts may accentuate or enhance individual differences arising from genetically based variations. In the mental health field in particular, investigators have highlighted the importance of gene–environment correlations—processes whereby genetically influenced traits in parents affect the environments they provide for children, or individually based traits contribute to the 'selection' of environments that function to reinforce existing behaviours—that are likely to offer major advances in life course studies of the development of disease risk.

1.3.4 Cohort effects

Many chronic diseases (see, for example, Strachan and Perry[85]) and psychosocial disorders[86] have shown marked and sometimes dramatic variations in reported prevalence over recent decades. Though often difficult to interpret because of associated changes in reporting and recording practices, where reliable underlying trends can be documented they have the potential to make important contributions to the understanding of life course influences on health. Two prime sources of effects may be involved: *period effects*, evident when changes in rate occur for individuals in different age groups at the same historical period, and *cohort effects*, evident when age-specific rates rise and fall when plotted by year of birth (cohort). When changes in prevalence are steady and linear, it is not feasible to distinguish these two sources of influence; non-linear variations can, however, more confidently be interpreted as either period or cohort effects.

Cohort effects may be associated with delayed consequences of biological programming or variations in developments at critical periods. Equally, variations in later life exposures may also be involved: cohort-related sex differences in lung cancer incidence in Britain, for example, relate to the fact that women took up smoking several decades after men.[85] Cohort differences can provide opportunities for hypothesis testing; for instance, the marked differences in breastfeeding and diet in infancy (protective factors against infant pulmonary illness, itself a long-term risk to adult respiratory health) in post-war British cohorts, as well as in exposure to atmospheric pollution from coal burning, should bring corresponding differences in later risk of respiratory illness.[87,88]

1.3.5 Analytic strategies

Life course epidemiology is concerned with two kinds of outcomes. First are events, such as the onset of illness or disability, or the occurrence of death, that can be seen in relation to age at onset and to exposure to risk and protective factors before onset. Second are incremental health changes, for example in the processes of development and in ageing. Risk and protective factors are, similarly, seen in terms of age at exposure and length of exposure, and the outcomes and the risk and protective factors are seen in a changing social context.

These dynamic aspects of measures and risk and protective factors greatly extend the analyst's opportunities. Information on sequence of risk and protective exposure, on the timing of events and the duration of episodes makes it possible to hypothesize causal effects, and pathways from initial exposure to onset or to a specific degree of change, for instance in cognitive function. Information on sequence also makes it possible to hypothesize how exposure to risk develops, whether an initial risk effect on an outcome distant in life history terms (such as the hypothesized effect of low weight at birth on adult blood pressure) intensifies or decays with age and/or time elapsed, and whether an initial effect acts equally on all sample members or whether an interaction with another factor is required for the outcome to occur. Information about many years of the individual's life makes it possible to compare patterns of development (such as height growth or bladder control) in relation to later health events and to health change in relation to age, and to heterogeneity of such outcomes. It allows us also to consider and sometimes to test for alternative explanations. Consideration of processes of risk development and heterogeneity of outcome encourage the study of individual differences. Genetic information about individuals should now enhance that possibility.

The changing social context is a source of analytic opportunity and of natural experiment. Inter-cohort comparison is a useful method, in so far as comparability of measures used by the different studies concerned allow it,[89] and can be used for a range of reasons. For example, comparison of cohorts that experienced different educational opportunities or different risks associated with the reduction of atmospheric pollution by policy change can be used to assess the impact of policy change. Within a continuing life course study, social change experienced by the sample can be used to show degree of success in adaptation to new circumstances, and the effectiveness of sample members' agency.[2] Natural experiments are discussed in Section 4.1 below.

Life course theory in the social and biological sciences provides essential guidelines for analytic strategy.[2,5,11,79] For example, Caspi, in discussing a key analytical question of whether 'social circumstances alter individual psychology or … psychological characteristics lead people into their social circumstances', outlines the importance of awareness by the analyst of social causation and selection theories.[90] Rutter et al.[16] in discussion of testing hypotheses about environmental effects on behaviour, emphasize the importance of identifying processes that lead to risk exposure, and the need to 'compare and contrast alternative causal mechanisms …. That involves an articulated theory of the different ways in which psychopathology might arise and, more specifically, of the possible different explanations for the particular pattern of risk associations that has been found'.

Almost all of the analytic opportunities outlined above require new statistical methods, and they are described in Chapters 6, 8 and 9.

1.4 The reality of life course research

Beginning a new life course investigation is expensive in time and money; as a result, the art of life course studies is to find existing data sources that most closely match the requirements of the research. Although it may seem that the ideal design is a prospective study from birth to adulthood, in practice life course analysis is often complicated by the nature of the data available, by missing data and missing sample members; innovative and opportunistic designs have been used to address those problems. As we shall see, no design is perfect, and all typically have limitations that need to be balanced against their advantages.

1.4.1 Innovative methods

Innovative methods have been used in epidemiology to access data in accelerated life course designs, mostly through sample selection. These designs make opportunistic use of routinely published statistics, or existing research or clinic samples, or events.

For example, demographic data in the form of published national statistics have been used to provide ready access to many years of life, both for the study of relationships of ecological factors and mortality and for the study of individual risk. Barker's initial studies used infant and maternal mortality statistics in areas of poor SES in the 1920s and related data on specific causes of mortality in the same areas 50 years later, in the 1970s.[13] Secular trend in height was confirmed using data from medical records of Norwegian military conscripts over a period of 40 years (Udjus 1964 quoted in Tanner et al.[91]). In many countries, census records for a sample of the population have been linked, to provide life course data on individuals. In Britain a sample of approximately 500 000 people provides information from censuses since 1971 that has been linked to vital registration data to provide information on births to and mortality in that sample.[20] While they make it possible to cover long periods of historical time and many years of life, these designs also have inevitable limitations, most notably that they offer little information about individuals and their context.

Catch-up designs that find members of samples originally studied for health purposes at an earlier time, or on whom earlier health records exist, make it possible to short-circuit the wait for ageing to take place. Barker, for instance, found adults whose birth records detailing size at birth had been stored for periods of up to 70 years, measured blood pressure and other aspects of health in the survivors and examined causes of death in non-survivors.[10,13] Frankel and colleagues[92] found medical and dietary records of a sample studied during the British pre-war economic depression, and discovered the survivor population in which to measure adult health. Populations of adolescents studied in both the Oakland Growth Study and in the Terman study of those with high IQ have been traced in later life for health study purposes.[93] Robins studied later health, social functioning and criminality among adults identified from child guidance clinic notes.[52] McCance and colleagues[94] studied adult risk of diabetes in a sample of North American Indians whose birth records were known, because they were at genetically determined raised risk. Such catch-up designs offer the advantage of information on health in early life and potentially many years of elapsed time; their inevitable 'downsides' involve reliance on retrospective reporting of events and exposures in the intervening years.

Exposure to particular risks thought to affect child health and development, and in turn to affect health in adulthood, has also been studied using catch-up methods. That offers the opportunity to study effects of exposures that cannot be introduced experimentally. For example, Stein et al.[95] and later Roseboom et al.[96] identified adults born during a famine experienced in a Dutch province during the Second World War, and whose birth and antenatal records had survived, and studied their adult health in order to investigate the long-term effects of malnutrition at different stages of development *in utero*. A similar study was undertaken on those exposed in early life to the siege of Leningrad in 1941–1942.[97] Rutter et al.[18] studied recovery in children released from exposure to severe psychological and physical deprivation in Romanian orphanages, and Lucas et al.[98] randomized premature infants to feeding regimes in order to study their effects on the development of cognitive function, in a design that is unlikely now to be ethically acceptable.

Migrant samples are used to examine the effects of environment, and to ask whether early life exposure can be modified by change of environment. For instance, the study of migrants from the Tokelau Islands to urban New Zealand showed that blood pressure rose with age in the migrants but not in those who did not migrate, indicating that the process associated with change was not biologically deterministically programmed in early life.[99] An important aspect of the argument for biological programming was that poor organ development in early life would be a powerful source of risk if that organ was unduly stressed in adulthood. That was confirmed in samples born in rural subsistence economies that migrated to Britain.[100] Findings from migrant studies require cautious interpretation, however, because of possible selection effects in migrant populations.

1.4.2 **The long-term prospective design**

The long-term prospective design can offer advantages of data collection consistently over many years of life, for the detailed study of pathways from suspected risk onset to outcome. In practice, however, it also has intrinsic problems. Sampling and all data collections are undertaken within the science and the practicalities of the day, and over time sample loss has to be managed.

Sampling that is regionally restricted may be an initial economy, but presents the dilemma as the study progresses of how far to follow those who leave the area, with consequent loss of representation if they are not followed. In this design, if all sample members are to be followed-up, the choice is ultimately between visiting sample members wherever they live, or paying for them to visit the study centre, and there is an example from New Zealand of how the latter course can be very successful.[101] Sample size is likely to be calculated at the outset to be adequate for anticipated loss, by contemporary standards, through death, migration, loss of contact and refusal. However, in a long-running study and at some periods in the life course, losses can be unexpectedly high, for instance in adolescence and early adulthood, or during periods when migration is higher than when the study began. Sample size in long-running investigations may have been restricted by the contemporary data handling capabilities, as in the British national birth cohort study begun in 1946.[102]

The nature of the sample is also related to the nature of data collections that can be undertaken. Large sample size tends to reduce the frequency of data collection (for financial reasons) and the quality and the nature of data collected, because either large numbers of data collectors (observers) will be necessary or self-reporting will be the preferred method. A geographically representative sample may be necessary for some purposes but, even in a small country such as Britain, is expensive in terms of data collection.

Considerable cost and effort is required in a long-running study to maintain response, and it is likely that feedback to participants about the use of the information they have provided helps to maintain interest and participation.[102] Providing feedback about the individual's health may also been seen by participants as a benefit, particularly in childhood and at older ages, but that may increase the risk of altering health related behaviour. How far that is so has yet to be systematically investigated. Increasingly, ethical requirements are likely to make this kind of feedback mandatory. They will also emphasize the essential 'duty of care' associated with health measurement, so that researchers are obliged to advise a participant about, for instance, a measured raised blood pressure, and the nature of advice has to be proportional to the degree of risk. Although in strict methodological terms this is an interference with the observation of progression of risk, the ethical considerations are paramount.

A further key consideration is that even in prospective studies, the nature of the data available to address life course questions is likely to be incomplete. In long-running studies, the scientific questions that drive later data collections can differ from those that informed the original design. When use of life course data is in this sense retrospective, there has to be an accommodation between the aims of analysis and the original aims of the data collectors.

Differences between the original aims and the current concerns can sometimes be resolved by making new combinations of the data. For example, the 1946 birth cohort pre-dated the development of the standardized parent and teacher questionnaires now widely used to assess emotional and behavioural problems in childhood, and so teacher's assessments of behaviour at school (collected for a different purpose) were used to assess adolescent depression.[103] Some kinds of data about individuals can be collected in retrospect from sources outside the study (e.g. geographical data about areas, information about qualifications awarded, hospital admissions). Other kinds of retrospective information can be collected using instruments developed for that purpose, such as the Parker questionnaire on adults' views of their relationships with their parents,[104] and the life grid method, in which key dates in respondents' biographies are used to prompt recollection.[105,106] The latter method has the problem that only those responding at the later date will provide information. In recent years, this has also become a particular problem with the addition of DNA samples to data collections begun before the availability of DNA. The greatest irreplaceable absence is likely to be in measures of biological and cognitive function, and temperament, that cannot be made in retrospect.

In addition, although repeated measures are the ideal in long-running studies, in practice measurement methods change. The preferred method of measuring blood pressure, for example, was the random zero mercury sphygmomanometer in the 1980s, but a decade later an electronic instrument was preferred. Studies spanning that period had to undertake comparative work to adjust to that change.[107] In a two-generation study, it was decided to use the same cognitive measures in a study of the cohort offspring as had been used in the study of the cohort almost 20 years earlier, but they had to be recalibrated to be 'generation fair'.[108]

Data about the social contexts through which a long-running study has passed may be only available in retrospect, such as contexts described by demographic statistics, policy reviews and research on attitudes and aspirations. That kind of information is required in order to understand, for example, social exclusion, influences to conform, perceptions of opportunity and of self in relation to others. Chapter 3 reviews methods concerned with these topics.

In very long-running studies, recoding becomes necessary from time to time as new classification systems become widely used (e.g. of SES or nutrients), so that comparisons can be made with other contemporary studies.

Finally, data collected over many years inevitably have missing values, and some members of the populations of such studies will have dropped out of the study, been available for data collections on some occasions and not others, or died before the outcome of interest could have occurred. Statistical methods for handling missingness by imputation are available, and statistical/epidemiological methods for dealing with varying periods of exposure to risk include proportional hazard techniques. These aspects of method are reviewed in Chapters 7 and 9.

1.5 **The future**

1.5.1 **Use of existing data**

Life course data will continue to be in great demand, and will be used far more than at present in aggregated, pooled and inter-cohort forms for comparative studies of health effects of the changing social context; for research into the long-term effects of treatment innovations and health-related behaviours; for studies of gene–environment and gene–gene interactions; and for epigenetic investigation across generations.

Some of the British studies begun in early life will soon have data throughout life, up to and including the later years (Table 1.1), providing new possibilities for the study of ageing. Facilities for making data accessible from such sources are being developed in Britain and in the USA.[109–111]

The existing studies that have measures of early life physical and cognitive development, and physical and cognitive function throughout life, offer a unique and new perspective for research into the processes of ageing. Those studies are already beginning to show how pathways to such indicators of the rate of ageing as cognitive decline, originate in early life, and how they are influenced by the social context.[112] Analytic techniques for handling the complexity of these kinds of analyses are discussed in Chapters 6, 8 and 9.

Understanding of health treatment will also be enhanced by the availability of clinically validated measures of, for example depression, covering long periods of the life course, together with information on treatments. That provides data on cases that are treated and cases not treated, so that comparisons of long-term treatment efficacy and other effects may be made. Over the long periods of time covered (Table 1.1), these investigations also have records of exposure to treatments that have changed considerably, for instance the pharmacological treatment of depression, and oral contraception.

Table 1.1 Examples of health studies that form the national resource of large long-term cohorts

Age at data collection	Birth years and sample size at first data collection						
	ELSA 1900–1951 (n = 16 000)*	Whitehall 2 1930–1950 (n = 10 308)*	NSHD 1946 (n= 5362)*	NCDS 1958 (n = 17 414)*	BCS70 1970 (n = 17 198)	ALSPAC 1991–1992 (n = 14 000)*,†	Millennium 2000–2001 (n = 20 000)
Birth							
1–5 years							
6–16 years							
Early adulthood 17–30 years							
Early middle adulthood 31–45 years							
Later middle adulthood 46–65 years							
Later life 66+							

*DNA resource available.

†Started in pregnancy.

Health-related behaviour has also changed considerably over time, and analyses of changing eating, smoking and exercise habits in life course data sources show the nature of change and of differences between cohorts,[87,113] as well as the social influences on change.[114]

The changing social context brings differences in health-related influences that can be examined in long-term follow-up investigations.[66,115] For example, it has already been shown in life course studies that chronic childhood exposure to parental separation is associated with slowed height growth,[44] and inter-cohort comparison should show whether that effect increases with rising rates of parental separation. Similarly, the effects of changing environmental influences on weight at birth such as atmospheric pollution from coal burning, maternal exercise, smoking and alcohol consumption can also be examined in inter-cohort analysis. Other kinds of social change, including, for instance, increasing educational qualifications in women, the changing nature and availability of work and of societal cohesion, can also be examined for their long-term health effects. Shanahan and Hofer have stressed the importance of capturing the dynamic and complex nature of social context for research on the interaction of genes and environment.[84] Epigenetic analyses concerned with transgenerational responses to environmental exposures exemplify the need for new, possibly combined sources of data on the social environment, which cover long periods of time.[116] Measurement of the social context is discussed in Chapter 3.

1.5.2 Development of new data sources

Despite the attractions of pooling existing data, it is inescapable that new data resources are needed on a scale appropriate for addressing new questions about genetic effects, and gene–environment and gene–gene interactions, and for the simultaneous assessment of disease–gene and intermediate phenotype (or disease risk)–gene interactions. Davey Smith *et al.* report that adequate statistical power requires at least 5000 and ideally 10 000 cases, of the disease concerned, and thus population samples of 500 000 and more will be required.[37] New studies of this kind, known as *biobank* studies because of their systematic storage of biological material, and intended to investigate specific disease outcomes, have been started in samples in middle and later life in order to minimize time to disease onset. For example, new studies intending to investigate early life course effects have been started recently in Britain (http://www.ukbiobank.ac.uk), Norway (http://www.fhi.no) and Denmark (http://www.serum.dk/sw9314.asp). Stoltenberg and Pickles describe in Chapter 4 the design and value of these new kinds of very large investigations singly and pooled. A difficult question facing designers of these large biobank studies is whether in the long run it will prove best to have a large study with a wide range of phenotypic data collected or a large study with a reduced range of phenotypic information. Clayton and McKeigue argue for case–control studies rather than cohort designs to provide adequate statistical power to detect modest risk ratios in gene–environment interactions.[117]

1.6 Conclusions

Development of data sources and of methods of data collection, measurement and analysis has been rapid and extensive in life course epidemiology. Continuing challenges include, in all types of life course epidemiology, the development of methods of measurement and analysis to characterize pathways over long periods of life, increasing the accessibility of data, and design of studies and analysis, as well as presentation of findings, in ways that are sensitive to the needs of clinical and policy practice.

References

1. Terman LM, Oden MH (1959). *Genetic studies of genius, volume 5. The gifted group at midlife: thirty five years' follow-up of the superior child.* Stanford University Press, Stanford, CA.
2. Elder GH, Shanahan MJ (2006). The life course and human development. In: Lerner RM, ed. *Handbook of child psychology, Vol 1, 6th edn: Theoretical models of human development.* Wiley and Sons, New York, pp. 665–715.
3. Douglas JWB (1964). *The home and the school.* McKibbon & Kee, London.
4. Baltes PB, Brim OG, ed. (1979). *Life-span development and behaviour.* Academic Press, New York.
5. Magnusson D, ed. (1996). *The lifespan development of individuals.* Cambridge University Press, Cambridge.
6. Murphy JM, Horton NJ, Laird NM, Monson RR, Sobol AM, Leighton AH (2004). Anxiety and depression: a 40-year perspective on relationships regarding prevalence, distribution, and co-morbidity. *Acta Psychiatrica Scandanavica* 109, 355–375.
7. Rutter M, Kim-Cohen J, Maughan B (2006). Continuities and discontinuities in psychopathology between childhood and adult life. *Journal of Child Psychology and Psychiatry* 47, 276–295.
8. Illsley R, Kincaid JC (1963). Social correlations of perinatal mortality. In: Butler NR, Bonham DG, ed. *Perinatal mortality.* Churchill Livingstone, Edinburgh, pp. 270–286.
9. Dubos R, Savage D, Schaedler R (1966). Biological Freudianism: lasting effects of early environmental influences. *Pediatrics* 38, 789–800.
10. Barker DJP (1998). *Mothers and babies and health in later life*, 2nd edn. Churchill Livingstone, Edinburgh.
11. Kuh D, Ben-Shlomo Y, ed. (2004). *A life course approach to chronic disease epidemiology*, 2nd edn. Oxford University Press, Oxford.
12. Forsdahl A (1977). Are living conditions in childhood and adolescence an important risk factor for arteriosclerotic heart disease? *British Journal of Social and Preventive Medicine* 31, 91–95.
13. Barker DJP (1992). *Fetal and infant origins of adult disease.* BMJ Press, London.
14. Berkman LF, Kawachi I, ed. (2000). *Social epidemiology.* Oxford University Press, Oxford.
15. Brunner E, Marmot MG (2006). Social organisation, stress, and health. In: Marmot MG, Wilkinson RG, ed. *Social determinants of health*, 2nd edn. Oxford University Press, Oxford, pp. 17–43.
16. Rutter M, Pickles A, Murray R, Eaves L (2001). Testing hypotheses on specific environmental causal effects on behaviour. *Psychological Bulletin* 127, 291–324.
17. Baltes PB, Mayer KU (1999). *The Berlin ageing study.* Cambridge University Press, Cambridge.
18. Rutter M, the ERA research team (1998). Developmental catch-up and deficit following adoption after severe global early privation. *Journal of Child Psychology and Psychiatry* 39, 465–476.
19. Finch CE, Crimmins E (2004). Inflammatory exposure and historical changes in human life-spans. *Science* 17, 1736–1739.
20. Hattersley L, Creeser R (1995). *Longitudinal study 1971–1991, history, organisation and quality of data.* Her Majesty's Stationery Office, London.
21. Leon DA, Koupilova I, Lithell HO, Berglund L, Mohsen R, Vagero D (1996). Failure to realise growth potential *in utero* and adult obesity in relation to blood pressure in 50 year old Swedish men. *British Medical Journal* 312, 401–406.
22. Goldberg DP, Hillier VF (1979). A scaled version of the General Health Questionnaire. *Psychological Medicine.* 9, 139–145.

23. Lewis G, Pelosi AJ, Dunn G (1992). Measuring psychiatric disorder in the community: a standardised assessment for use by lay interviewers. *Psychological Medicine* 22, 465–486.

24. Bebbington PE, Nayani T (1995). The psychosis screening questionnaire. *International Journal of Methods in Psychiatric Research* 5, 11–19.

25. Stern Y, ed. (2006). *Cognitive reserve.* Psychology Press, New York.

26. Huppert F, Baylis N, Keverne B (2006). *The science of well-being.* Oxford University Press, Oxford.

27. Kawachi I, Berkman LF, ed. (2001). *Neighbourhoods and health.* Oxford University Press, New York.

28. Wadsworth MEJ, Bartley MJ (2006). Social inequality, family structure, and health in the life course. *Koelner Zeitschrift fur Soziologie und Sozialpsychologie* 46, 125–143.

29. Leeson C, Kattenhorn M, Morley R, Lucas A, Deanfield JE (2001). Impact of low birth weight and cardiovascular risk factors on endothelial function in early adult life. *Circulation* 103, 1264–1268.

30. Muthen B (2001). Latent variable mixture modelling. In: Marcoulides G, Schumaker R, ed. *New developments and techniques in structural equation modelling.* Erlbaum, New Jersey pp. 1–33.

31. Goldstein H (1995). *Multilevel statistical models,* 2nd edn. Edward Arnold, London.

32. Schafer JL (1997). *Analysis of incomplete multivariate data.* Chapman & Hall, London.

33. Brick JM, Kalton G (1996). Handling missing data in survey research. *Statistical Methods in Medical Research* 5, 215–238.

34. Rubin D (1976). Inference and missing data. *Biometrika* 63, 581–592.

35. Caspi A, McClay J, Moffitt TE, Mill J, Martin J, Craig IW, *et al.* (2002). Role of genotype in the cycle of violence in maltreated children. *Science* 297, 851–854.

36. Wadsworth MEJ, Vinall LE, Jones AL, Hardy RJ, Whitehouse DB, Butterworth SL, *et al.* (2004). Alpha1-antitrypsin as a risk for infant and adult respiratory outcomes in a national birth cohort. *American Journal of Respiratory Cell and Molecular Biology* 31, 559–564.

37. Davey Smith G, Ibrahim S, Lewis S, Hansell AL, Palmer LJ, Burton P (2005). Genetic epidemiology and public health: hope, hype and future prospects. *Lancet* 366, 1484–1498.

38. Morris JN (1967). *Uses of epidemiology.* Churchill Livingstone, Edinburgh.

39. Marmot MG, Brunner E. (2004). Cohort profile: the Whitehall II study. *International Journal of Epidemiology* 33, 1–6.

40. Dawber TR (1980). *The Framingham study: the epidemiology of atherosclerotic disease.* Harvard University Press, London.

41. Marmot MG, Syme SL, Kagan A (1975). Epidemiologic studies of CHD and stroke in Japanese men living in Japan, Hawaii and California. *American Journal of Epidemiology* 102, 514–525.

42. Beaglehole R, Eyles E, Prior I (1979). Blood pressure and migration in children. *International Journal of Epidemiology* 8, 5–10.

43. Wadsworth MEJ, Cripps HA, Midwinter RA, Colley JRT (1985). Blood pressure at age 36 years and social and familial factors, cigarette smoking and body mass in a national birth cohort. *British Medical Journal* 291, 1534–1538.

44. Montgomery SM, Bartley MJ, Wilkinson RJ (1997). Family conflict and slow growth. *Archives of Disease in Childhood* 77, 326–330.

45. Berkman LF, Glass T, Brisette I, Seeman TE (2000). From social integration to health: Durkheim in the new millennium. *Social Science and Medicine* 51, 843–857.

46. Stansfeld SA, Marmot MG, ed. (2002). *Stress and the heart.* BMJ Books, London.

47. Whincup PH, Cook DG, Geleijns, JM (2004). A life course approach to blood pressure. In: Kuh D, Ben Shlomo Y, ed. *A life course approach to chronic disease epidemiology,* 2nd edn. Oxford University Press, Oxford, pp. 218–239.

48. Harris T, Brown GW, Bifulco A (1990). Loss of parent in childhood and adult psychiatric disorder: a tentative overall model. *Development and Psychopathology* 2, 311–328.

49. Kim-Cohen J, Caspi A, Moffitt TE, Harrington HL, Milne BS, Poulton R (2003). Prior juvenile diagnoses in adults with mental disorder: developmental follow-back of a prospective-longitudinal cohort. *Archives of General Psychiatry* 60, 709–717.

50. Jaffee SR, Moffitt TE, Caspi A, Fombonne E, Poulton R, Martin J (2002). Differences in early childhood risk factors for juvenile-onset and adult onset depression. *Archives of General Psychiatry* 58, 215–222.

51. Monroe SM, Harkness KL (2005). Life stress, the 'kindling' hypothesis, and the recurrence of depression: considerations from a life stress perspective. *Psychological Review* 112, 417–445.

52. Robins LN (1966). *Deviant children grown up*. Williams & Wilkins, Baltimore, MD.

53. Wadsworth MEJ (1979). *Roots of delinquency: infancy, adolescence and crime.* Martin Robertson, Oxford.

54. Moffitt TE (1993). Adolescence-limited and life-course persistent antisocial behavior: a developmental taxonomy. *Psychological Review* 100, 674–701.

55. Laub JH, Sampson R. (2003). *Shared beginnings, divergent lives: delinquent boys to age 70.* Harvard University Press, Cambridge, MA.

56. Greenhough WT, Black JE, Wallace CS (1987). Experience and brain development. *Child Development* 58, 539–559.

57. Bateson P, Martin P (1999). *Design for a life.* Jonathan Cape, London.

58. Caldji C, Diorio J, Meaney MJ (2000). Variations in maternal care in infancy regulate the development of stress reactivity. *Biological Psychiatry* 48, 1164–1174.

59. Boyce WT, Keating DP (2004). Should we intervene to improve childhood circumstances? In: Kuh D, Ben Shlomo Y, ed. *A life course approach to chronic disease epidemiology*, 2nd edn. Oxford University Press, Oxford, pp. 415–445.

60. Feinstein L (2003). Inequality in the early cognitive development of British children in the 1970 cohort. *Economica* 70, 73–98.

61. Werner E (1995). Resilience in development. *Current Directions in Psychological Science* 32, 159–162.

62. Rodgers B (1994). Pathways between parental divorce and adult depression. *Journal of Child Psychology and Psychiatry* 35, 1289–1308.

63. Bifulco A, Moran P (1998). *Wednesday's child.* Routledge, London.

64. Ryff CD, Singer B, Love GD, Essex MJ (1998). Resilience in adulthood and later life. In: Lomranz J, ed. *Handbook of aging and mental health*. Plenum Press, New York, pp. 69–96.

65. Marmot M, Siegrist J, Theorell T. (2006). Health and the psychosocial environment at work. In: Marmot M, Wilkinson RG, ed. *Social determinants of health*, 2nd edn. Oxford University Press, Oxford, pp. 105–131.

66. Ben-Shlomo Y, Kuh D (2002). A life course approach to chronic disease epidemiology: conceptual models, empirical challenges and interdisciplinary perspectives. *International Journal of Epidemiology* 31, 285–293.

67. Lawlor DA, Ben Shlomo Y, Leon DA (2004). Pre-adult influences on cardiovascular disease. In: Kuh D, Ben Shlomo Y, ed. *A life course approach to chronic disease epidemiology*, 2nd edn. Oxford University Press, Oxford, pp. 41–76.

68. Kuh D, Ben-Shlomo Y, Lynch J, Hallqvist J, Power C (2003). Life course epidemiology. *Journal of Epidemiology and Community Health* 57, 778–783.

69. Maughan B, Rutter M (2001). Antisocial children grown up. In: Hill J, Maughan B, ed. *Cambridge monographs in child & adolescent psychiatry: conduct disorders*. Cambridge University Press, Cambridge, pp. 507–552.

70. Nagin DS, Land KC (1993). Age, criminal careers, and population heterogeneity: Specification and estimation of a nonparametric, mixed Poisson model. *Criminology* 31, 327–362.

71. Broidy LM, Nagin DS, Tremblay RE, Bates JE, Brame B, Dodge KA (2003). Developmental trajectories of childhood disruptive behaviors and adolescent delinquency: a six-site, cross-national study. *Developmental Psychology* 39, 222–224.

72. Croudace TJ, Jarvelin MR, Wadsworth MEJ, Jones PB (2003). Developmental typology of trajectories to night time bladder control: epidemiologic application of longitudinal latent class analysis. *American Journal of Epidemiology* 157, 834–842.

73. Colman I, Croudace TJ, Wadsworth MEJ, Ploubidis GB, Jones PB (2006). Longitudinal phenotypes of mental disorder from age 13 to 53: a latent class analysis. *Journal of Affective Disorders* 91 Suppl. 1, S89–S89.

74. Graber JA, Lewinsohn PM, Seeley JR, Brooks Gunn J (1997). Is psychopathology associated with the timing of pubertal development? *Journal of the American Academy of Child and Adolescent Psychiatry* 36, 1768–1776.

75. Moffitt TE, the E-Risk Study Team (2002). Teen-aged mothers in contemporary Britain. *Journal of Child Psychology and Psychiatry* 43, 727–742.

76. Stouthamer-Loeber M, Wei E, Loeber R, Masten AS (2004). Desistance from persistent serious delinquency in the transition to adulthood. *Developmental Psychopathology* 16, 897–918.

77. Krieger N (2001). Theories for social epidemiology. *International Journal of Epidemiology* 30, 668–677.

78. Rothman KJ (1981). Induction and latent periods. *American Journal of Epidemiology* 114, 253–259.

79. Rutter M, Moffitt TE, Caspi A (2006). Gene–environment interplay and psychopathology: multiple varieties but real effects. *Journal of Child Psychology and Psychiatry* 47, 226–261.

80. Wizemann TM, Pardue M-L (2001). *Exploring the biological contributions to human health: does sex matter?* National Academy Press, Washington, DC.

81. Tai ES, Corella D, Deurenberg-Yap M, Cutter J, Chew SK, Tan CE, *et al.* (2003). Dietary fat interacts with the-514C>T polymorphism in the hepatic lipase gene promoter on plasma lipid profiles in a multiethnic Asian population: the 1998 Singapore National Health Survey. *Journal of Nutrition* 133, 3399–3408.

82. Ordovas JM (2006). Genetic interactions with diet influence the risk of cardiovascular disease. *American Journal of Clinical Nutrition*. 83 (Suppl) 443S–446S.

83. Caspi A, Sugden K, Moffitt TE, Taylor A, Craig IW, Harrington H, *et al.* (2003). Influence of life stress on depression: moderation by a polymorphism on the 5-HTT gene. *Science* 301, 386–389.

84. Shanahan M, Hofer S (2005). Social context in gene–environment interactions: retrospect and prospect. *Journal of Gerontology* 60B, 65–76.

85. Strachan DP, Perry IV (1997). Time trends. In: Kuh D, Ben Shlomo Y, ed. *A life course approach to chronic disease epidemiology*. Oxford University Press, Oxford, pp. 201–219.

86. Rutter M, Smith DJ (1995). *Psychosocial disorders in young people: time trends and their causes*. Wiley, Chichester.

87. Wadsworth MEJ, Butterworth SL, Montgomery SM, Ehlin A, Bartley MJ (2003). Health. In: Ferri E, Bynner J, Wadsworth MEJ, ed. *Changing Britain, changing lives: three generations at the turn of the century*. Institute of Education Press, London, pp. 207–236.

88. Prynne CJ, Paul AA, Price GM, Day KC, Hilder WS, Wadsworth MEJ (1999). Food and nutrient intake in a sample of four year old children in 1950: comparison with the 1990s. *Public Health Nutrition* 2, 537–547.

89. Ferri E, Bynner J, Wadsworth MEJ, ed. (2003). *Changing Britain, changing lives: three generations at the turn of the century*. Institute of Education, London.

90. Caspi A (2004). Life course development: the inter-play of social selection and social causation within and across generations. In: Chase-Lansdale PL, Kiernan K, Friedman RJ ed. *Human development across lives and generations*. Cambridge University Press, Cambridge, pp. 8–27.

91. Tanner JM, Hayashi T, Preece MA, Cameron N (1982). Increase in length of leg relative to trunk in Japanese children and adults from 1957 to 1977. *Annals of Human Biology* 9, 411–423.

92. Frankel S, Davey Smith G, Gunnell D (1999). Childhood socioeconomic position and adult cardiovascular mortality: the Boyd Orr cohort. *American Journal of Epidemiology* 150, 1081–1084.

93. Schwartz JE, Friedman HS, Tucker JS, Tomlinson-Keasey C, Wingard DL, Criqui MH (1995). Sociodemographic and psychosocial factors in childhood as predictors of adult mortality. *American Journal of Public Health* 85, 1237–1245.

94. McCance DR, Pettit DJ, Hanson RL, Jacobsson LT, Knowler WC, Bennett PH (1994). Birth weight and non-insulin dependent diabetes: thrifty genotype, thrifty phenotype, or surviving small baby genotype? *British Medical Journal* 308, 942–945.

95. Stein Z, Susser M, Saenger G, Marolla F (1975). *Famine and human development: the Dutch hunger winter of 1944–45.* Oxford University Press, Oxford.

96. Roseboom TJ, van der Meulen JH, Ravelli AC, van Montfrans GA, Osmond C, Barker DJP (1999). Blood pressure in adults after prenatal exposure to famine. *Journal of Hypertension* 17, 325–330.

97. Stanner SA, Bulmer K, Andres C, Lantsava OE, Borodina V, Poteer VV (1997). Does malnutrition *in utero* determine diabetes and coronary heart disease in adulthood? Results from the Leningrad siege study. *British Medical Journal* 315, 1342–1348.

98. Lucas A, Morley R, Cole TJ, Lister G, Leeson-Payne C (1992). Breast milk and subsequent intelligence quotient in children born preterm. *Lancet* 339, 261–264.

99. Salmond CE, Joseph JG, Prior IAM, Stanley DG, Wessen F (1985). Longitudinal analysis of the relationship between blood pressure and migration: the Tokelau Islands migrant study. *American Journal of Epidemiology* 122, 291–301.

100. McKeigue PM, Pierpoint T, Ferrie JE, Marmot MG (1992). Relationship of glucose intolerance and hyperinsulinaemia to body fat pattern in south Asians and Europeans. *Diabetologia* 21, 1414–1431.

101. Silva PA, Stanton WR, ed. (1996). *From child to adult: the Dunedin multidisciplinary health and development study.* Oxford University Press, Auckland.

102. Wadsworth MEJ, Kuh D, Richards M, Hardy R (2006). Cohort profile: the 1946 national birth cohort. *International Journal of Epidemiology* 35, 49–54.

103. Van Os J, Jones P, Lewis G, Wadsworth MEJ, Murray R (1997). Developmental precursors of affective illness in a general population birth cohort. *Archives of General Psychiatry* 54, 625–631.

104. Rodgers B (1996). Reported parental behaviour and adult affective symptoms. *Psychological Medicine* 26, 51–61; 63–77.

105. Belli RF (1998). The structure of autobiographical memory and the event history calendar. *Memory* 6, 383–406.

106. Berney L, Blane D (2003). The life grid method of collecting retrospective information from people at older ages. *Research Policy and Planning* 123, 204–209.

107. Rogers S, Davey Smith G, Doyle W (1988). Field evaluation of the Copal UA-123 automatic sphygmomanometer. *Journal of Epidemiology and Community Health* 42, 321–324.

108. Wadsworth MEJ (1986). Effects of parenting style and preschool experience on children's verbal attainment. *Early Childhood Research Quarterly* 1, 237–248.

109. Lowrance WW (2006). *Access to collections of data and materials for health research.* The Wellcome Trust, London.

110. National Archive of Computerized Data on Aging. nacda@icpsr.umich.edu.

111. National Research Council of the National Academies (2005). *Expanding access to research data: reconciling risks and opportunities.* National Academy of Sciences, Washington, DC.

112. Richards M, Wadsworth MEJ (2004). Long-term effects of early adversity on cognitive function. *Archives of Disease in Childhood* 89, 922–927.

113. Schoon I, Parsons S (2003). Life style and health related behaviour. In: Ferri E, Bynner J, Wadsworth MEJ, ed. *Changing Britain, changing lives: three generations at the turn of the century.* Institute of Education Press, London, pp. 237–260.

114. Schooling MJ (2001). *Health behaviour in a social and temporal context.* PhD thesis, University of London.

115. Hertzman C, Power C (2006). A life course approach to health and human development. In: Heymann J, Hertzman C, Barer ML, Evans RG, ed. *Healthier societies: from analysis to action.* Oxford University Press, Oxford, pp. 58–82.

116. Pembrey ME, Bygren LO, Kaati G, Edvinsson S, Northstone K, Sjostrom M, *et al.* (2006). Sex-specific, male-line transgenerational responses in humans. *European Journal of Genetics* 14, 159–166.

117. Clayton D, McKeigue P (2001). Epidemiological methods for studying genetic and environmental factors in complex disease. *Lancet* 358, 1356–1360.

Chapter 2

Measurement and design for life course studies of individual differences and development

Jane Costello and Adrian Angold

Abstract

This chapter reviews methods for studying individual differences across the life course. It starts from the position that even when a life course study is basically observational or descriptive, there is an underlying concern to understand more about causality. Thus, the discussion of methods pays attention to the implications of different research designs and aspects of measurement for drawing causal conclusions. There are two aspects of research methods that have to be considered in designing a life course study: study design and measurement of individuals. Under the first heading the chapter describes observational and quasi-experimental designs for life course research. A section on genetically informative designs describes a range of options for increasing the genetic information that can be obtained from life course research. The section on capturing individual differences discusses continuous versus categorical measurement, the timing of measurements, the range of information that can be collected, from census data to biodata, and non-intrusive methods for collecting individual life course information. A section on biological information discusses applications of molecular genetics and psychoneuroendocrinology to life course research. The aim of the chapter is to encourage researchers involved in life course research to obtain the greatest possible value from this expensive and time-consuming enterprise.

2.1 Introduction

There are enormous differences in people's chances of survival at birth, their quality of life and their life expectancy, from one century to another and from one part of the world to another. Explanations for these differences have varied from those that affect everyone living in a time or place, such as climate or nutrition, to those that affect some people more than others, such as vulnerability to stressors. Hobbes[1] believed that 'the difference between man and man is not so considerable', and that when external conditions were poor, as in times of war, the life of man was universally 'solitary, poor, nasty, brutish, and short'. However, the more we study the human life course the more we see that individual differences, some of them beginning at conception and others acquired over development, can have a dramatic effect on both survival and quality of life, even when the environment is harsh. These individual differences can also be shown to interact with environmental differences, so that the life course of any individual becomes more and more 'canalized'[2] over time by the interaction of individual and environmental characteristics.

This chapter on methods for studying individual differences across the life course has three parts. First, we describe the *model of individual development* that underpins the discussion. Secondly, we describe different kinds of *study design* that have been used to capture individual differences and development. Thirdly, we look at some principles guiding the *choice of measures* to capture individual differences and development.

2.2 What do we mean by 'development'?

Central to the view of development taken in this chapter is the concept of epigenesis. As summarized by Gilbert Gottlieb:

> Individual development is characterized by an increase of complexity of organization (i.e., the emergence of new structural and functional properties and competencies) at all levels of analysis (molecular, subcellular, cellular, organismic) as a consequence of horizontal and vertical coactions among the organism's parts, including organism–environment coactions. Horizontal coactions are those that occur at the same level (gene–gene … organism–organism), whereas vertical coactions occur at different levels (cell–tissue, … behavioral activity–nervous system) and are reciprocal, meaning that they can influence each other in either direction, from lower to higher or from higher to lower levels of the developing system[3] (p. 7).

This epigenetic view of development (1) presupposes change and novelty; (2) underscores the importance of timing in behavioural establishment and organization; (3) emphasizes multiple determination; and (4) leads us *not* to expect invariant relationships between causes and outcomes across the span of development.[4] The challenge, as set out by the developmentalist Uri Bronfenbrenner, is to find ways to describe

> the progressive, mutual accommodation, throughout the life span, between a growing human organism and the changing immediate environment in which it lives, as this process is affected by relations obtaining within and between these immediate settings, as well as the larger social contexts, both formal and informal, in which the settings are embedded.[5] (p. 514).

Bronfenbrenner uses a four-level terminology to simplify the myriad nested systems of human development: the *microsystem*, the complex of relationships between the developing person and the immediate environment (internal biology, home, school, workplace, etc.); the *mesosystem*, the complex of relationships among microsystems, e.g. among family, school and church; the *exosystem*, extensions of the mesosystem that do not contain the developing individual, but impinge on the settings in which that person is found (the legal system, agencies of local, state, and national government, and so on); and the *macrosystem*, referring to the institutional patterns of the culture that function as 'carriers of information and ideology that … endow meaning and motivation to particular agencies, social networks, roles, activities, and their interrelations'[5] (p. 515).

For this chapter, we concentrate on methods to measure what Bronfenbrenner calls the *microsystem*: characteristics of developing individuals in their immediate environments. However, we know to our cost that changes at one level in a bioecological system can have unintended consequences elsewhere in the system. To give a single example, cultural pressures at the macrosystem level to be 'tough on crime' in the USA have created a vast prison industry that eats up increasingly large proportions of state and national budgets (exosystem), affecting what is available for other tasks such as education (mesosystem), which in turn may reduce a child's chance of going to a decent school, and thus change that individual child's life course (microsystem).

2.3 The choice of *study design* to capture individual differences and development across the life course

However complex the idea of epigenesis, we can design studies that will illuminate the various parts of the puzzle. The design of any particular study, however, needs to be tailored to the particular question to which it seeks an answer. To take a few examples:

Are you interested in the causes of a particular outcome?

You will need individuals who vary on outcome, e.g. cardiovascular disease, and have measures of possible causal factors. e.g. childhood poverty.

Are you interested in secular change (period effects; effects of calendar time, controlling for developmental stage)?

You will need individuals of different generations measured at the same age, e.g. 11 year olds and then their children when they reach 11.

Are you interested in effects of a particular event (cohort/year of birth effects, controlling for age)?

You will need people who did/did not experience the key event, e.g. Hurricane Katrina.

Are you interested in change as a function of age or developmental stage?

You will need individuals who contribute multiple data points encompassing the key ages/developmental stages, e.g. puberty, retirement.

Are you interested in the effects of a particular risk factor/exposure?

You will need individuals who vary on exposure, e.g. poverty, and have measures of putative effects, e.g. cardiovascular disease.

Are you interested in combinations of these questions (e.g. are there secular changes in the impact of childhood poverty on death from cardiovascular disease)?

You will need individuals of different generations with and without risk exposure, with measures of the outcome of interest.

Another characteristic of life course research is that, at some level, it is concerned not just to describe phenomena but to explain them. Even if the research design is, on the surface, purely observational, we want to use the correlational patterns that emerge over time to explore *why* women live longer than men in industrialized societies, or *why* low birth weight predicts insulin resistance in middle age.[6] So this section on choice of study design begins with a brief discussion of causality and its measurement in life course research. We then discuss three important aspects of a life course study that have implications for study design: whether you have an experimental component in the study; the duration of the study; and the level of measurement. We describe some of the most common designs used for studies of individual differences across development, and discuss their implications for sampling, duration and measurement.

2.3.1 The search for causality

How can we *know* that something was the effect of a certain cause? We know clearly enough in everyday life, but people have argued for centuries about the true definitions of cause and effect. Attempts to define them rapidly become circular. For the empirical researcher, the question is how to demonstrate this in a given situation. However strongly I believe that childhood poverty is the cause of the early mortality that I observe in my life course study, how can I show that the relationship is causal, and not because the children being born into poor families are less healthy at birth?[7]

An approach that has gained popularity since the 1960s is based on an idea of the eighteenth century philosopher David Hume: 'We may define a cause to be *an object followed by another, ... where, if the first object had not been, the second never had existed*'[8] (Section VII).

The prototypical test involves the idea of a *counterfactual*. If we expose a child to a fearful stimulus, and *at the same time* do not expose the same child to the same stimulus, we can argue that the difference in the same child's response to the two situations was caused by the fearful stimulus. As demonstrated by Maldonado and Greenland,[9] the counterfactual approach to causal inference applies equally to observational and experimental research designs, and is structurally equivalent to other systems of reasoning about cause and effect. However, of course, this is an impossible research model because we cannot both expose and not expose the same child at the same time. However, the counterfactual metaphor is a useful one, because the comparison it describes comes close to the ideal experiment, to which all the other causal research designs are approximations. In the real world, we generally follow John Stuart Mill's more practical approach, which states that that a causal relationship is more likely if (1) the cause preceded the effect; (2) we can assume some sort of relationship between cause and effect; and (3) our identified cause is the only logical explanation we can find for the effect.[10] The famous Henle–Koch principles,[11] elaborated by Hill,[12] Susser[13] and for psychiatry by Robins and Guze,[14] impose additional requirements such as biological plausibility and a dose–response gradient.

The randomized controlled experiment is the highest standard of comparison for research that aims to establish causality. In a randomized experiment, subjects' assignment to one research condition or another (e.g. treatment or no treatment) is based on chance. This procedure makes it easier to ascribe causality to an intervention because (given a reasonable number of study subjects) it (1) distributes threats to validity randomly across treatment conditions; (2) permits the assumption that at pre-test the expected value of all variables (measured or not) will be the same across treatment conditions; and (3) allows the researcher to compute a valid estimate of error variance. Thus, the great strength of the randomized design is that it provides an unbiased estimate of the average treatment effect.[15] The challenge for life course research is to develop causal models in the absence of randomized trials.

2.3.2 Observational or non-experimental studies in life-course research

Since the basic design of most life course research is observational, this section begins by considering how we can use non-experimental designs to infer causality. It is helpful to think of there being two dimensions to non-experimental designs. The key axes are *selection* (cohort versus case–control) and *direction* (prospective versus retrospective). Cohort studies tend to have a forward direction, examining the effects of putative risk factors in the population on the disease of interest, while case–control designs work backwards, using a comparison between people with and without the disease of interest to explore the impact of one or more risk factors. Not surprisingly, cohort studies have often been prospective and case–control studies retrospective, but this is not inevitable. As Rothman and Greenland[16] point out, 'Both cohort and case–control studies may employ a mixture of prospective and retrospective measurements, using data collected before and after the disease occurred' (p. 74).

2.3.2.1 Cohort studies

The cohort study, which is the format of most life course studies, rarely sets out as a rigorous test of a causal hypothesis. More often, the primary goal is descriptive, although the underlying questions are causal. A cohort study moves intellectually from putative cause to outcome. An example of a hugely influential cohort study is the Framingham Heart Study, begun in 1948 as a study of the population of a New England town. A group of people representative of the population of interest (people at risk of heart disease) has been followed through time, from risk exposure to disease onset, or death from other causes. In other studies, both the causes and the outcomes are quite non-specific; for example, a birth cohort study may simply collect a range of data [birth weight, birth complications, growth trajectories, illness and accidents, life events, education, socio-economic status (SES), and so on] in the hope that some of this information can be linked down the road to causes of later illness and death. Put like that, the cohort design is about as far from a strict experimental design as one could possibly get. Nevertheless, cohort studies have been important in at least suggesting important causal pathways and, just as importantly, eliminating others. One of the investigators on the Framingham study describes such a situation:

> At the initiation of the Framingham Study, it was held that a single etiology for atherosclerotic disease would be found to be essential, and in most instances sufficient, to produce the pathology … The Framingham Study successfully identified or documented major contributors to cardiovascular disease including atherogenic personal attributes, living habits that promote these, indicators of preclinical disease and innate susceptibility to these influences … From the prospective of

epidemiologic investigations carried out, the study has accumulated information on the incidence of cardiovascular disease, the undistorted full clinical spectrum of all who have it, its importance as a force of morbidity and mortality, clues to pathogenesis and the chain of circumstances leading to its occurrence[17] (pp. 206, 211).

One important point to note about this candid comment is that the researchers were *completely wrong* in the hypotheses that guided the study at the beginning: there was no single, necessary and sufficient cause of heart disease. Elsewhere the author cheerfully acknowledges several other quite mistaken hypotheses that the original researchers held, such as the belief that, for those at risk of heart attacks, exercise is dangerous. Paradoxically, given the state of knowledge at the time, Framingham was almost certainly a more productive use of public funds to explore the causes of heart disease than the equivalent amount spent on rigorous clinical trials. These might have disproved current aetiological ideas, but they could not have generated such a rich stew of new ideas and research methods.

Birth cohorts In a *birth cohort* study, the sample is selected at birth (or before). Cohort studies may, however, start at a later age. For example, all the 140 000 participants for the Women's Health Initiative (see below) were recruited after menopause. When subjects are recruited later in life, it is common to exclude from the sample everyone who already has any disease that is an object of research interest, so that it can be assumed that the direction of causality runs from risk exposure to disease, and that all the cases are newly occurring (incident cases). For example, the Framingham Study excluded from its sample anyone who had coronary heart disease at the initial examination.[18]

Selective sampling Another modification of the cohort design involves selectively oversampling some subgroups of a general population sample. If this is done carefully, so that the sampling fraction of the various groups is known, then it is possible to calculate the population prevalence rate of both diseases and risk factors by weighting each observation by the reciprocal of the probability with which each participant was sampled. For example, in our study of children living in an 11-county area of North Carolina, we wanted to oversample the American Indian children who lived on a federal reservation in the middle of the study area, to be able to look in detail at this smaller but interesting group of children. We therefore recruited every Indian child in the study's age range, but only a subsample of Anglo children living in the area, so that the final sample has 350 Indians and 1071 non-Indians; enough of each group to make statistically powerful comparisons. However, by giving each child an appropriate weight proportional to their chance of being selected, we could also calculate prevalence rates for the whole study area, where Indians make up only 3 per cent of the population.

Overlapping cohorts Another variant of the simple cohort study that has been used a lot in developmental studies is the 'general model'[19] or overlapping cohorts design, which uses a series of cohorts of different ages, followed over time. For example, for the Great Smoky Mountains study, we recruited children aged 9, 11 and 13 in 1993. This design allows the researcher to deal to some extent with the problem that a single cohort experiences a historical event at the same age. Cohorts of different ages will experience a historical event at different ages, and conversely will go through the same developmental stage in different historical climates.[20] An example familiar to life course researchers is Elder's study of the impact of drastic income loss during the depression of the 1930s on two groups, one born early in the 1920s and one at the end of the 1920s.[21] The children (especially the boys) who were younger at the time that disaster struck were more strongly affected by family hardship than were the older ones; Elder found age differences in effects on work, family relations and psychological health that endured into middle age. This *cohort effect* can be contrasted with a *period effect* that we found in the Great Smoky Mountains study when we examined the impact of September 11, 2001 on the 19 and 21 year olds whom we were interviewing that year. In this case, those interviewed after September 11 reported a different pattern of drug use from that seen in those interviewed before September 11; drug use and abuse was higher in women, and lower in men, after that date, but we found no cohort effect; the same effect was seen in both 19 and 21 year olds.[22] Maughan and Lindelow[23] used two birth cohorts, one born in 1958 and one in 1970, to see whether the characteristics of women who became mothers in their teens differed over time. They found that the predictors of teen parenthood did not differ much between the cohorts, but that current levels of adversity in adulthood, including broken marriages and multiple partners, was higher in the younger cohort.

Pros and cons of cohort studies Researchers interested in a life course approach to disease are likely to be attracted to a cohort-based (prospective), hypothesis-light design that leaves as much room as possible for serendipitous findings. A great deal of important knowledge has been generated by cohort studies, but it has to be acknowledged that they are an expensive form of research; too expensive for most funding agencies to contemplate, given the commitment to tie up resources far into the future. This is particularly true of birth cohort studies. A second problem is that researchers age along with their subjects, and studies can falter when the first generation of investigators retire. Thirdly, a cohort by definition consists of people born within a defined time period, and moving through history together. Thus, 30 year olds from a 1920 birth cohort will have experienced a different world from cohorts from a 1970 birth cohort. For example, Collishaw and colleagues used data from children born almost 30 years apart to compare adolescents from three cohorts born in 1958, 1970 and 1984. They found considerable differences in levels of behavioural problems, and lesser differences in emotional symptoms.[24] The differences in Maughan and Lindelow's study of two generations of teen mothers[23] is another example of the dangers of generalizing from a single cohort. However, serious and usually government-level funding is needed to support multiple birth cohorts, as well as careful planning to ensure that measures are comparable across the generations.

For causal research, cohort studies are a mixed blessing. They usually give rise to more causal questions than they answer, but this is not necessarily a bad thing, if they inspire other, more focused experimental studies. They can also be used to disprove hypotheses, as in the case of the value of hormone replacement therapies (HRTs) in the Women's Health Initiative (discussed in more detail in Section 2.3.3 below).

2.3.2.2 Case–control studies

Case–control studies also begin with general population samples, but they select subgroups of interest, and control groups, in whom to explore the causes of disease. This can be done backwards in time, by selecting cases of disease and looking back to the causes, or forwards, by selecting on the basis of a putative risk factor and following cases and controls through time.

Retrospective case–control studies Retrospective case–control studies select people with the disease of interest, and a disease-free control group, from an identified population, in order to calculate the relative level of risk exposure in the two groups. What can be concluded about risk factors from case–control studies depends a great deal on how the controls were selected. For example, Brent and colleagues[25] compared the psychiatric histories of 67 adolescents who killed themselves with an equal number of adolescents from the same city, matched on the median income, population density, racial composition and age distribution of the community they lived in. Within this level of community sampling, cases and controls were individually matched on age, sex, SES and county of residence. Compared with these closely matched controls, the cases had a much worse history of depression, substance abuse, conduct disorders and earlier suicide attempts. Brent *et al.* used this to argue that 'research, treatment, and prevention efforts should target particularly those with mood disorders, but also youth with substance abuse, conduct disorder, and a history of suicidal behavior.' (p. 527).

Prospective case–control studies Here we consider studies that select people from a general population sample on the basis of putative risk for a disease that is not yet manifest, and a control group, and follow them over time to test the validity of the causal hypothesis. This is different from an experimental design in that the groups are not assigned the risk factor of interest, but selected because they have it or do not. A famous example is Doll's prospective study of the smoking habits of doctors.[26] He divided them into groups on the basis of amount of daily smoking, age at onset of smoking and duration of smoking, and observed lung cancer rates over time relative to those of non-smokers. He found strong effects of amount and duration of smoking, but not of age at onset. The study strongly implicated smoking in the causal pathway to lung cancer, but could not prove conclusively that some third factor was not the cause of both smoking and cancer.

In life course research, it is sometimes possible to move both backwards and forwards using a case–control approach. For example, current work on the relationship between birth weight and glucose intolerance started with suggestive clinical observations on adults, used existing cohort studies to look back to infancy, and is now working forward to the disease end-point, diabetes.[27] In our cohort study beginning in childhood, we were able to use retrospective data on birth weight to compare adolescents of low and normal birth weight,[28] finding that low birth weight predicted adolescent depression in girls. Moving forward in time, we were then able to show that the risk was specific to puberty, and disappeared by the time the girls were 19. So we were able to refine the range of possible causal hypotheses to those that reflected effects of puberty rather than maturation in general.

In recent years, the case–control design has come to the fore in linkage studies of genetic risk, and in particular in studies of gene–environment interactions. 'Discordant' monozygotic (identical) twins, one of whom has a given disease and the other does not, provide naturally occurring case–control designs. For example, when Breitner and colleagues compared the medical histories of elderly male monozygotic twin pairs discordant for Alzheimer's disease, they found that 'sustained use of nonsteroidal anti-inflammatory drugs (NSAIDs) was associated with delayed onset and reduced risk' of Alzheimer's disease, but not of other common illnesses such as arthritis or diabetes.[29] This finding has led to several trials of the use of NSAIDS to prevent Alzheimer's disease, with cautiously optimistic results so far,[30] and an increase in prophylactic NSAID use in the population.

Pros and cons of case–control community studies Nested case–control studies are especially useful if cases and controls are to be examined using methods too expensive to use on the whole sample. However, it is important that controls are selected very carefully, especially in terms of the amount of time that they have been exposed to known risk factors or the disease in question. If controls are poorly selected, all the advantages of the case–control nested design will be lost. Readers are referred to Rothman and Greenland's *Modern epidemiology*[16] for detailed instructions on selecting controls from observational studies.

2.3.2.3 Reducing the time demands of observational life course research

Within both observational and experimental studies, there are many ways in which time can be manipulated to increase efficiency and reduce cost. The simplest design is to follow subjects from conception or birth, at least across the life course, preferably from one generation to the next. However, it is extremely hard to engage funding agencies in commitments to keep such studies going. Other designs worth considering capitalize on memory or already collected data. For example, many studies concerned with death from cancer or cardiovascular disease have recruited subjects in mid-life and relied on recall for estimates of such risk factors as smoking or toxic exposures. Sometimes it is possible to monitor cohort members' health outcomes indirectly, through cancer registries or death certificates. Occasionally, an old cohort study can be revived for a new purpose. For example, the Collaborative Perinatal Project, a 14-site cohort of 60 000 pregnant women recruited in the late 1950s and early 1960s,[31] has acquired a new lease of life as a source for studies of early risk for adult disorders such as depression,[32] schizophrenia[33] and tobacco dependence.[34] Sometimes such studies involve following-up a whole sample, as Robins did when she tracked down adults who had attended a child guidance clinic.[35] Sometimes it is possible to embed a case–control study within such a follow-forward design; for example, Niendam and colleagues identified 32 people with schizophrenia from the Collaborative Perinatal Project sample, and matched them with 25 non-schizophrenic siblings and 201 comparison subjects to test for differences on the Wechsler Intelligence Scale for Children administered at age 7.[33]

Many studies have used retrospective recall to fill in gaps in the life history. Sometimes this information can be remarkably accurate. For example, Buka and colleagues[36] compared mothers' recall of aspects of their pregnancy and childbirth with hospital records, and found that even over 30 years mothers were highly accurate reporters of the child's birth weight, although other details, such as gestational age, were much less consistent with written records. Lifetime retrospective recall has also been used to compile lifetime medical and psychiatric histories. These are much more problematic. In the first National Comorbidity Study, a representative survey of psychiatric disorders in the USA,[37] rates were reported for current, 1-year and lifetime prevalence of disorders. Across a wide range of diagnoses, 1-year rates were about twice current rates, and lifetime rates were about twice 1-year rates. Two explanations for this are (1) there was an epidemic of psychiatric disorders close to the time of the survey; or (2) people forgot or failed to report episodes occurring earlier in life. The marked increase in age-specific rates of the disorder in younger cohorts is consistent with either explanation.

2.3.3 Experimental studies in life course research

The essence of an experiment or clinical trial is that the researcher manipulates the situation in some way.[15] Ideally, only one factor is manipulated, in a manner that tests its role in the aetiology of a disease. Even in the laboratory it is hard to keep all but a single factor constant across study groups, and in the real world it is almost impossible. Very occasionally properly *randomized experimental studies* are feasible in the context of life course research. Other kinds of less rigorous experiments that can be conducted in the context of life course research are *field trials*, and *community trials*. It is sometimes possible to use genetically informative samples as 'natural experiments' that control at least some of the potential confounds. *Twin studies* are one of the most important 'natural experiments' of this kind; others are *family studies*, *adoption studies* and *migration studies*. Finally, we discuss the exciting developments in causal life course research made possible by the fall in cost and difficulty of *molecular genetic studies*.

It is quite rare for experimental studies to be embedded in life course research projects. This is a pity, because there are benefits for both kinds of research. For example, the ongoing Women's Health Initiative, a cohort study of 140 000 post-menopausal women in the USA, has embedded some important experimental studies of the impact of hormone replacement on women's health. Some 16 000 women have been randomly assigned to various combinations of oestrogen and progesterone, and already the findings have blown apart several assumptions underlying the use of HRT by millions of women. Randomization to oestrogen plus progestin resulted in no significant improvements in general health, vitality, mental health, depressive symptoms or sexual satisfaction,[38] whereas after 5 years there were significantly increased hazard ratios for coronary heart disease, breast cancer, stroke and pulmonary embolism.[39] Despite a significantly lower risk of colorectal cancer and fractures in women on hormones, the absolute increase in risk was equivalent to 19 excess deaths in 10 000 women. It would have been extremely difficult to assemble a reasonably representative sample of 16 000 women willing to be randomly assigned to HRT. However, it was relatively less difficult to assemble 140 000 women willing to take part in an observational study of ageing (one of us among them), and from there to take the next step of recruiting volunteers for the experimental part of the project.

2.3.3.1 Field trials

'Field trials differ from clinical trials in that they deal with subjects who have not yet gotten disease and therefore are not patients'[16] (p. 70). In the standard field trial, the number of people studied compared with the number getting the disease tends to be large. Also, participants are not already attending a clinical facility, as they usually are in clinical trials, so the research team may have to go out into the community to recruit and follow them. All of this can make field trials very expensive. For example, Rothman[16] estimates that the Multiple Risk Factor Intervention Trial (MRFIT), which tested several prevention strategies for myocardial infarction, required over 12 000 subjects and cost more than half a billion dollars in today's money. Not surprisingly, field trials tend to have fairly limited lives, falling short of a life course perspective.

Field trials tend to be used for studies of prevention programmes, i.e. studies of groups that have not necessarily been exposed to a risk factor for a disease, or are at high risk but have not yet shown signs of disease. MRFIT, which selected middle-aged men at known risk for heart disease, is an example of a targeted[40] prevention field trial.

Sometimes it is possible to use naturally occurring groups or clusters to reduce the cost of field trials. Schools or classrooms within schools make natural units for studying the effects of experimental interventions on children. An example of such a 'cluster randomized trial' is the work done by Kellam and colleagues in Baltimore.[41] Classrooms within a large number of schools were randomly assigned to receive, or not to receive, two interventions designed to help children to improve success in school: one designed to improve school achievement, and another, the 'Good Behavior Game', designed to improve behaviour. Unusually for an intervention of this kind, the 6-year-olds in this study have been followed-up for several years, and the researchers have been able to study the effects of the interventions on the life course of the participants. For example, the authors found that the 'Good Behavior Game' reduced the likelihood that boys, but not girls, would begin to smoke by age 14.[42]

2.3.3.2 Community trials

Sometimes it is possible to carry out field trials using larger units of measurement than individuals. For example, whole cities could be used as units in a field trial of the effectiveness of an anti-smoking intervention.[43] Water fluoridation trials in cities necessarily have to be community interventions, since everyone drinks from the same supply. In these cases, researchers do not track results at the level of individuals, but of communities; for example, they might use death certificates to test the effectiveness of an intervention to reduce pollution levels, or to increase seat belt use.

Pros and cons of field trials and community trials These are often the closest that life course research gets to experimental testing. However, the direct causal link between intervention and outcome is threatened unless the intervention sites are comparable on all other potential risk factors, and this is often hard to prove. In practice, large-scale community intervention trials tend to be expensive and hard to keep funded over an extended period.

2.3.4 Genetically informative designs as natural experiments in life course research

Life course studies present extraordinary opportunities for exploring how our genetic predispositions interact with our environments to produce the people we are, the things we do and the deaths we die. These issues can best be explored in situations that 'pull apart' the standard state of things in which our genetic parents also provide our rearing environment. Here we briefly discuss three such 'natural experiments': twin studies; adoption and fostering studies; and migration studies.

2.3.4.1 Twin and family designs

For a long time, people have puzzled over why some twins are more alike than other twins. The stoic philosopher Posidonius (first century BCE) attributed the similarities of identical twins to shared astrological circumstances, although later St Augustine of Hippo (fourth century CE) pointed to the differences in fraternal twins as a disproof of this causal explanation, and the early physician Hippocrates (fifth century BCE) attributed similar diseases in twins to shared material circumstances. It was not until the nineteenth century that Francis Galton saw the value of twins as an experimental paradigm for exploring the 'nature versus nurture' issue.[44] His method was to see if twins who were similar at birth diverged in dissimilar environments, and whether twins dissimilar at birth converged when reared in similar environments. There are now several twin cohorts being studied over time to explore more sophisticated versions of the same questions. Natural experimental twin designs relevant to life course research include the following.

Comparisons of monozygous and dizygous twin pairs If a characteristic is to some extent 'genetic', then twins who are genetically identical (MZ pairs) should look more similar than twins who share only half their genes (DZ pairs). A huge amount of work over the past 40 years has shown that this is the case for the majority of human traits (although there are some curious exceptions, e.g. some types of cancer[45] and overall life expectancy[46]). Longitudinal twin studies have begun to elucidate the extent of genetic influences on characteristics such as cognitive and physical abilities, but also on the rates at which such abilities decline with age.[47] For example, repeated studies of a subgroup of the Swedish Twin Registry showed changes in the genetic and environmental variance of some measurements with age, such that for motor functioning, mean arterial pressure and forced expiratory volume the percentage of genetic variance increased with increasing age, while the proportion of variance attributable to environmental factors hardly changed. In the case of measures of grip strength and well-being, in contrast, the proportion of genetic variance remained constant from age 50 to 90.[48]

Despite its great power, the standard twin design has several problems.[49] Most importantly, when the twins are both brought up by their biological parents it is impossible to disentangle the effects of a similar nurturing environment from the effects of similar genes.

Also, it cannot be assumed that twins are "the same" as singletons, or that that the environments of MZ twins, in the womb or out of it, are identical. However, if care is taken to rule out alternative explanations, this design can be very fruitful.[50]

Twins reared separately The Swedish Twin Registry of 25 000 twin pairs includes several hundred pairs, both MZ and DZ, who were not brought up together. This provides a powerful design for teasing out the effects of environment versus genes. For example, by comparing these groups with a matched sample of MZ and DZ twins reared together on several personality traits,[51] the investigators were able to show that the similarity of MZ twins on the 'agreeableness' trait of the NEO personality inventory[52] was in fact more the result of rearing environment than of genetics. Despite the attractions of the design, however, few studies will be large enough to be able to make use of it; there were only about 100 MZ pairs reared apart in the huge Swedish sample.

Children of twins Although the children of MZ twins are perceived as cousins, they are genetically half-siblings, whereas the children of DZ twins are, as Rutter puts it, 'cousins both genetically and socially'.[53] Although the genetic difference between cousins and half-sibs is quite small, the design can be valuable because the children of twins reared apart share genes but not environment. For example, d'Onofrio and colleagues showed that although smoking during pregnancy was influenced by genetic factors, it has a direct environmental influence on the birth weight of the fetus which genetic and shared environmental confounds could not account for.[54] However, this is another design that needs a large population or background sample to produce enough children of twins.

Discordant twins If MZ twins differ on a key characteristic, the difference can be used to test for a causal relationship in a way that controls for several potential confounders. For example, Silvertoinen and colleagues[55] used four large twin studies to identify twin pairs of whom one had died of coronary heart disease (CHD), and compare the heights of the twins. They found a clear inverse relationship between height and CHD death even in the MZ pairs. This suggests that the association is due to non-familial environmental factors.

2.3.4.2 Adoption and fostering studies

Children reared by non-biological parents provide another 'natural experiment' that can pull apart nature and nurture. Adoption studies were used to establish that there was a genetic component to alcoholism, criminality, personality disorders, antisocial personality, somatization disorder, affective disorder, hyperactivity and schizophrenia.[56] They have considerable methodological problems, the primary one for life course research being that the social meaning of adoption is very different in different times and places. So a community sample with a wide age span or with participants from different cultures could not assume that adoption or fostering had the same significance for all.

An important component of the adoption design is being able to compare the birth mother with the adoptive mother. This became very difficult for a period, but may be less so nowadays with the increase in 'open' adoptions. Information about birth fathers has always been very hard to obtain. A problem for research with recent adoptions is that birth mothers are increasingly involved in the raising of their child after adoption, so the nature–nurture split is not a clean as it used to be.

The recent influx of Romanian children into the UK has provided an opportunity to study the effects of environment at the group level, by comparing children brought to the UK at different ages with same-aged children still in orphanages, and with children born and adopted within the UK.[57] These studies showed starkly that there was a critical period (6 months) beyond which deprivation in infancy had a marked and irreversible effect on cognitive functioning lasting at least into adolescence. Children adopted before 6 months, however, showed no later effects of their early deprivation.[58] Since it is highly unlikely that the infant adoptees were genetically different from the later adoptees, this is evidence for an environmental effect on cognitive development.

2.3.4.3 Migration studies

Situations in which people undergo rapid environmental change can provide tests of the extent to which a characteristic is under genetic control. An interesting example is puberty, which has been shown to be strongly genetic within stable societies[59,60] However, when a community in Papua New Guinea moved from living in the mountains, where food was scarce and boys were fed before girls, to the coastal plain, where food was abundant, the median age at menarche fell from 18 years to 15.8 years in two decades.[61] Another example showing that apparently 'genetic' conditions are under environmental control is the case of schizophrenia in first- and second-generation immigrants to and from many countries, including Caribbean and African immigrants to Europe, and Finnish immigrants to Sweden.[62–64]

Adult children of migrants to Israel from Europe and North Africa were studied by Dohrenwend in a classic paper that asked whether the association between mental illness and poverty was a function of 'social causation', the stresses of life, or 'social selection', the downward drift of people with mental illness.[65] He predicted that if social causation were operating, then the North Africans, who are discriminated against in Israel, would show more mental illness. On the other hand, if social selection were operating, then the children of European immigrants, whose families had been in Israel longer, would show an excess, since all the 'healthy' ones would have moved out of poverty by now. The authors reported that

> ... rates of schizophrenia are higher for respondents of European background with SES controlled, as would be expected if sorting and sifting processes function to hold down more healthy persons of disadvantaged North African background while leaving behind a residue of severely ill persons of advantaged European background. This outcome implies that social selection processes are more important than social causation processes in the relation between SES and schizophrenia. By contrast, holding SES constant, we found that rates of major depression in women and antisocial personality and substance use disorders in men are higher in Israelis of North African background, as would be expected if an increment in adversity attaching to disadvantaged ethnic status produces an increment in psychopathology. These results suggest that social causation processes are stronger than social selection processes in inverse relations between SES and these disorders[65] (p. 951).

This study ingeniously used a two-generational life course design to address one of the most vexing questions in psychiatry.

Migration studies have been enormously valuable for studying the effects on health of changes in diet, life stress and healthcare. However, they face the problem that migrant groups are rarely representative of the community they leave behind. They may be exceptionally healthy and adventurous, or they may be the most desperate and stressed of their country's citizens. For example, Verhulst and colleagues[66] compared self-report psychiatric symptoms of Turkish youth whose families had migrated to the Netherlands with those of two comparison groups: native-born Dutch youth and Turkish youth living in Turkey. The immigrant Turkish youth reported more delinquency, aggression and attention problems than the Turkish youth living in Turkey, but not more anxiety and depression. However, they showed more anxiety and depression than Dutch youth living in the Netherlands. The author's explanation is that 'Turkish families give higher value to obedience and conformity than to autonomy, which may induce anxiety in children. This is especially true for Turkish immigrant families in Europe, because they represent the more traditional, rural society in Turkey rather than the society at large'[66] (p. 138). This may be true, but the quotation illustrates another problem with many non-experimental designs: our urge to explain our findings plausibly.

2.3.4.4 Pros and cons of genetically informative designs for life course research

Twins, adoptees and migrants are uncommon, and any general population sample is unlikely to have enough of them for statistically powerful analysis. The influx of Romanian adoptees was an extraordinary 'natural experiment' born of a tragedy. Over the life course of its subjects, it will doubtless, like other studies born of tragedy, such as the Dutch famine study, be informative about the impact of early deprivation on adult chronic diseases.

In the case of twins, it is sometimes possible to oversample them as part of the original sample selection, as is proposed, for example, for the Swedish LifeGene cohort study. If so, twins can greatly strengthen the power of a life course study to test causal hypotheses about mechanisms of action. At first, genetically informative designs were used to demonstrate to a doubtful world that many human characteristics and diseases had a genetic component. More recently, however, their great value has been to explore the environments within which genes are expressed. The height and CHD study is an example. It is well known that height is strongly heritable. Therefore, if there is a marked discordance in the heights of MZ twins, and this discordance is associated with a disease outcome (in this case CHD), this is suggestive evidence that the circumstances that caused the height differential, such as different intrauterine conditions leading to different birth weights, may also have created different levels of risk for CHD decades later.

In summary, there are dozens of ingenious ways of doing life course research; not all of them require national governments to commit untold millions, or for researchers to commit their entire lives. However, the more ingenious designs tend to have their own drawbacks. Follow-forward designs constrain the analyses to areas on which information was collected in the earlier study, while 'passive' prospective studies, such as those using death certificates, tend to have a limited range of outcome measures. Case–control studies can only estimate risk relative to the control group, while none of these designs has the potential of the cohort longitudinal study to throw up serendipitous findings that can change the way we look at the world. For example, the link between low birth weight and adult blood pressure and cardiovascular mortality[67] was not dreamed of when the National Survey of Health and Development began in 1946.

An example of serendipity in our own work occurred when a gambling casino was opened on an Indian reservation whose children we had been studying for years as part of the Great Smoky Mountains study.[68] Under the contract agreed between the tribe and the casino management, every tribal member received a small proportion of the casino's profits; the children's shares going into savings accounts until they left school. Of course, no such income supplement came to non-Indian families in the study. This gave us an opportunity to look at the impact of an addition to family income on children's emotional and behavioural problems in a 'natural experiment' that got around the problem that families whose incomes rise are often different in some ways from those whose incomes do not rise. We found a marked improvement in the behavioural problems of children whose families moved out of poverty, but a much smaller effect on emotional symptoms (anxiety and depression). The results were replicated in non-Indian families that moved out of poverty, which was reassuring, as we would expect the same findings, although we could not attribute them to the income change in White families as securely as we could in the Indian families.

The opportunity to move in new directions, undreamed of when a study began, is one of the pleasures of life course research.

2.4 Capturing individual differences and development at different *levels of measurement*

Life course research makes use of an enormously wide range of methods for measuring everything from environmental pollutants to individual genes. In the remainder of this chapter, we focus on a small part of this range: the assessment of individual characteristics—biological, psychological and behavioural—across the life course. We concentrate on the questions that each researcher has to answer when choosing how to measure individual differences at the level of observable or reportable states of the individual, and of the biological systems that mediate the impact of the world on the individual.

2.4.1 Issues in measuring individual differences at the phenomenological/behavioural level

One of the strengths of life course research has been its interest in moving easily between medical and psychiatric conditions as both predictors and outcomes. Recent research showing, for example, the increased all-cause mortality associated with depression[69] highlights the importance of doing so. However, the need to know what is going on in the individual at both the medical and the psychiatric levels (not to mention at the level of cognitive and general functioning) creates major problems of cost and participant burden. There is no single, or simple, answer, but some general principles are worth consideration.

2.4.1.1 Using continuous versus categorical measures

Individual difference research in biology and psychology has tended to use continuous measures (height, weight, IQ, temperament scales), while the medical sciences have traditionally used categories (measles, depression, cancer) and, even when they use continuous measures, tend to dichotomize them (high blood pressure, high cholesterol). The problem with categorical definitions, for life course research, is that the criteria tend to change over time.

For example, 'high blood pressure' has a much lower threshold now than it did a decade ago. In practice, this conflict of styles is not as dramatic as it looks, because most dichotomous classifications are made by collecting a number of symptoms. Depression using the current American diagnostic classification, for instance, requires five or more of a list of nine symptoms. It is simple enough to convert the diagnostic classification into a scale score, so long as all the data have been preserved.

There are more problems in going in the other direction if, as with many psychiatric and medical diagnoses, there are additional criteria that are not included in the scale score. Depression in DSM-IV,[70] for example, requires that the symptoms be present together during the same 2-week period, that they represent a change from previous functioning, are not caused by drug abuse or a medical condition or by bereavement, and cause significant distress or functional impairment. Most depression scales do not cover these topics. It is not yet clear how much is lost, in terms of predictive power or associated morbidity, by using 'pseudo-diagnoses' based on scale scores alone. It may be that the additional criteria matter more as guides to treatment than as predictors of functioning over time, and that pseudo-diagnoses based on scale scores may often be quite adequate for life course research.

It is often valuable to be able to examine the range over which a risk factor or intervention has its effect, in which case continuous measures are valuable. For example, a study of the effects on adults of having been exposed prenatally to the Dutch famine of 1944–1945 found an increase in systolic blood pressure of 2.7 mmHg for each kilogram decrease in birth weight.[71] Our study of the effects of birth weight on risk for adolescent depression found a significant linear decrease of 0.2 of a standard deviation in mean number of adolescent girls' depressive symptoms with each pound increase in birth weight, but no effect at all for boys.[28]

On the other hand, life course studies may lose the attention of the medical community if they cannot communicate in the same language, which is the language of diseases. Some epidemiological studies get around the problem by asking for self-report of illnesses ('has a doctor told you that you have X?') or using registries of various sorts, but these entail their own forms of inaccuracy.

2.4.1.2 Measuring at the appropriate level of complexity

There are two aspects to this principle: the *timing* of measurement and the *intensity* of measurement.

Timing of measurement   Some phenomena (e.g. heart rate) change in seconds in response to changing environmental stimuli, while others (e.g. hair colour) change quite slowly over the life span. Yet others (e.g. height) change relatively rapidly at some developmental stages, and slowly at others. The timing of measurement in life course research needs to reflect the velocity of change of the phenomena under study.[72] For example, to estimate the relationship between oestrogen levels and peak growth velocity, researchers needed to assess children every 4 months to capture the changes in growth rate.[73] Using a different degree of resolution, Larson[74] 'beeped' children every few minutes throughout the day to measure the relationship between social situation and depression across childhood and adolescence. At the other extreme, a crude test of the hypothesis that low birth weight predicts cardio-vascular mortality would require only birth weight and mortality records.

Often the challenge for researchers is to work out a contact schedule for study partici-pants that meets competing needs of several kinds of measurement that have differing time frames. For example, until recently, nutritional epidemiologists were stuck at the level of ecological or correlational studies of the effects of diet on disease, because they lacked the tools to link individual nutrition, which is best measured using daily dietary information, to life course outcomes.[75] However, they have developed several kinds of interlinked measures that enable them to make reasonably reliable estimates of food eaten, and nutrients ingested, using relatively simple tools such as food frequency ques-tionnaires.[76] This means that a questionnaire can be used to approximate much more detailed and burdensome measurements, and that information on food can be collected as part of a package of different measures, perhaps at an annual interview.

Another aspect of the timing of measurement is that it needs to be sensitive to major changes in the individual or the environment. The annual or biennial assessments that we tend to use rather mindlessly may miss a lot of activity around a key event: marriage, birth of a child, death of a parent; events whose timing the researcher cannot predict in the way that, for example, the timing of puberty is somewhat predictable. What are needed here are adaptations of the 'sentinel event' methodology used in surveillance epidemiology.[77] The occurrence of a sentinel event (e.g. marriage, or admission to hospital) would trigger a special assessment. Clearly there are difficulties with ensuring that participants report key events, but some (births, marriages, deaths, imprisonment) are matters of public record, and improvements in computerized record linkage may make this approach more feasible in the future.

Intensity of measurement It sometimes seems as though researchers are born with an irrational preference for a certain type of measurement; I insist on using diagnostic inter-views, you think questionnaires are better, while she believes only in the results of magnetic resonance imaging (MRI). It is surprising that so little work has been done to compare the cost and efficiency of different types of data collection against one another. One argument often used by life course researchers is that limits on time and money force them to use short, simple methods that collect relatively low intensity data. However, this begs the question of what sort of data can adequately be collected using quick and easy methods, and which really need more intensity of measurement. For example, some studies take great care to weigh and measure participants using the latest equipment and carefully trained research staff, while others simply ask people their height and weight.

Which method is the more cost efficient? Assuming that the more labour-intensive method is more accurate, how much of a decrement in accuracy is acceptable before self-report becomes unacceptable?

In our studies of puberty, we have gone to great lengths to obtain blood samples, self-report Tanner staging and responses to questions about the child's perceptions of being 'early', on time or delayed in pubertal development relative to other children. As described earlier, the hormone measures from the blood samples proved essential to understanding the role of puberty in depression.[78] However, in the case of substance abuse, hormonal measures were not predictive, whereas age at first use of alcohol or tobacco (which was not related to hormonal development) predicted drug abuse.[79] Thus, the most cost-efficient intensity of measurement of puberty varied with the outcome: hormonal assays for depression, age for substance abuse.

2.4.1.3 Thinking about the best source(s) of information

Informants Until quite recently it was assumed in mental health research that children could not provide reliable or valid information about their own mental states. In the 1960s, clinicians and researchers began to test this assumption,[80,81] and found that children's reports were not markedly less reliable or valid than those of parents about their children. The problem that quickly arose, however, was the discovery that parents and children responded very differently to questions about the same phenomena.[82,83] It is quite common for parent and child to agree less than 10 per cent of the time on the presence or absence of psychiatric symptoms, even when the reports of each individual show a high test–re-test reliability. The same thing can be found when parent reports are compared with those of teachers,[84] or even fathers with mother.[85–87] Twin studies have shown that the heritability of different psychiatric disorders varies with informant.[88–90]

This lack of agreement is far from being specific to psychiatric symptoms; informants disagree markedly on such topics as the amount of pain someone is experiencing,[91,92] the child's level of physical health and well-being,[93] and success in managing diabetes.[94]

The issue often is not so much who is right, as how to choose what information to use in reaching a decision about someone's health or illness, or, in a clinical setting, about what treatment should be provided. Practice guidelines[95] often recommend collecting information from at least one parent, the child and a teacher, and weighting conflicting evidence towards believing positive reports more than negative ones.[96] This is an expensive procedure for large longitudinal studies. On the basis of interviews with multiple sources, some researchers[97,98] have recommended that children can be used as the single best source of information about fears and anxieties, and possibly about depression. It is generally agreed that children's information about their own hyperactivity or attentional deficits has little value, while the value of their reports of conduct and oppositional problems may change with age; parents can tell us about younger children's temper tantrums and overt rule breaking, but may know little about their adolescents' covert stealing and drug abuse.

Adults have generally been the single source of information about their own mental health, unless they suffer from dementia or psychosis. It would be interesting to know whether the degree of non-agreement seen in studies of children would be mirrored in studies of adults, and what the effect of having only one informant would be on, for example, adult genetic studies.

There will be the usual problems of lack of agreement among information sources, but sometimes a different source can add a valuable insight. For example, in Loeber *et al.*'s study of young men in Pittsburgh, even using the combined report of the participant, parent and teacher only identified 54 per cent of youth who had a record of criminal delinquency from the juvenile court records.[99] The authors believe that there are very few 'false positives' from any data source, so combining information from all these sources might produce a more accurate estimate of juvenile delinquency than choosing among them.

Alternative sources of information The discussion so far has dealt with interview or questionnaire methods for collecting information about study participants, but there may be areas of psychopathology for which other methods can be used in some countries. Hospital admissions, or even out-patient diagnoses or drug prescriptions, can sometimes be identified at the individual level. The same is true of criminal records. Births, marriages and deaths are public access records in most places. Sometimes it is possible to link records held by different agencies. For example, Bata and colleagues[100] linked hospital records to national mortality records for two periods: 1984–1988 and 1989–1993, to see whether changes in therapeutic methods had improved 5-year survival, controlling for differences in the severity of cases admitted to hospital. They found that there was a 5 per cent increase in 5-year survival that was associated with changes in the treatments used, and was not due to differences in patient characteristics.

Here too there will be lack of agreement among records, as well as doubt about the quality of matches, and ethical questions about combining publicly accessible and study-specific data. However, electronic databases have made record linkage infinitely easier, and as time goes on this may be one of the most fruitful new sources of data for life course research.

2.4.1.4 Thinking about the range of uses of the information

Some life course research is begun with long-term follow-up in mind; many other studies start with quite other goals, and then wake up one morning to find that they have become life course studies. It makes sense for anyone embarking on a longitudinal study to ask some what-if questions: if this study went on longer than we originally planned, what data should we be collecting now? Or, if this data set became useful for purposes beyond its immediate goals, what data should be there to help other researchers? To give a couple of examples, we started a 5-year study (now in its 12th year) to look at children's need for and access to mental health services in a rural area. Because the USA has not supported birth cohort studies like those in the UK and other European countries, this small study has since become an important source of basic information about prevalence and risk factors. By good fortune, the investigators' interest in the impact of puberty led us to collect small blood samples from the subjects each year. Over time, this has proved to be tremendously important for looking not only at puberty, but also at stress and obesity.

However, there are several things that, had we seen the study as a life course one, we would have included, most notably measures of temperament and IQ.

In the end, whether you have collected the right data for the questions that emerge down the road is going to be a matter of luck. However, luck can be invited through a judicious selection of measurement domains and intensity of measurement. Sometimes alternating between labour-intensive methods (e.g. interviews) and cheaper methods (e.g. questionnaires) can be cost efficient, providing that you know what the relationships are between the different levels of measurement.

2.4.2 Issues in measuring individual differences at the intra-organismic level

Life course research is seldom concerned with individual differences solely at the level of behavioural phenomena; usually the goal is to make links from the phenomenologic to the intra-organismic level, in the hope of identifying 'mechanisms', if not 'causes', of differences in behavioural or health outcomes. For example, in our studies of the effects of puberty on depression,[78,101,102] we examined separately the relationship between depression and not only standard 'observable' phenomena such as menarche, body morphology and self-image, but also a range of the hormones involved in reproductive maturity [follicule-stimulating hormone (FSH), luteinizing hormone (LH), oestradiol, testosterone, androstenedione and dehydroepiandrosterone (DHEA-S)]. The goal was to see if we could pinpoint more closely the 'mechanism' driving the extraordinary increase in depression in girls that begins at around age 13. In multiple regression models that included the hormone measures, along with age and several morphological measures of puberty, it was the steroid hormones oestradiol and testosterone that predicted depression, controlling for all the other measures. Clearly, this does not mean that these levels of steroid hormones by themselves cause depression across the reproductive life span; if it did, all women of child-bearing age would be depressed. What it does suggest is that a change at the intra-organismic level (steroid hormone secretion) at this developmental stage of life is a better marker of increased risk for depression than the markers that have previously been used: age, morphological development ('Tanner stage'[103]) or age at menarche.

In 2001, the National Academy of Sciences in the USA published a report: *Cells and surveys: should biological measures be included in social science research?* [104] The title is something of a misnomer, because it is clear that the contributors thought that biological measures certainly should be included in social research, and that they would be in future in any case, whatever the committee thought.

The book provides helpful insights into how, why and when to include intra-organismic measures in large longitudinal research projects. For example, one chapter describes how the MacArthur Study of Successful Aging has repeatedly generated information on 10 biological parameters reflecting the functioning of four biological systems: the hypothalamic–pituitary–adrenal (HPA) axis (cortisol, DHEAS), the sympathetic nervous system (epinephrine, norepinephrine), the cardiovascular system (blood pressure) and metabolic processes (body mass index, cholesterol, homocysteine, glycosylated haemoglobin),[105] using data collected during home visits to around 1000 elderly people. In another example, the ongoing National Health and Nutrition Examination Survey collects elaborate biological measures on a nationally representative sample of the non-institutional population of the USA, employing mobile examination centres (e.g. Giles *et al.* [106]). So the technologies exist, and have been field-tested. We focus here on some of the issues that arise in incorporating biological measures of this kind into long-term longitudinal studies, whether as genetic markers or as indicators of stress exposure.

2.4.2.1 Collecting genetic information in life course research

Earlier we discussed genetically informative designs for life course research. Here we discuss some methodological and ethical issues in collecting and using genetic information, particularly DNA.

The role of families in shaping human development has been a central interest of life course research. So the potential to include genetic information in life course research has long been of interest. Until recently, the only way to do this was to select non-representative samples that were genetically informative: high-risk families, adoptive families, families with twins or populations that had migrated from their native country. Few studies using genetically informative designs have been longitudinal. Few have sampled from the general population in ways that make their findings generalizable far beyond their own sample. Even twin studies have often relied on volunteer or low-response samples that raise problems of response bias. The other major problem with most of these designs is that they rely on statistical models to measure the relative amounts of the variance in the outcome measure that can be attributed to genes, but cannot pinpoint the precise gene or genes responsible, or the precise individuals at risk.

All this has changed with the development of cheaper technologies for examining candidate genes in large populations. DNA can now been obtained from very small samples of body fluids or tissues (blood, cheek scrapes). This raises questions for every life course study: should we collect material for DNA analysis, and what should we do with it, given the constraints of ethics and science?

Readers are referred to the National Academy of Science volume mentioned earlier[104] for a thoughtful and thorough discussion of both issues. The answer to the first question is clearly yes, and the discussion of ethical issues is encouraging,[107] but the authors raise many valuable points about the likely usefulness of DNA information for social research over the short and long term. Ewbank[108] identifies the following major uses that are relevant for life course research: (1) predicting individual differences in outcomes (e.g. disease, length of life); (2) as controls when estimating the effects of other variables (e.g. the effect of diet on a certain cancer; (3) controlling for genetic risk; (4) as effect modifiers (gene–gene or gene–environment interactions); and (5) as instrumental variables (genes as stand-ins for much more complex constructs such as health status).

Wallace[109] looks at the question the other way around: how can population studies be useful for genetic research? He notes the following uses: (1) assessing the distribution of known gene markers in demographically defined populations; (2) exploring associations between gene markers and phenotypes using entire cohorts or nested case–control designs; (3) using cohort studies to examine the relationship between a gene and multiple possible outcomes; (4) using cohort studies as a source of families for a range of within-family linkage studies, such as sib-pair, trio (two parents and offspring), co-twin, half-sib and other combinations; and (5) studies of gene–environment interactions. Examples of the latter use have shown a genetic component in the regulation of environmentally acquired infections[110] and, in the area of psychopathology, evidence that a functional polymorphism in the promoter region of the serotonin transporter (5-HTT) gene moderated the influence of stressful life events on depression.[111]

Pros and cons of collecting genetic information for life course research A big advantage of DNA as a research tool is that, for all practical purposes, it need only be collected once, and that once can be any time. Longitudinal research presents the opportunity for participants to change their mind about consenting to DNA analyses, even if they refused at first. Researchers often fear that asking for blood or cheek scrapes will reduce participation or, even more troubling for life course research, cause participants to drop out. This has not been our experience, or that of many other researchers.[105,112,113] Indeed, some of our participants are delighted that finally we are doing 'real science'. However, it is important to offer participants the opportunity to refuse to provide biodata and still continue with the rest of the study, and to use minimally invasive methods. It is also important to ensure that lay interviewers are adequately trained to collect, label, store and transmit biodata safely and with appropriate respect for the participant's 'gift'[114] to the study. For example, cheap and simple bar code printers are very useful for labelling cheek scrape samples in the participant's home, and logging them safely into the laboratory. A further problem with DNA is the understandable nervousness of ethical review boards. We discuss this later, in the context of other types of biodata.

2.4.2.2 Using biodata for the study of stress in life course research

Studies of the impact of stressors over the life course often have to make a leap of faith: the individual was exposed to a stressor; the individual suffered a degradation of mental or physical health; therefore, the former caused the latter. If it were possible to identify a psychological or physiological change following stressor exposure that could be construed as an intra-organismic cost of coping with the stressor ('stress'), and the latter could be linked in turn to medical or mental illness, then the causal connection would be stronger.

There is a vast laboratory-based literature on biomarkers of stress, but only recently have either the theories or the methods appeared that could relate this type of work to life course or epidemiological studies.

Effects of stressors have been studied in four main systems: the autonomic nervous system; the metabolic system; the immune system; and the neuroendocrine system. All of these systems assist in maintaining the body's physiological (and psychological) integrity in the presence of a changing environment. Depending on the goals of the study, it will be important to decide whether to measure the system in a baseline state, or under challenge, or both. For example, time to recovery following a stressor can be as important a measure of stress as the degree of response under challenge.[115]

Autonomic nervous system The effects of stressors have long been measured in altered autonomic balance characterized by increased sympathetic nervous system (SNS) tone and reactivity and by decreased parasympathetic nervous system (PNS) tone. It is possible to obtain both heart rate and blood pressure readings using automated equipment that is portable and does not require any expertise of the interviewer. For example, in a community study of children and adolescents, we used a portable Dina MAP automatic blood pressure monitor, and a Zymed Holter monitor to provide a continuous electrocardiogram reading during a variety of physical and mental stress tasks. Both worked perfectly well in the home setting, and can be used continuously for several days, at least by adults.[116]

Metabolic system Among the many aspects of the metabolic system, some that have been studied in the context of stress are body mass index (BMI) or hip to waist ratio, cholesterol, and glucosylated haemoglobin as a measure of glucose levels. The first is easily obtained in field studies, although accurate equipment (scales and stadiometers) must be used, and a standard protocol for clothing observed. The use of calipers to measure skin fold thickness is sometimes feasible, but in some cultures it is not possible for hip or buttock skin fold measures to be taken, especially if the interviewer is not of the same sex as the subject.

Other measures require blood samples. This is relatively simple if participants come to a central site for evaluations, as in the Dunedin longitudinal study, for example. If this is not possible, or if travelling laboratories are not available, it will be necessary to send out trained phlebotomists to subjects' homes (as in the MacArthur Study of Successful Aging). This can be an expensive addition to a life course study. Sometimes it may be feasible to conduct a smaller case–control study; for example, to select a group under high stress and a control group, and recruit them to come into the laboratory for additional testing, including blood work.

Neuroendocrine system The HPA axis plays a central role in homeostatic regulation of the body.[117] HPA activity can be measured in blood or saliva; for example, the glutocorticoid hormone cortisol can be assayed in both whole blood samples and dried blood. The latter technique is well adapted to field studies for which phlebotomy is an expensive option. Cortisol release is pulsatile and episodic, and shows strong diurnal variation. Thus, it is important to obtain multiple measures, and to record the time of day when a sample is obtained. Cortisol reflects the impact of recent experience, roughly within the past hour. Because the environment in the home can usually not be controlled, as that of a laboratory can, to ensure a standard environment for baseline measures, cortisol is probably most useful in field studies in the context of a challenge task, where the response to a known stressor can be assessed. So far, efforts to develop screens for psychopathology based on endocrine measures (e.g. cortisol/DHEA ratio as a screen for depression[118]) have not shown sufficiently high predictive values to be useful in the real world.[119]

Immune system The stress response may deplete cellular energy and immune reserves, and these energy reserves have to be replenished to provide for immunity, growth and other functions. Psychoneuroimmunology has documented pervasive inter-connections between psychosocial stressors and immune function (see, for example[120–122]). Animal and clinical studies indicate that early stressor exposure influences the development of the immune system and can lead to diminished activation and maintenance capacities.[123,124] Both transient stressors, such as social conflict, exam taking or performance anxiety,[125–128] and chronic stressors, such as a poor marital relationship or caring for a relative with Alzheimer's disease,[129] result in altered immune function.

Given the complexity of psychoneuroimmunological relationships, an overall physiological index of chronic stress has been difficult to derive. The cardiovascular, neuroendocrine and other autonomic systems that mediate the stress response operate in milliseconds to minutes, and are subject to diurnal variation, pulsatile or episodic fluctuation, and acute contextual effects as well as developmental change. This makes them difficult to track under natural conditions.

The challenge for life course research is to find methods that permit repeated measurement of stress, whether at fixed intervals or in response to specific events. In the Great Smoky Mountains study, we took advantage of the fact that capillary blood samples were already being collected to test whether Epstein–Barr virus (EBV) antibodies could be used as a stress marker in a field study. Antibodies to resident viruses reflect immunocompetence in keeping the virus in check, a capacity that is eroded by psychosocial stress. In individuals infected with the EBV, circulating levels of viral antibody have been consistently linked to daily stress levels[125,126,129,130] and negative mood.[131] On the other hand, social integration, support and stress management interventions are reflected in lower EBV antibodies[132,133] Over all, the internal burden of stress indexed by EBV titres has been shown to correspond to recent ongoing exposure and responses to stressors.[134,135]

Pros and cons of collecting biodata This very brief look at a few biomarkers that have potential use in life course research aims to encourage researchers to enlist expert colleagues and explore with them the costs and benefits of what is, for most psychosocial researchers, a new area. One thing that you will discover is the tremendous value of your life course data to biomedical science. Molecular genetics, for example, is in need of well characterized, representative population samples in which to test candidate genes. Where once 'experiments of nature' such as twins or adoptees were needed for genetic research, now hypotheses can be tested directly on individuals. Equally important is good information about the individual's environment, especially their environmental history across childhood and adolescence. Caspi *et al.*'s landmark study of men from the Dunedin longitudinal study[136] showed that there was no main effect of either the gene or of early adversity on young adult conduct disorder, but a clear interaction of gene and early environment. It is notable that this and other ground-breaking papers on gene–environment interaction came not from a genetics laboratory but from a multidisciplinary group working on a birth cohort study. There are many life course studies that could contribute, like the Dunedin study, to important breakthroughs in our understanding of individual differences in the long-term impact of stressors.

We have mentioned earlier that study participants often value the ability to contribute biodata to do 'real science'. However, ethical review boards will want strong assurances that such materials are being treated with the care and concern that the participant's 'gift' deserves. If significant amounts of blood are to be drawn, a trained phlebotomist will be needed. Finger-stick blood spots, cheek scrapes and saliva can be collected by lay personnel, but they must be carefully trained. There is a big difference between talking to people and touching them, and staff need to be trained to respect the person's body as they handle it. Procedures for stabilizing biodata, transmission to the laboratory, record keeping, and so on must be carefully specified in applications for ethical approval, and in Standard Operating Procedure manuals for staff.

The question of how to handle feed-back to study participants will be answered differently in different studies and countries. This too must be carefully set out in ethical approval applications, following the institution's guidelines. In the USA, a federal Certificate of Confidentiality can be obtained, which protects data from subpoena by any court. This should shield subjects' DNA information from the eyes of insurance companies. Sometimes subjects want information, especially about genetics. It is for individual investigators to decide how to handle this, but they need to remind participants that once any information has been shared, even with the participant, the investigator can no longer be responsible for its continuing confidentiality.

2.5 Conclusions

This chapter has focused on methods for studying individual differences in life course research. In one section, we have talked about research designs, and in another about measurement issues. There is no room in a single chapter to be specific about the huge range of designs and measures available for different purposes. We have tried to raise some questions for you, the researcher, to think about.

If there is a take home message, it is *prepare for serendipity*. No-one embarking on a longitudinal study can know what will be the key questions tomorrow, or the day after tomorrow. The best we can do is to ensure that we have covered as many bases as possible. Since we always want to get more information than we can afford to collect, and more than participants can tolerate our collecting, then we need to be cunning and flexible in our methods. Do we need these annual interviews, or could we alternate them with something different: a real-time study of loneliness using hand-held minicomputers,[137] or a case–control functional MRI study of brain effects of early trauma? Can we monitor participants' life events (births, imprisonments, deaths) from a distance using public access records? Can we use a historical event to study stress response?[22]

Representative longitudinal data sets are national treasures. With new questions arising all the time, it is our job to see that they become ever more valuable as time passes.

Acknowledgements

This work was supported by grants DA11301 and MH57761 and Independent Scientist Award MH01167 from the National Institutes of Health.

Further reading

Bronfenbrenner U (1977). Toward an experimental ecology of human development. *American Psychologist* 32, 513–531.

Dohrenwend BP, Levav I, Shrout PE, Schwartz S, Naveh G, Link BG, *et al.* (1992). Socioeconomic status and psychiatric disorders: the causation–selection issue. *Science* 255, 946–952.

Maldonado G, Greenland S (2002). Estimating causal effects. *International Journal of Epidemiology* 31, 422–429.

Rothman KJ, Greenland S (1998). *Modern epidemiology*, 2nd edn. Lippincott-Raven, Philadelphia.

Shadish W, Cook T, Campbell D (2002). *Experimental and quasi-experimental designs for generalized causal inference.* Houghton Mifflin, Boston.

Susser M (1991). What is a cause and how do we know one? A grammar for pragmatic epidemiology. *American Journal of Epidemiology* 33, 635–648.

References

1. Hobbes T (1651). *Leviathan.* Clarendon Press, Oxford.

2. Waddington CH (1957). *The strategy of genes.* Allen and Unwin, London.

3. Gottlieb G (1991). Experiential canalization of behavioral development: theory. *Developmental Psychopathology* 27, 4–13.

4. Cacioppo JT, Tassinary LG (1990). Inferring psychological significance from physiological signals. *American Psychologist* 45, 16–26.

5. Bronfenbrenner U (1977). Toward an experimental ecology of human development. *American Psychologist* 32, 513–531.

6. Phillips DIW, Barker DJP, Fall CHD, Seckl JR, Whorwood CB, Wood PJ, *et al.* (1998). Elevated plasma cortisol concentrations: a link between low birth weight and the insulin resistance syndrome? *Journal of Clinical Endocrinology and Metabolism* 83, 757–760.

7. DiLiberti JH (2000). The relationship between social stratification and all-cause mortality among children in the United States: 1968–1992. *Pediatrics* 105, e2.

8. Hume D (2000). *An enquiry concerning human understanding.* Oxford University Press, New York.

9. Maldonado G, Greenland S (2002). Estimating causal effects. *International Journal of Epidemiology* 31, 422–429.

10. Mill J (1856). *A system of logic: ratiocinative and inductive.* Reprint. London: Rutledge, 1892.

11. Koch R (1882). Dei Aetiologie der Tuberculose. *Berl Klin Wochenschr* 19, 221–230.

12. Hill AB (1965). Environment and disease: association or causation? *Proceedings of the Royal Society of Medicine* 58, 295–300.

13. Susser M (1991). What is a cause and how do we know one? A grammar for pragmatic epidemiology. *American Journal of Epidemiology* 33, 635–648.

14. Robins E, Guze SB (1970). Establishment of diagnostic validity in psychiatric illness: its application to schizophrenia. *American Journal of Psychiatry* 126, 107–111.

15. Shadish W, Cook T, Campbell D (2002). *Experimental and quasi-experimental designs for generalized causal inference.* Houghton Mifflin, Boston.

16. Rothman KJ, Greenland S (1998). *Modern epidemiology*, 2nd edn. Lippincott-Raven, Philadelphia.

17. Kannel WB (1990). Contribution of the Framingham Study to preventive cardiology. *Journal of the American College of Cardiology* 15, 206–211.

18. Kannel WB, Castelli WP (1972). The Framingham study of coronary disease in women. *Medical Times* 100, 173.

19. Schaie KW (1965). A general model for the study of developmental problems. *Psychological Bulletin* 64, 92–107.

20. Schaie KW (1986). Beyond calendar definitions of age, time, and cohort: the general developmental model revisited. *Developmental Review* 6, 252–277.

21. Elder GH (1996). Human lives in changing societies: life course and developmental insights. In: Cairns R, Elder GH Jr, Costello EJ, ed. *Developmental science*. Cambridge University Press, Cambridge, MA, pp. 31–62.

22. Costello EJ, Erkanli A, Keeler G, Angold A (2004). Distant trauma: a prospective study of the effects of 9/11 on rural youth. *Applied Developmental Science* 8, 211–220.

23. Maughan BM, Lindelow M (1997). Secular change in psychosocial risks: the case of teenage motherhood. *Psychological Medicine* 27, 1129–1144.

24. Collishaw S, Maughan B, Goodman R, Pickles A (2004). Time trends in adolescent mental health. *Journal of Child Psychology and Psychiatry* 45, 1350–1362.

25. Brent DA, Perper JA, Moritz G, Allman C, Friebd A, Roth C, *et al.* (1993). Psychiatric risk factors for adolescent suicide: a case–control study. *Journal of the American Academy of Child and Adolescent Psychiatry* 32, 521–529.

26. Doll R, Peto R (1976). Mortality in relation to smoking: 20 years' observations on male British doctors. *British Medical Journal* ii, 1525–1536.

27. Barker DJP (2005). The developmental origins of insulin resistance. *Hormone Research* 64, 2.

28. Costello EJ, Worthman C, Erkanli A, Angold A (2007). Low birthweight predicts female adolescent depression: a test of competing hypotheses. *Archives of General Psychiatry* 64, 338–344.

29. Breitner J, Welsh K, Helms MJ, Gaskell PC, Gau BA, Roses AD, *et al.* (1995). Delayed onset of Alzheimer's disease with nonsteroidal anti-inflammatory and histamine H2 blocking drugs. *Neurobiology of Aging* 16, 523–530.

30. Etminan M, Gill S, Samii A (2003). Effect of non-steroidal anti-inflammatory drugs on risk of Alzheimer's disease: systematic review and meta-analysis of observational studies. *British Medical Journal* 327, 128.

31. Hardy J (2003). The Collaborative Perinatal Project: lessons and legacy. *Annals of Epidemiology* 13, 303–311.

32. Gilman S, Kawachi I, Fitzmaurice G, Buka SL (2003). Family disruption in childhood and risk of adult depression. *American Journal of Psychiatry* 160, 939–946.

33. Niendam T, Bearden C, Rosso I, Sanchez LE, Hadley T, Nuechterlein KH, *et al.* (2003). A prospective study of childhood neurocognitive functioning in schizophrenic patients and their siblings. *American Journal of Psychiatry* 160, 2060–2062.

34. Buka S, Shenassa E, Niaura R (2003). Elevated risk of tobacco dependance among offspring of mothers who smoked during pregnancy: a 30-year prospective study. *American Journal of Psychiatry* 160, 1978–1984.

35. Robins L (1988). Data gathering and data analysis for prospective and retrospective longitudinal studies. In Rutter M, ed. *Studies of psychosocial risk: the power of longitudinal data*. Cambridge University Press, Cambridge, MA, pp. 315–324.

36. Buka SL, Goldstein J, Spartos E, Tsuang M (2004). The retrospective measurement of prenatal and perinatal events: accuracy of maternal recall. *Schizophrenia Research* 71, 417–426.

37. Kessler RC, McGonagle KA, Zhao S, Nelson CB, Hughes, M, Eshleman S, *et al.* (1994). Lifetime and 12-month prevalence of DSM-III-R psychiatric disorders in the United States: Results from the National Comorbidity Study. *Archives of General Psychiatry* 51, 8–19.

38. Hays J, Ockene J, Brunner R, Kotchen JM, Manson JE, Patterson RE, *et al.* (2003). Effects of estrogen plus progestin on health-related quality of life. *New England Journal of Medicine* 348, 1839–1854.

39. Rossouw J, Anderson GL A, Prentice R, LaCroix AZ, Kooperberg C, Stefanik ML, *et al.* (2002). Risks and benefits of estrogen plus progestin in healthy postmenopausal women: principal results from the Women's Health Initiative randomized controlled trial. *Journal of the American Medical Association* 288, 321–333.

40. Gordon RS (1983). An operational classification of disease prevention. *Public Health Reports* 98, 107–109.

41. Kellam SG, Rebok G, Ialongo N, Mayer L (1994). The course and malleability of aggressive behavior from early first grade into middle school: results of a developmental epidemiology-based preventive trial. *Journal of Child Psychology and Psychiatry* 35, 259–291.

42. Kellam SG, Anthony JC (1998). Targeting early antecedents to prevent tobacco smoking: findings from an epidemiologically-based randomized field trial. *American Journal of Public Health* 88, 1490–1495.

43. Syme SL (1998). Social and economic disparities in health: thoughts about intervention. *The Milbank Quarterly* 76, 493–505.

44. Galton F (1875). The history of twins as a criterion of the relative powers of nature and nurture. *Journal of the Royal Anthropological Institute* 5, 391–406.

45. Baker SG, Lichtenstein P, Kaprio J, Holm N (2005). Genetic susceptibility to prostate, breast, and colorectal cancer among Nordic twins. *Biometrics* 61, 55–63.

46. Christensen K, Vaupel JW (1996). Determinants of longevity: genetic, environmental and medical factors. *Journal of Internal Medicine* 240, 333–341.

47. Finkel D, Reynolds CA, McArdle JJ, Pedersen NL (2005). The longitudinal relationship between processing speed and cognitive ability: genetic and environmental influences. *Behavior Genetics* 35, 535–549.

48. Finkel D, Pedersen NL, Reynolds CA, Berg S, de Faire U, Svartengren M (2003). Genetic and environmental influences on decline in biobehavioral markers of aging. *Behavior Genetics* 33, 107–123.

49. Rutter ML, Simonoff E, Silberg JL (1994). How informative are twin studies of child psychopathology? In: Bouchard TJ, Propping P, ed. *Twins as tools of behavioral genetics.* John Wiley & Sons, Inc., Chichester, pp. 179–184.

50. Rutter M, Thorpe K, Greenwood R, Northstone K, Golding J (2003). Twins as a natural experiment to study the causes of mild language delay: I: design; twin–singleton differences in language, and obstetric risks. *Journal of Child Psychology and Psychiatry* 44, 326–341.

51. Bergeman CS, Chipuer HM, Plomin R, Pedersen NL, McClearn GE, Nesselroade JR, *et al.* (1993). Genetic and environmental effects on openness to experience, agreeableness, and conscientiousness: an adoption/twin study. *Journal of Personality* 61, 159–179.

52. Costa PT Jr, McCrae RR (2000). NEO personality inventory. In: Kazdin AE, ed. *Encyclopedia of psychology*, Vol. 5. American Psychological Association, Washington, DC, pp. 407–409.

53. Rutter M (2006). Proceeding from correlation to causal inference: the use of natural experiments. (*Submitted*).

54. D'Onofrio BM, Turkheimer EN, Eaves LJ, Corey LA, Berg K, Solaas MH, *et al.* (2003). The role of the children of twins design in elucidating causal relations between parent characteristics and child outcomes. *Journal of Child Psychology and Psychiatry* 44, 1130–1144.

55. Silventoinen K, Zdravkovic S, Skytthe A, McCarron P, Herskind Am, Koskenvuo M, *et al.* (2006). Association between height and coronary heart disease mortality: a prospective study of 35,000 twin pairs. *American Journal of Epidemiology* 163, 615–621.

56. Cadoret RJ (1986). Adoption studies: historical and methodological critique. *Psychiatric Developments* 4, 45–64.

57. Rutter M, O'Connor TG, English and Romanian Adoptees Study Team (2004). Are there biological programming effects for psychological development? Findings from a study of Romanian adoptees. *Developmental Psychology* 40, 81–94.

58. Beckett C, Maughan B, Rutter M, Castle J, Colvert E, Groothues C, *et al.* (2006). Do the effects of early severe deprivation on cognition persist into early adolescence? Findings from the English and Romanian adoptees study. *Child Development* 77, 696.

59. Kaprio J, Rimpela A, Winter T, Viken RJ, Rimpela M, Rose RJ (1995). Common genetic influences on BMI and age at menarche. *Human Biology* 67, 739–753.

60. Loesch D, Huggins R, Rogucka E, Hoang N, Hopper J (1995). Genetic correlates of menarcheal age: a multivariate twin study. *Annals of Human Biology* 22, 479–490.

61. Worthman CM (1999). Evolutionary perspectives on the onset of puberty. In: Trevathan WR, McKenna JJ, Smith EO, ed. *Evolutionary medicine*. Oxford University Press, Oxford, pp. 135–163.

62. Leao TS, Sundquist J, Frank G, Johansson L, Johansson S, Sundquist K (2006). Incidence of schizophrenia or other psychoses in first- and second-generation immigrants: a national cohort study. *Journal of Nervous and Mental Disease January* 194, 27–33.

63. Harrison G, Glazebrook C, Brewin J, Cantweel R, Dalkin T, Fox R, *et al.* (1997). Increased incidence of psychotic disorders in migrants from the Caribbean to the United Kingdom. *Psychological Medicine* 27, 799–806.

64. Fossion P, Ledoux Y, Valente F, Servais L, Staner L, Pelc I, *et al.* (2002). Psychiatric disorders and social characteristics among second-generation Moroccan migrants in Belgium: an age- and gender-controlled study conducted in a psychiatric emergency department. *European Psychiatry* 17, 443–450.

65. Dohrenwend BP, Levav I, Shrout PE, Schwartz S, Naveh G, Link BG, *et al.* (1992). Socioeconomic status and psychiatric disorders: the causation–selection issue. *Science* 255, 946–952.

66. Janssen MM, Verhulst F, Bengi-Arslan L, Erol N, Salter C, Crijnen AM (2004). Comparison of self-reported emotional and behavioral problems in Turkish immigrant, Dutch and Turkish adolescents. *Social Psychiatry and Psychiatric Epidemiology* 39, 133–140.

67. Wadsworth ME, Capps HA, Midwinter RE, Colley JR (1985). Blood pressure in a national cohort at the age of 36 related to social and familial factors, smoking, and body mass. *British Medical Journal* 291, 1534–1538.

68. Costello EJ, Compton SN, Keeler G, Angold A (2003). Relationships between poverty and psychopathology: a natural experiment. *Journal of the American Medical Association* 290, 2023–2029.

69. Cuijpers P, Smit F (2002). Excess mortality in depression: a meta-analysis of community studies. *Journal of Affective Disorders* 72, 227–236.

70. American Psychiatric Association (1994). *Diagnostic and statistical manual of mental disorders fourth edition (DSM-IV)*. American Psychiatric Press, Inc., Washington, DC.

71. Painter RC, Roseboom TJ, Bleker OP (2005). Prenatal exposure to the Dutch famine and disease in later life: an overview. *Reproductive Toxicology* 20, 345.

72. Carolina Consortium on Human Development (1996). *Developmental science: a collaborative statement*. Cambridge University Press, Cambridge, MA.

73. Klein K, Martha P, Blizzard R, Herbst T, Rogol A (1996). A longitudinal assessment of hormonal and physical alterations during normal puberty in boys II. Estrogen levels as determined by an ultrasensitive bioassay. *Journal of Clinical Endocrinology* 81, 3203–3207.

74. Larson RW, Raffaelli M, Richards MH, Ham M, Jewell L (1990). Ecology of depression in late childhood and early adolescence: a profile of daily states and activities. *Journal of Abnormal Psychology* 99, 92–102.

75. Willett W (1998). Nutritional epidemiology. In: Rothman K, Greenland S. *Modern epidemiology*, 2nd edn. Lippincott-Raven, Philadelphia, pp. 623–642.

76. Sampson L (1985). Food frequency questionnaires as a research instrument. *Clinical Nutrition* 9, 171–173.

77. Buehler J (1998). Surveillance. In: Rothman K, Greenland S. *Modern epidemiology*, 2nd edn. Lippincott-Raven, Philadelphia, pp. 435–457.

78. Angold A, Costello EJ, Worthman CM (1999). Pubertal changes in hormone levels and depression in girls. *Psychological Medicine* 29, 1043–1053.

79. Sung M, Erkanli A, Angold A, Costello E (2004). Effects of age at first substance use and psychiatric comorbidity on the development of substance use disorders. *Drug and Alcohol Dependence* 75, 287–299.

80. Graham P, Rutter M (1968). The reliability and validity of the psychiatric assessment of the child: II. Interview with the parent. *British Journal of Psychiatry* 114, 581–592.

81. Rutter M, Graham P (1968). The reliability and validity of the psychiatric assessment of the child: I. Interview with the child. *British Journal of Psychiatry* 114, 563–579.

82. Costello AJ, Edelbrock CS, Dulcan MK, Kalas R, Klaric SH (1984). *Development and testing of the NIMH diagnostic interview schedule for children in a clinic population: final report* (contract no. RFP-DB-81-0027). NIMH Center for Epidemiologic Studies, Rockville, MD.

83. Edelbrock C, Costello AJ, Dulcan MK, Conover MC, Kalas R (1986). Parent–child agreement on child psychiatric symptoms assessed via structured interview. *Journal of Child Psychology and Psychiatry* 27, 181–190.

84. Achenbach TM, McConaughy SH, Howell CT (1987). Child/adolescent behavioral and emotional problems: implications of cross-informant correlations for situational specificity. *Psychological Bulletin* 101, 213–232.

85. Ivens C, Rehm LP (1988). Assessment of childhood depression: correspondence between reports by child mother and father. *Journal of the American Academy of Child and Adolescent Psychiatry* 27, 738–741.

86. Kazdin AE, French NH, Unis AS (1983). Child, mother, and father evaluations of depression in psychiatric inpatient children. *Journal of Abnormal Child Psychology* 11, 167–180.

87. van den Oord EJ, Verhulst FC, Boomsma DI (1996). A genetic study of maternal and paternal ratings of problem behaviors in 3-year-old twins. *Journal of Abnormal Psychology* 105, 349–357.

88. Topolski TD, Hewitt JK, Eaves L, Myer JN, Silberg JL, Simonoff E, *et al.* (1999). Genetic and environmental influences on rating of manifest anxiety by parents and children. *Journal of Anxiety Disorders* 13, 371–297.

89. Eaves LJ, Silberg JL, Myer JM, Maes HH, Simonoff E, Pickles A, *et al.* (1997). Genetics and developmental psychopathology: 2. The main effects of genes and environment on behavioral problems in the Virginia Twin Study of adolescent behavior development. *Journal of Child Psychology and Psychiatry* 38, 965–980.

90. Thapar A, McGuffin P (1995). Are anxiety symptoms in childhood heritable? *Journal of Child Psychology and Psychiatry* 36, 439–447.

91. Stone A, Broderick J, Shiffman S, Schwartz J (2004). Understanding recall of weekly pain from a momentary assessment perspective: absolute agreement, between- and within-person consistency, and judged change in weekly pain. *Pain* 107, 61–69.

92. Cremeans-Smith J, Stephens M, Franks M, Martire L, Druley J, Wojno W (2003). Spouses' and physicians' perceptions of pain severity in older women with osteoarthritis: dyadic agreement and patients' well-being. *Pain* 106, 27–34.

93. Waters E, Stewart-Brown S, Fitzpatrick R (2003). Agreement between adolescent self-report and parent reports of health and well-being: results of an epidemiological study. *Childrens Care Health and Development* 29, 501–509.

94. Freund A, Johnson S, Silverstein J, Thomas J (1991). Assessing daily management of childhood diabetes using 24-hour recall interviews: reliability and stability. *Health Psychology* 10, 200–208.

95. Shueman SA, Troy WG (1994). The use of practice guidelines in managed behavioral health programs. In: Shueman SA, Troy WG, Mayhugh L, ed. *Managed behavioral health care: an industry perspective*. Charles C. Thomas Publishing, Springfield, IL, pp. 149–164.

96. Angold A (1994). Clinical interviewing with children and adolescents. Rutter M, Taylor E, Hersov L, ed. *Child and adolescent psychiatry: modern approaches.* Blackwell Scientific Publications, Oxford, pp. 51–63.

97. Goodman R, Ford T, Richards H, Gatward R, Meltzer H (2000). The Development and Well-being assessment: description and initial validation of an integrated assessment of child and adolescent psychopathology. *Journal of Child Psychology and Psychiatry* 41, 645–656.

98. Reich W, Earls F (1987). Rules of making psychiatric diagnoses in children on the basis of multiple sources of information: preliminary strategies. *Journal of Abnormal Child Psychology* 15, 601–616.

99. Farrington DP, Loeber R, Stouthamer-Loeber M, Van Kammen WB, Schmidt L (1996). Self-reported delinquency and a combined delinquency seriousness scale based on boys, mothers, and teachers: concurrent and predictive validity for African-Americans and Caucasians. *Criminology* 34, 501–525.

100. Bata IR, Gregor RD, Wolf HK, Brownell B (2006). Trends in five-year survival of patients discharged after acute myocardial infarction. *Canadian Journal of Cardiology* 22, 399–404.

101. Angold A, Worthman CW (1993). Puberty onset of gender differences in rates of depression: a developmental, epidemiologic and neuroendocrine perspective. *Journal of Affective Disorders* 29, 145–158.

102. Angold A, Costello EJ, Worthman CM (1998). Puberty and depression: the roles of age, pubertal status, and pubertal timing. *Psychological Medicine* 28, 51–61.

103. Marshall WA, Tanner JM (1969). Variations in pattern of pubertal changes in girls. *Archives of Disease in Childhood* 44, 291–303.

104. National Research Council (2001). *Cells and surveys: should biological measures be included in social science research?* National Academy Press, Washington, DC.

105. Crimmins E, Seemen T (2001). Integrating biology into demographic research on health and aging (with a focus on the MacArthur Study of Sucessful Aging). In: Finch A, Vaupel J, Kinsella K, ed. *Cells and surveys: should biological measures be included in social science research?* National Academy Press, Washington, DC, pp. 9–41.

106. Giles W, Croft J, Greelund K, Ford E, Kittner S (2000). Association between total homocyst(e)ine and the likelihood for a history of acute myocardial infarction by race and ethnicity: results from the Third National Health and Nutrition Examination Survey. *American Heart Journal* 139, 446–453.

107. Durfy S (2001). Ethical and social issues in incorporating genetic research into survey studies. In: Finch A, Vaupel J, Kinsella K, ed. *Cells and surveys: should biological measures be included in social science research?* National Academy Press, Washington, DC, pp. 303–328.

108. Ewbank D (2001). Demography in the age of genomics: a first look at the prospects. In: Finch A, Vaupel J, Kinsella K, ed. *Cells and surveys: should biological measures be included in social science research?* National Academy Press, Washington, DC, pp. 64–109.

109. Wallace R (2001). Applying genetic study designs to social and behavioral population surveys. In: Finch A, Vaupel J, Kinsella K, ed. *Cells and surveys: should biological measures be included in social science research?* National Academy Press, Washington, DC, pp. 229–249.

110. Garcia A, Abel M, Cot P, Richard P, Ranque S, Feingold J, *et al.* (1999). Genetic epidemiology of host predisposition to microfilaraemia in human loiasis. *Tropical Medicine and International Health* 4, 565–574.

111. Caspi A, Sugden K, Moffitt T, Taylor A, Craig IW, Harrington H, *et al.* (2003). Influence of life stress on depression: moderation by a polymorphism in the 5-HTT gene. *Science* 301, 386–389.

112. Weinstein M, Willis R (2001). Stretching social surveys to include bioindicators: possibilities for the health and retirement study, experience from the Taiwan Study of the Elderly Series. In: Finch A, Vaupel J, Kinsella K, ed. *Cells and surveys: should biological measures be included in social science research?* National Academy Press, Washington, DC, pp. 250–276.

113. Christensen K (2001). Biological material in household surveys: the interface between epidemiology and genetics In: Finch A, Vaupel J, Kinsella K, ed. *Cells and surveys: should biological measures be included in social science research?* National Academy Press, Washington, DC, pp. 42–63.

114. Titmuss R (1971). *The gift relationship, from human blood to social policy.* Pantheon Books, New York.

115. McEwen BS, Stellar E (1993). Stress and the individual. Mechanisms leading to disease. *Archives of Internal Medicine* 153, 2093–2101.

116. Halter J, Reuben D (2001). Indicators of function in the geriatric population. In: Finch A, Vaupel J, Kinsella K, ed. *Cells and surveys: should biological measures be included in social science research?* National Academy Press, Washington, DC, pp. 156–179.

117. McEwen BS, Mendelson S (1993). Effects of stress on the neurochemistry and morphology of the brain: counterregulation versus damage. In: Goldberger L, and Breznitz S, ed. *The handbook of stress.* 2nd edn. The Free Press, New York, NY, pp. 101–26.

118. Goodyer IM, Herbert J, Tamplin A (2003). Psychoendocrine antecedents of persistent first episode major depression in adolescents: a community based longitudinal inquiry. *Psychological Medicine* 33, 601–610.

119. Angold A (2003). Adolescent depression, cortisol and DHEA. *Psychological Medicine* 33, 573–581.

120. Boyce WT, Chesney M, Alkon A, Tschann JM, Adams S, Chesterman G, *et al.* (1995). Psychobiologic reactivity to stress and childhood respiratory illnesses: results of two prospective studies. *Psychosomatic Medicine* 57, 411–422.

121. Cacioppo JT, Berntson GG, Malarkey WB, Kiecolt-Glaser JK, Sheridan JF, Poehlmann KA, *et al.* (1998). Autonomic, neuroendocrine, and immune responses to psychological stress: the reactivity hypothesis. *Annals of the New York Academy of Sciences* 840, 664–673.

122. Moynihan JA (2003). Mechanisms of stress-induced modulation of immunity. *Brain, Behavior, and Immunity* 17, S11–S16.

123. Coe C, Lubach G (2003). Critical periods of special health relevance for psychoneuroimmunology. *Brain, Behavior, and Immunity* 17, 3–12.

124. McDade TW, Beck MA, Kuzawa C, Adair LS (2001). Prenatal undernutrition, postnatal environments, and antibody response to vaccination in adolescence. *American Journal of Clinical Nutrition* 74, 543–548.

125. Glaser R, Pearl DK, Kiecolt-Glaser JK, Malarkey WB (1994). Plasma cortisol levels and reactivation of latent Epstein–Barr virus in response to examination stress. *Psychoneuroendocrinology* 19, 765–772.

126. Sarid O, Anson O, Yaari A, Margalith M (2001). Epstein–Barr virus specific salivary antibodies as related to stress caused by examinations. *Journal of Medical Virology* 64, 149–156.

127. Sgoutas-Emch SA, Cacioppo JT, Uchino BN, Malarkey W, Pearl D, Kiecolt-Glaser JK, *et al.* (1994). The effects of an acute psychological stressor on cardiovascular, endocrine, and cellular immune response: a prospective study of individuals high and low in heart rate reactivity. *Psychophysiology* 31, 264–271.

128. Benschop RJ, Geenen R, Mills PJ, Naliboff BD, Kiecolt-Glaser JK, Herbert TB, *et al.* (1998). Cardiovascular and immune responses to acute psychological stress in young and old women: a meta-analysis. *Psychosomatic Medicine* 60, 290–296.

129. Kiecolt-Glaser JK (1999). Norman Cousins Memorial Lecture 1998. Stress, personal relationships, and immune function: health implications. *Brain, Behavior, and Immunity* 13, 61–72.

130. Kiecolt-Glaser JK, Malarkey WB, Chee M, Newton T, Caioppo JT, Mao HY, *et al.* (1993). Negative behavior during marital conflict is associated with immunological down-regulation. *Psychosomatic Medicine* 55, 395–409.

131. Esterling BA, Antoni MH, Kumar M, Schneiderman N (1993). Defensiveness, trait anxiety, and Epstein–Barr viral capsid antigen antibody titers in healthy college students. *Health Psychology* 12, 132–139.

132. Esterling BA, Antoni MH, Schneiderman N, Carver CS, LePerriere A, Ironson G, *et al.* (1992). Psychosocial modulation of antibody to Epstein–Barr viral capsid antigen and human herpesvirus type-6 in HIV-1-infected and at-risk gay men. *Psychosomatic Medicine* 54, 354–371.

133. Lutgendorf SK, Antoni MH, Kumar M, Schneiderman N (1994). Changes in cognitive coping strategies predict EBV-antibody titre change following a stressor disclosure induction. *Journal of Psychosomatic Research* 38, 63–78.

134. Herbert TB, Cohen S (1993). Stress and immunity in humans: a meta-analytic review. *Psychosomatic Medicine* 55, 364–379.

135. Herbert CP, Cohen S (1993). Depression and immunity: a meta-analytic review. *Psychological Bulletin* 113, 472–486.

136. Caspi A, McClay J, Moffitt TE, Mill J, Martin J, Craig IW, *et al.* (2002). Role of genotype in the cycle of violence in maltreated children. *Science* 297, 851–854.

137. Larson R, Moneta G, Richards M, Wilson S (2002). Continuity, stability, and change in daily emotional experience across adolescence. *Child Development* 73, 1151–1165.

Chapter 3

Measurement and design for life course studies of the social environment and its impact on health

Barbara Maughan and Michael Wadsworth

Abstract

This chapter discusses issues in the measurement of the social environment, and in the interpretation of health–environment associations, in life course studies. It differentiates measures of individuals' 'micro' social worlds—typically deriving from the family, the workplace and close social relationships—from 'macro' influences deriving from the broader social and cultural context, and provides examples of how each can be used in testing hypothesized associations between environmental influences and health. In addition, it examines practical issues in the use of such indicators in life course studies, and outlines both the challenges and the opportunities for life course epidemiology that arise from the recent rapid pace of social change.

3.1 Introduction

Health outcomes depend not only on individual endowments, but also upon the environments that individuals encounter across the life course; health change is hypothesized to be the result of interactions between individuals' biological and social capital and the current contexts, exposures and demands that they face.[1] Wilkinson[2] summarizes findings from social epidemiology as showing the adverse health effects of 'low social status, lack of friends, and a difficult start in life', and reminds us that there are biological explanations for each of these effects. He concludes that 'If this is indeed what the social epidemiology is telling us, then it fits well with what many of the great sociologists have identified as the basis of our sensitivity to the social environment', including the ways in which individuals come to perceive and evaluate the social world, and the self in relation to that world, and how those perceptions and evaluations affect action and expectation.[3,4]

Against that background, life course studies need to be as concerned with assessing the social environment and individuals' responses to it as they are with tracing individual characteristics. This chapter complements Chapter 2 by focusing on issues in the measurement of the social environment, and approaches to assessing its effects on health. Environmental measurement is central to life course studies for two main reasons. The first and most basic is shared with all other branches of epidemiological enquiry: to further our understanding of those aspects of individuals' environments that are salient for health and disease outcomes, and to learn more about the ways in which they have their effects. Cross-sectional studies have identified a plethora of links between individuals' health status and the environments they experience. Such associations may index a variety of processes: social factors may constitute relatively direct causal influences on health, may index increased exposure to more biological risk factors, may moderate the effects of biological risks, or may even mediate their effects. The key role of life course studies is to add a developmental dimension to those findings, exploring such issues as effects of the *timing* of environmental exposures, the impact of their *accumulation* across development, and the ways in which they act in conjunction with other vulnerabilities to influence later health. Is exposure to poverty, for example, only deleterious for health if it occurs at certain stages in development; if it is persistent rather than transitory; or if it is accompanied by other adverse experiences? Does parental divorce act as a direct risk factor for psychological well-being, or is its primary impact one of increasing psychological vulnerability to later stress, or exposure to subsequent socio-economic hardship? Do those babies who grow poorly in early life but appear to escape later risks to health[5] do so because of some protective environmental factor, or the interaction of genetic and environmental effects? The life course perspective, and the structure of life course studies, can offer unique strengths in addressing questions of this kind.

The second key reason for a concern with the social environment centres on tracking the effects of social change and, where possible, capitalizing on such changes to extend our understanding of environmental impacts on health. In most urbanized societies, the extent and pace of change is now considerable: individuals will experience marked variations in their environments at different stages in the life course, and contrasts across generations are yet more stark. In Britain, for example, the physical demands of the workplace and the security of tenure of occupations have greatly reduced over recent decades, with important consequences for both mental and physical health. Family structure has changed, with the postponement of ages at marriage and child-bearing, rising rates of separation, divorce and re-partnering, and changing patterns of many traditional social bonds. Although the distribution of wealth and purchasing power has broadened, and standards of living have risen, poverty and economic insecurity have not been greatly reduced. The various forms of social capital and their distribution have also changed, as too has their likely impact on health. Health-related habits of diet, exercise, smoking and consumption of alcohol and recreational drugs have all changed; and expectations of social and economic circumstances, and of access to education and occupations, have all increased. Healthcare has become increasingly effective, and increasingly concerned with the management of disease risk as well as with disease. The changing age structure of the population has also brought new health challenges associated with longer life, including the prevention and care of mental and physical frailty, disability and disease.

Changes of this kind present challenges for life course studies, but they also offer important opportunities: in particular, as cohort comparative data become increasingly available, historical trends of this kind can be used—in common with international comparisons and migration studies—as 'natural experiments' to tease out the impact of the environment on health. Chapter 5 explores the role of planned experiments—interventions studies—in testing hypotheses about environmental mediation. This chapter complements that approach by focusing on issues in the measurement and testing of environmental influences in naturalistic, observational designs, ranging from those based entirely on aggregate data to those building on individually based longitudinal studies (whether retrospective or prospective) to test environmentally based hypotheses. In the physical health arena, such approaches have concentrated on designs that compare environmental exposures, and use differences in those exposures as essential elements of quasi-experimental design. Once associations have been established, hypothesized biological pathways for effects have been tested (in particular in studies of the effects of stress on neuroendocrine systems), and animal models have been used to explicate the likely processes involved. In the mental health field, epidemiological studies have increasingly moved to the use of genetically informative designs to highlight environmental as well as heritable influences on health. Twin and adoption studies have been used to estimate the overall impact of environmental influences, and their changes with age and developmental stage, and studies of measured genes and environments are now beginning to be used to explore specific hypothesized aspects of gene–environment interplay.[6,7]

Health-related social influences may arise throughout the life course—from the pre-natal period onwards—and at a variety of levels, some relatively proximal to the individual, others more distal. One of the most influential conceptualizations of these varying levels of influence is Bronfenbrenner's[8] bioecological model (see also Chapter 2), which identified four environmental 'system' levels: the microsystem (encompassing the individual's immediate environments—family, school, friendship groupings and workplace); the mesosystem (encompassing connections among those immediate environments); the exosystem (encompassing influences on microsystem elements, but not directly on the individual); and the macrosystem, encompassing wider social and cultural contexts: educational and occupational opportunities, prevailing attitudes to and expectations of health and education, and contemporary expectations of behaviour and conformity that influence population health through, for instance, variations in age at first birth, or the likelihood of experiencing divorce.

We use a simplified version of that model here, contrasting 'micro' and 'macro' aspects of environmental exposures. At the micro level, we include influences associated with the family (including family lifestyle, family health-related behaviours such as diet, relationships within the family and emotional response styles); the peer group; the school and work environments; and also relevant aspects of social status and material and financial circumstances. At the macro level, we include the wider cultural context, opportunity structures and expectations, and systems of health and social care provision as they impact on the health of individuals and of generations (Table 3.1).

Table 3.1 Examples of sources of social environmental impacts on health

	Infancy and the pre-natal period	School years	Working life	Retirement
Micro social environment	Family of origin, kindergarten, neighbourhood circumstances	Family of origin, school and adolescent peers, educational attainment, personal and family socio-economic, and neighbourhood circumstances	New family formation, occupational peers, adult friendships, occupational satisfaction, personal and family socio-economic and neighbourhood circumstances	Family and friends, personal and family socio-economic and neighbourhood circumstances
Macro social environment	Healthcare availability, concepts of family life and of health	Educational opportunity, and perceived value of education, perception of obligations	Occupational opportunity, perceived social obligations	Pension and healthcare provision, family care of the elderly

3.2 Measurement of micro social factors

Health-related impacts of micro social contexts may themselves arise at a variety of levels: in terms of variations in social statuses and material conditions; as a result of patterns of interactions with others; and in terms of individuals' perceptions of and responses to their social situations. Data for life course analyses thus need to measure the social environment and its change at all three levels differentiated in Table 3.2.

3.2.1 Use of micro social measures in life course research

Measures at *Level 1* are used to indicate social status, and to compare social status and its stability and change within and between generations. Continuous exposure to poor home circumstances and low status in the community and at work, for example, have been shown to be associated with raised risk to health in the form of symptoms of persistent mental stress,[9–11] and chronic poor physical health, [5,12–14] in both childhood and adult life. Interpretations of such findings have then implicated not only aspects of material deprivation (Level 1), but also less than optimal interactions with others (Level 2), and perceived low self-efficacy (Level 3).[9,15–17]

Biological pathways for such effects may run through a variety of routes, including raised risk of infection and chronic inflammation associated with poor hygiene and inadequate nutrition,[18] and suggestions that 'Disturbance of usual homeostatic equilibrium by the repeated activation of the fight-or-flight response may be responsible for social differences in neuroendocrine, physiological, and metabolic variables which are precursors of ill health and disease.'[16] Social pathways for such findings suggest that health can be adversely affected by an accumulation of risk, whereby adverse childhood circumstances

Table 3.2 The micro social environment

	Examples of purpose	Topic area	Data sources
Level 1	Description of socio-economic status, home, school and work physical environments, the neighbourhood environment	Parental and own occupational status, income and educational attainment, home crowding and availability of amenities, neighbourhood type, school (private or public), teacher/student ratios, student attainment, student socio-economic status, school amenities	Self-report, published statistics, reports from school and educational authorities, neighbourhood dis/advantage indicators
Level 2	Interactions with others	Parent–child interactions, partner and peer relationships, assessments of conformity to peer norms	Psychometric measures, self-reports, reports of others, e.g. teachers
Level 3	Perceptions of self in relation to social circumstances	Parental and child perceived opportunities in education and occupation, perceived social obligations	Self-reports

increase later risks of unemployment, poor coping skills, poor self-perceptions and deleterious health-related behaviours.[19–21] In contrast, childhood acquisition of good health habits, and attainment of educational qualifications may have long-term beneficial effects on health.[22]

Level 2 measures are well exemplified by work on parenting in childhood, and on social integration and support in adult life. The basic hypotheses are that lack of adequate parental care in childhood, or exposure to abusive or emotionally inconsistent parenting, are risks for a wide range of later disorders,[23,11] while in adulthood those who experience 'good' social integration and support have a raised likelihood of better mental health.[24,25] The longitudinal models hypothesize that childhood and adolescent experiences of effective care within the family offer long-term protection against minor mental health problems (including depression and anxiety) because of associated feelings of security and trust[26] and the development of positive attitudes and relationship capacities. Mediators of adverse early experiences may run through both biological and psychological vulnerabilities set up in childhood, or through selection into later risk-prone environments. Adverse physical health outcomes of childhood maltreatment, for example, suggest that chronic early stress has effects on the cardiovascular system, the immune system and on neurobiological functioning,[27] and pre-clinical studies now provide persuasive models for the ways in which a range of early experiences, both pre- and post-natal, may influence the brain.[28] Social stressors and supports may also moderate, or be moderated by, genetically based vulnerabilities. In adulthood, for example, Ryff and Singer[29] speculate that social supports may be protective against genetic risk, while Caspi *et al.*[30] have shown that genetic factors can moderate the effects of maltreatment on risk for antisocial outcomes at different stages in the life course.

Level 3 measures—concerned with self-perceptions—are integral to many uses of measures at Level 2. Systematic development of measures describing the nature of interactions at work, for example, has been undertaken in relation to the effort–reward and demand–control paradigms. Reports of work demands in relation to perceived control have been associated with risk of heart disease in longitudinal studies over periods of 5 years and more, and work in the Whitehall II study shows that effort–reward imbalance and perceived low job control act independently.[31] In those not employed, measures of self-efficacy and self-esteem concerned with belonging and approval have comparable effects.[13] Measures of positive well-being and happiness have also been developed,[32] and shown to be associated with good health, and are beginning to be explored in life course studies.[33] The work of life course studies in this respect is to ask not only how and when positive self-perceptions develop, but also how they are maintained, and in what circumstances they are robust or vulnerable to challenge.

Level 3 measures tapping the concept of agency—individuals' sense of autonomy, intention and capacity to carry actions forward[34]—have been less well used in health-related studies to date. Schooling,[35] however, showed that health-related behaviour was influenced by an interaction between public and private images of particular activities. When the public image of smoking, for example, was of a mildly rebellious and machismo activity, those who wished to present that image were most inclined to smoke; but when the prevailing image of smoking changed, and it was regarded it as an unpleasant habit with a serious health risk, then those who wished to present themselves as healthy and responsible were less likely to smoke. Doyal and Gough[36] showed that agency that is continually blocked by unemployment is a risk for poor mental health outcomes. McMunn and colleagues[37,38] studied perceived quality of social roles in women, in terms of both motherhood and paid work outside the home. They concluded that multiplicity of roles and quality of roles were associated with health, and the relationships were not explained by health selection.

3.2.2 Interpreting associations with micro social measures

While the initial phases of work using micro social measures centre on establishing associations with health outcomes, the eventual aim will be to determine the causal status of such links, and to delineate risk pathways for their effects. Several issues need to be considered here. First, because adverse social circumstances tend to cluster, tracking effects of any specific risk inevitably presents challenges: have we identified the key risk indicator, or effects stemming from a closely related confounder? In the behavioural domain, for example, there is now extensive confirmation of links between maternal smoking in pregnancy and antisocial outcomes in offspring,[39] and pre-clinical studies provide clear evidence of effects of nicotine exposure on development of the fetal brain. Despite this, uncertainties over the causal role of smoking in pregnancy remain, in part because pre-natal smoking co-occurs so strongly with other risks for poor child outcomes—young maternal age, low maternal education, antisocial traits in parents, poor material conditions, and so forth. Adequate measurement of, and tests for the effects of, plausible confounders of this kind are thus key issues for consideration at the stage of study design. Confounding may present fewer difficulties in relation to post-natal exposures, but problems of interpretation can still arise. In some instances, these relate to accurate identification of the key elements of risk: for some outcomes, for example, evidence suggests that associations with relatively 'distal' risk factors such as family poverty in childhood are largely mediated through more proximal indicators of family functioning or the quality of parent–child relationships.[40] In other instances, the key need may be to differentiate social selection from social causation: do observed patterns of association indeed reflect impacts of adverse social circumstances on health, or might pre-existing individual vulnerabilities function in part to 'select' individuals into more risk-prone environments? In recent years, the importance of selection/causation issues has been especially highlighted by findings from behaviour genetic research. In the psychiatric field in particular, studies of this kind have provided important correctives to unquestioning 'environmentalist' assumptions by showing that social contexts and adverse life experiences are not randomly distributed: both parents' and individuals' own genes contribute to susceptibility to environmental adversity, but they also affect variations in *exposure* to adverse environmental effects.

Taking child development issues as one core focus, behaviour genetic studies have shown that gene–environment correlations (rGE) of this kind can arise in three main ways.[41] The first (*passive* rGE) involves parental genotypes, and arises when the environments that parents provide for their children (pre- as well as post-natally) reflect aspects of their own genetically influenced traits. Other forms of rGE reflect effects of children's genes on the experiences they encounter. *Evocative* rGE arises when genetically influenced child characteristics evoke particular patterns of response from others—so that, for example, a temperamentally difficult child may evoke more negative responses from parents than a child with equable temperamental traits. *Active* rGE occurs when genetically influenced traits lead individuals to 'select' environments consonant with their own characteristics; here, for example, temperamental factors might lead some individuals to experience more 'stress-prone' environments than others, or to vary in their likelihood of access to social support. Cumulated across the life course, genetically mediated processes of this kind could clearly have powerful effects.

At times, findings of this kind have been taken to imply that many putative 'environmental' risk factors reflect genetically rather than environmentally mediated effects. In practice, generalizations of this kind are unlikely to be warranted on either side of the argument; what is needed is systematic studies designed to test them out. In the child development field, Terrie Moffitt and colleagues' Environmental Risk twin study[6] represents an exemplary programme of this kind. Building on the strengths offered by a longitudinal twin study, this programme has set out to test how far a range of well-replicated 'environmental' correlates of childhood conduct problems do indeed reflect environmentally mediated effects. This group has shown, for example, that within identical twin pairs, the twin receiving more maternal negativity and less warmth at age 5 had higher rates of conduct problems 2 years later;[42] that both genetic and environmental processes are involved in the increased risk for conduct problems shown by young children of depressed mothers;[43] and that variations in relatively normative approaches to discipline (such as smacking) involve genetic mediation, while more severely negative parenting (such as maltreatment) does not.[44] Over time, strategies of this kind should offer important advances in our understanding of both the sources of environmental risk exposures, and the mechanisms through which they have their effects.

3.2.3 Practical aspects of using micro social measures in life course studies

Like the measurement of individual characteristics (discussed in Chapter 2), the selection and use of micro environmental measures raises a number of issues in life course research. At Level 1, these turn in part on the need for the most objectively accurate, well-validated and reliable measures to investigate the impact of such exposures as material or financial circumstances on indices of growth or attainment. Triangulation of measures—gaining others' reports as well as those of the index individual—offer one approach to validation here and, with appropriate consents, information on individual attributes such as educational attainment or patterns of healthcare use can be confirmed and augmented (and burdens on respondents reduced), through linkage with administrative records. Objective data on the immediate social context can be obtained from published statistical sources in terms, for example, of indices of neighbourhood deprivation or features of the school environment. However, information on many other apparently 'objective' issues (such as, for example, partnership status, or fertility or occupational histories) will inevitably rely heavily on the accuracy of individual informant's reporting. Though measures of current status or conditions at the time of a study contact will generally be well reported, researchers also frequently want to 'fill in the gaps' since the last study contact, to produce as complete as possible a longitudinal record. Here, lack of recall or the tendency to 'telescope' events can constitute major difficulties in generating accurate event histories, or in detailing the timing of past status changes, in studies with widely spaced follow-up intervals. Techniques to aid recall over longer time intervals include life course calendars or assisted diary grids,[45,46] where individually 'meaningful dates' (dates of marriage, children's births, and so on) are initially established with respondents, then used to anchor the dating of other events. More generally, appropriate levels of measurement need to be selected in light of the specific hypotheses to be addressed, and the follow-up intervals to be covered; the level of detail that can be achieved reasonably accurately across a 1-year follow-up will simply not be feasible when study members are contacted on a much less frequent basis.

The second key challenge in the use of indicators at Level 1 arises from the effects of social change: across an individual life course, and more markedly across generations, both the measures and the phenomena being investigated also frequently vary. The nature of employment, for example, has changed greatly in most Western societies over recent years, as have theoretical approaches to classifying the status of occupations; as a result, the approaches used to ascertain the skill level of particular occupations, or to classify socio-economic status (SES), have also inevitably changed, and data collected at earlier time points may not be consistent with those required at later stages. In the British 1946 national birth cohort study, for example, socio-economic data were collected from the cohort members' parents during the period 1946–1961, and from the cohort themselves from 1961 to 2006. During that time, measures and coding systems for SES changed considerably; as a result, comparisons across extended periods of time typically can only be made using simplified, aggregated groupings (e.g. non-manual versus manual). In a similar way, comparisons of school-leaving attainments in three national birth cohorts spanning a 24-year period have been complicated by marked changes in the proportions of young people completing formal qualifications, and by changing classification systems in the educational domain.[47] While it is clearly impossible to anticipate changes of this kind entirely, experience to date highlights the utility of collecting as detailed measures as possible at each study time point, to allow for maximum flexibility in re-casting earlier data in the light of emerging new demands.

The greatest difficulty in collecting data for Level 2 measures for use in life course epidemiology is the inclusion of time. Many life course hypotheses suggest that, in order to be damaging to health in the long term, exposure to adverse social circumstances needs to be chronic, and/or to occur at sensitive or critical periods in development. Particular attention thus needs to be paid to the timing of environmental measurements, and to assessing duration and severity of exposures. When, as with Level 2 measures, the focus is on relationship qualities, contemporaneous, prospective assessments are almost always to be preferred over retrospective reports. Measures are typically collected via self-reports; where more detailed data collection is feasible, direct observational procedures may be employed, and some studies have capitalized on the availability of existing materials, such as home movies. Once again, however, the long time frame of life course studies poses challenges here. As new knowledge emerges, so attention may focus on new constructs not seen as relevant at earlier stages of a study, or new and more reliable methods of assessment may be developed. As a result, information collected at earlier time periods may have omissions, may not be regarded as adequately detailed for subsequent analysis, and is very likely to be based on measurement methods that are no longer in use. In the British 1946 birth cohort, for example, no contemporaneous data were collected on the quality of parental relationships during the study members' childhoods, so that aspect of the family context—now widely regarded as crucial for many aspects of early development—can only be characterized in terms of broad indicators such as parents' presence or absence, and the child's exposure to parental separation or divorce. Some retrospective data collection has been possible to fill this gap at more recent waves, but it is clear that this can only function as a partial substitute for prospective reports. Evaluations of the adequacy of retrospective reporting[48] suggest that although the *timing* of past events or experiences may not be reliably reported, reporting on the *nature* of past exposures may be less subject to bias; pursuing our last example, it may thus be possible to establish retrospectively that an individual was exposed to some level of parental discord in childhood, even if it is not possible to date that exposure with any precision. In addition, while concerns over retrospective reporting have typically focused on the possibility that subjects in adverse current circumstances will exaggerate past difficulties, available evidence suggests that the reverse pattern (individuals who are currently functioning well showing a tendency to under-report early adversities) is often more common. For some hypotheses, judicious use of retrospective reports may thus be justified; and in some circumstances—such as, for example, in relation to reports of exposure to abuse or neglect, where ethical considerations often constrain contemporaneous questioning in childhood—it may be the only approach available. As we stress throughout this chapter, however, avoidance or prospective minimization of time problems requires imaginative concern for future analysis at each stage of study planning; the establishment of baseline measures with which later measures can be compared, to indicate direction and extent of change; and as much prospective data collection as possible.

Data collection for Level 3 measures relies heavily on self-report and self-assessment to assess, for example, the perceived stigma or sense of exclusion reported by individuals in a particular occupation, or with a particular standard of living. Here in particular, information collected in retrospect is not likely to be meaningful, and most reliance will need to be placed on prospectively ascertained reports. Verification of such information at the micro social level requires comparison of the individual's self-assessment with that from others in the same occupation and, ideally, data on mental health in order to disentangle poor self-perceptions from other factors that may affect reporting.

In reality, no life course study can achieve the perfect set of micro social data, and some compromises are always likely to be needed. In catch-up designs, or in prospective studies beginning in adulthood, long periods of the life course will of necessity have to be characterized using retrospective reports, or through measures available from records; in long-term prospective studies, information that at later times comes to be seen as necessary may have been omitted at early study contacts, or not been collected in an adequately detailed way. Lessons learned from the first generation of life course studies suggest that while it is impossible to circumvent these difficulties completely, the best way to reduce them is to collect data at the most detailed level feasible at each specific study contact, to allow maximum flexibility for later re-framing of measures.

3.3 Macro social data

Macro social data are used to compare age cohorts and populations over time and between countries, using information about societal circumstances at the varying levels illustrated in Table 3.3

Life course epidemiological studies have made three kinds of uses of macro social data—to develop, test and confirm hypotheses. Although we discuss these uses separately here for illustrative purposes, in practice they are strongly inter-related, and demonstrate well how life course work frequently crosses traditional subject boundaries.

3.3.1 Macro social data and hypothesis development

Epidemiologists sometimes refer to analysis of macro social data for hypothesis development as 'ecological analysis'—the use of aggregate data at the group or population level to generate hypotheses about associations affecting individuals. Barker[49] used this method in the development of the biological programming hypothesis to examine the long-term health effects of childhood exposure to poor socio-economic circumstances. Comparisons of towns and districts of serious poverty with more affluent areas revealed that areas with high infant mortality in the 1920s also had a high prevalence of premature adult death from ischaemic heart disease and bronchitis some 50 years later, in the 1960s and 1970s. Ischaemic heart disease is associated with prosperity; on the basis of these findings, Barker[49] suggested, as Forsdahl[50] had speculated, that poor nutrition in early life was likely to increase susceptibility to a rich diet later in the life course. In a similar way, childhood poverty was found to be a source of increased risk of infant pulmonary infection, a strong and independent source of risk for death from bronchitis in adulthood, even after adjustment for the effects of smoking. From these observations, Barker[49] and others developed the notion that the experience of poverty in early life has a long-lasting adverse effects on health, fundamentally because it impairs growth. This hypothesis, initially developed on the basis of aggregate data, has since been extensively verified in longitudinal studies of individuals.

In a related way, Berkman and her colleagues[51] drew together work from social theory concerning social integration and alienation, from psychology concerning attachment relationships, and from sociology concerning social networks, to develop a conceptual model linking social networks (or in our terms macro social factors) with health. They concluded that 'the social structure of the (social) network itself is largely responsible for determining individual behaviour and attitudes by shaping the flow of resources which determine access to opportunities and constraints on behaviour'.[51] Their model hypothesizes that macro social circumstances affect social networks and thus also such psychosocial mechanisms as social support and engagement, that are in turn associated with health behaviours, psychological pathways to outcomes such as depression, and physiological pathways to outcomes such as cardiovascular reactivity. The work of Siegrist[52] and of Marmot and his colleagues[13,53] has developed these hypothesized links between the

Table 3.3 Examples of macro social data

	Purpose	Indicators	Source
Level 1	Opportunity structure	Suffrage and voting, unemployment risk, years of compulsory schooling, occupational social mobility, percentage in higher education, percentage women in higher education, migrant flow	National and international statistics
Level 2	Economic structure	Distribution of wealth and purchasing power, home ownership, percentage of high earners who are women, economic depression and inflation	National and international statistics
Level 3	Family structure	Age at first birth, family size, marriage and stable partnership, divorce	National and international statistics
Level 4	Care structure	Pension provision, methods of care of elderly, prevalence of kindergarten, entitlement to healthcare, availability of key therapy (e.g. antenatal care), smoking control	National and international statistics
Level 5	Social organization	Social cohesion, crime prevalence, experience and stability of war	National and international statistics

macro and the micro social environments and health. The effectiveness of their models lies in their biological plausibility, as demonstrated in their work[16] and in comparison with animal models.[54]

3.3.2 Macro social data and hypothesis testing

Macro social data are also used for hypothesis testing, for example to verify that a relationship observed at the individual level is also found at the macro level. Most work on this topic has been undertaken to test hypotheses concerned with psychosocial risk, in particular social status and social vulnerability.[12] The characterization of populations that is necessary for undertaking inter-population or international comparisons, or comparisons of the same geographical area at different historical times, has generally been done using information on availability and distribution of financial assets[55] and on cultural styles and social cohesion.[56,57] The latter two studies were concerned with the health effects of observed changes in community cohesion. Decline in quality of social cohesion had an apparent adverse effect on heart disease,[56] while improving cohesion had an apparent beneficial effect on mental health.[57] Social cohesion has been measured by perceived trust and interaction, and was regarded as a partial confirmation of findings from micro social studies focusing on social support.

World Bank statistics show the reduction in infant mortality and other health measures as national income increases,[58] and Wilkinson[55] shows how indicators of a nation's equality of income distribution relate to health in terms of adult and infant mortality, as well as to expectation of life. Within nations it seems that social equity is an essential factor in understanding such differences. For example, the Indian state of Kerala '... has health indicators similar to those of the United States—despite a *per capita* income of 99 percent lower and annual spending on health of just $28 a person'.[59] Similarly, Cuba's infant mortality rate is similar to that of the USA despite major differences in per capita income. In both cases these variations are attributed to differences in social equity in spending on health and education, and to differences in gender equity in education, ownership rights and opportunities for occupation and earnings.[59] Further examples come from historical comparisons of health indicators in countries that have changed from a socially stable period under Communism to a period of social and economic disruption and uncertainty; here, results have highlighted the adverse health effects of that change in terms of fertility and mortality, particularly mortality from violence and alcohol-related disorders.[60,61]

Classification systems have also been developed to characterize the equity of nations based on social rather than economic indices. Esping-Andersen,[62] for example, classified countries in terms of the provision they make for the care of dependent citizens, and of the family's role in the care of the elderly, and comparable classifications have been made by others.[63,64] To an extent these kinds of social classifications relate to national health indices, for instance infant mortality[65,66] and expectation of life.[67] In countries where a higher proportion of the elderly live with their families, for example, indicators of health inequality are more favourable.[67] One international comparison of death rates from coronary heart disease used divorce rates to differentiate European countries in terms of marital stability, and showed that mortality rates from heart disease were higher in countries with high rates of divorce and lower in those with low divorce rates.[68] Bartley[67] suggested that perhaps such measures help to explain the associations of national differences in income inequality with national differences in health. Conclusions from such comparisons are always, however, subject to the continuing debate over whether such effects are partly the result of social selection, rather than the effects of stress.[10]

3.3.3 Macro social data and research design: natural experiments

Macro social data have also been used to valuable effect in identifying populations subject to life course health risks that cannot be ethically or artificially introduced, but that constitute key natural experiments for testing environmental hypotheses. It has been possible, for example, to investigate the long-term effects of starvation on the developing fetus in populations starved because of war: obstetric records from such a period were found in adulthood, and the current health or cause of death of those same individuals has been studied.[69] In a comparable way, investigation of the effects of extreme early social deprivation on cognitive, social and behavioural development has been possible through studies of children adopted from Romanian orphanages after the collapse of Communism.[70] Here, the radical change of environment following adoption allowed for assessments of the reversibility of effects, while careful attention to the initial research design made it possible to contrast outcomes across groups with differing lengths of exposure to early deprivation.

Migrant studies are further powerful designs for natural experiments, highlighting risk and protective effects associated with exposure at the place of origin, and the extent to which migrants carry health risks with them, or acquire them *de novo* in their new settings. Marmot *et al.*,[71] for example, showed that Japanese migrants to Hawaii and California increased their risk of ischaemic heart disease if they took on the lifestyle of native Hawaiians or Californians, but remained at the lower Japanese levels of risk if they did not. In a similar way, in the Tokelau Islands study, those who remained on the Islands experienced a much lower rise in blood pressure with age than is usual in the Western urbanized world, whereas those who migrated to urban New Zealand experienced the blood pressure rise with age characteristic of those who live in urbanized society.[72]

Further bases for epidemiological opportunism or natural experiments can be developed when samples already enrolled in longitudinal investigations pass through socially defined risk periods, or are exposed to new environmental opportunities or constraints. In Britain, for example, investigators have capitalized on the ongoing study of one of the British birth cohorts (individuals born in 1958), to examine the health impact of unemployment.[73] Members of this sample entered the labour market as national unemployment rates began to rise steeply, making it possible to investigate both early risk factors for selection into unemployment as well as the impact on later health of unemployment of varying periods.[73] In a similar way, Elder[74] studied the inter-generational impact of the American depression in a catch-up longitudinal study of the sons of men who had faced a radical loss of family earnings during adolescence, while Costello *et al.*[75] were able to investigate the impact of changed economic circumstances in an American Indian sample whose economic circumstances markedly improved over time.

3.3.4 Inter-cohort comparisons to assess health effects of macro social change

Since so many aspects of the macro social context changed over the last half of the twentieth century, as did all aspects of healthcare, it has also been of value to compare these effects in cohorts whose members experienced these differing exposures. Two kinds of questions can be addressed by this method, using either existing birth cohort studies or ecological level data. The first addresses the long-term health effects of change in healthcare systems or early nutrition; the second focuses on whether the pathways to health outcomes differ for differing birth cohorts.

An unusually long-term instance of the first kind comes from an epigenetic study of the effect of poor harvests on early nutritional status. Pembrey et al.[76] used data on harvests during the nineteenth century in a rural Swedish community to show that men's exposure to poor harvests during their period of slowest pre-pubertal growth (from 9 to 12 years) was associated with longevity in their grandsons; for women, exposure during fetal development and in infancy was associated with longevity in granddaughters. This evidence for trans-generational influence, particularly in men, provides striking support for what Shanahan and Hofer[77] have called contextual triggering. In a similar way, Finch and Crimmins[78] studied mortality in Swedish national cohorts born since 1751 to develop the hypothesis that reduced exposure to infection in childhood has been a vital aspect of the decline in premature adult mortality.

In contrast, in addressing the second kind of question, inter-cohort comparisons of samples studied over many years raise other opportunities. The sample populations of the first three British national birth cohort studies (initiated in 1946, 1958 and 1970) varied greatly not only in their exposures to healthcare, diet, exercise, nutrition, alcohol consumption and recreational drug use, but also in their experience of the macro social circumstances described in Table3.2.[79] Increasingly, comparisons of these variations in exposures and experiences are being used to study their impact on the health of individuals; for instance, cohort differences in exposure to atmospheric pollution from coal burning are being used to examine effect size differences in outcomes that include pulmonary disease in childhood and adult life, respiratory function in adulthood and weight at birth. Comparable inter-cohort comparisons will in future be used in studies that have the health of cohort, rather than the individual, as the outcome; they will use cohort differences in health and development, together with life course knowledge of pathways from early life to mid and later life outcomes, to model the health profile of each cohort as it is projected to be in future at, for instance, ages 60, 70 and 80 years.

Alongside these key opportunities, inter-cohort comparisons also bring analytical difficulties. As in the case of micro social measures, these centre on effects of change both in social environmental circumstances and in the scientific context. In Britain, birth cohort studies covering the greater part of the second half of the twentieth century provide extensive opportunities to address the effects of social change on succeeding generations.[79] Inevitably, however, both within and between studies, the measures used have been those current in scientific use at the time of each data collection. There are many examples of the consequent *post hoc* interpretative problems that have ensued. In the

1946 birth cohort study, for example, the measures of depression taken in adulthood were changed as the cohort aged for contemporary scientific reasons, and all of the measures taken on this early cohort differed from those used in the two subsequent cohort studies. Here, comparable percentile cut-off points can be imposed on differing measures to examine both within- and between-cohort differences in early predictors of high scores, but cohort comparisons of rates or levels *per se* are unlikely to be feasible. In a similar way, comparisons of other continuous measures (e.g. of height, income or blood pressure) have been achieved by aggregating results into percentile groups; when measures are not continuous (as, for example, in the case of socio-economic groupings or diagnoses), equivalents have to be sought using the criteria for each grouping within the measure. The opportunity to do this, however, may only be available when the original measures have been recorded and coded in sufficient detail.

Interpretative problems in the study of secular trends were examined in detail in one of the most stringent and comprehensive studies of this sort, concerned with psychosocial disorders that are a threat to individual as well as social well-being, and that peak at the end of the teenage years. Included were crime, depression, anorexia and bulimia, suicidal behaviour, and abuse of alcohol and psychoactive drugs.[80] Despite difficulties of interpretation associated with changing diagnostic criteria, changes in recording practices and limitations associated with retrospective reports, the investigators were nonetheless able to rule out some plausible hypotheses—important among them being that the increasing prevalence of psychosocial disorder could be accounted for by increasing unemployment rates at the societal level.

3.3.5 The measurement of societal context and its change

Contemporary attitudes and other aspects of the spirit of the times as expressed in expectations and customs are referred to by social scientists as Zeitgeist. Zeitgeist is important because it includes the standards by which individuals assess themselves, in terms, for example, of social status. Life course epidemiology increasingly requires indicators of the Zeitgeist, as the importance of social status in relation to health is recognized,[12,81] together with the nature of the individual's interaction with society. Ideally the investigator should know the contemporary pressures for conformity and expectations of behaviour in relation to social position prevalent at the time of a particular study, in order to adjust for and assess their effects. Where issues of this kind have not been adequately tapped in original data sources, however, other sources of data may prove valuable in interpreting effects.

In some instances, past attitude surveys may be of value here, provided they cover the required time frame and include constructs of interest. Other aspects of Zeitgeist, particularly those concerned with perceptions of opportunity and of ageing, can be captured by inference from policy innovations and official demographic statistics, though these need to be interpreted with care. Change in the proportions of men and women becoming students in higher education in Britain in the latter half of the twentieth century, for example, may be taken as a reflection of women's increasing demand for higher education, and thus evidence of a changing attitude towards education.[82] However, that would be to overlook the socio-economic differences in attitudes to education at the same era highlighted by Young and Willmott,[83] and the idea, prevalent in the 1960s, that women were not as capable as men of logical, deductive scientific argument.[84] In a similar way, increases in alcohol consumption by women, particularly those with higher qualification levels and in high status occupations, may be interpreted as evidence of women increasingly conforming to male norms,[85] but they may also reflect women's perceived increased freedom of social expression.

3.3.6 The effects of Zeitgeist on data collection

Some aspects of Zeitgeist, in particular the scientific assumptions of the time, may not be recognizable until later time points. For instance, Roche[86] notes that in the early days of the Fels Growth Study (begun in 1929), there was 'widespread scientific belief that a fetus was shielded from environmental effects'. These effects are inevitably reflected in data collections in life course studies. In a comparable way, the British 1946 birth cohort study did not collect data on parental smoking during the early years because it pre-dated the publication of evidence of its adverse health effects, and data collected on diet in 1950 (cohort age 4 years) was first coded many years later because no coding system was then available. That study also did not measure physical function in childhood (e.g. blood pressure) because at that time it was a measure associated with diagnosis, but by the time of the 1970 study birth cohort study blood pressure had become an accepted measurement of function in childhood.

3.4. Conclusions

Social context has an essential role in the life course study of health as an indicator of exposure, and of intensity and timing of exposure to social circumstances known to have adverse effects on development, health and ageing. Systematic work in aspects of life course epidemiology concerned with the health of individuals has achieved a progression of understanding of how exposures to micro level social stressors have their apparent effects, moving from inference to hypothesized biological processes. To an extent this progression has also been supported by work at the macro level but, beyond their use for sampling frames, macro level data have not been so systematically used. However, as life course epidemiology is increasingly concerned with meta analysis, analysis of pooled data and the comparison of sample populations born at different social times, work with macro social data is likely to increase.

Throughout this chapter, we have emphasized the need for life course studies to take as robust an approach as possible to testing environmental hypotheses, through imaginative use of study design and attempts to pit differing causal hypotheses against one another. As we have seen, some of the key issues here centre on paying careful attention to the possibility of confounding, and on differentiating social causation from social selection effects. Careful specification of hypotheses, and the use of designs capable of pitting alternative hypotheses against one another, are central needs if the life course processes underlying observed environmental associations are to be more fully explicated. Finally, we should note that while there has been a veritable explosion of potential biomedical measurements relating to the expanding range of biological mechanisms being elucidated, the development of social measures has, by comparison, remained quite limited. Social gradients in health show little evidence of diminishing, yet tests of pathways for these effects have tended to concentrate on a few conceptually well-motivated—and now strongly validated—examples. Elsewhere, we are still largely collecting social indicators that, while having clear prognostic power, are of uncertain theoretical status. One key task for the next generation of life course studies lies in the development of further models and related measurements to enable us to 'unpack' these effects.

References

1. Kuh D, Ben Shlomo Y, ed. (2004). *A life course approach to disease epidemiology*, 2nd edn. Oxford University Press, Oxford.
2. Wilkinson RG (2006). Ourselves and others—for better or worse: social vulnerability and inequality. In: Marmot M, Wilkinson RG, ed. *Social determinants of health*, 2nd edn. Oxford University Press, Oxford, p. 345.
3. Bourdieu P (1989). Social space and symbolic power. *Sociological Theory* 7, 14–25.
4. Eyerman R, Turner BS (1998). Outline of a theory of generation. *European Journal of Social Theory* 1, 91–106.
5. Barker DJP (1998). *Mothers and babies and health in later life*, 2nd edn. Churchill Livingstone, Edinburgh.
6. Moffitt TE (2005). The new look of behavioral genetics in developmental psychopathology: gene–environment interplay in antisocial behaviors. *Psychological Bulletin* 131, 533–554.
7. Rutter M (2005). Environmentally mediated risks for psychopathology: research strategies and findings. *Journal of the American Academy of Child and Adolescent Psychiatry* 44, 3–18.
8. Bronfenbrenner U (1979). *The ecology of human development: experiments by nature and design.* Harvard University Press, Cambridge, MA.
9. Stansfeld SA, Fuhrer R, Shipley M (1998). Types of social support as predictors of psychiatric morbidity in a cohort of British civil servants. *Psychological Medicine* 28, 881–892.
10. Bartley MJ, Ferrie J Montgomery SM (2006). Health and labour market disadvantage: unemployment, non-employment, and job insecurity. In: Marmot MG, Wilkinson RG, ed. *Social determinants of health*, 2nd edn. Oxford University Press, Oxford, pp. 78–96.
11. Maughan B (2002). Depression and psychological distress: a life course perspective. In Kuh DJ, Hardy RJ, ed. *A life course approach to women's health.* Oxford University Press, Oxford, pp. 161–176.
12. Marmot MG, Wilkinson RG, ed. (2006). *Social determinants of health*, 2nd edn. Oxford University Press, Oxford.
13. Marmot MG, Siegrist J, Theorell T (2006). Health and the pychosocial environment at work. In: Marmot M, Wilkinson RG, ed. *Social determinants of health*, 2nd edn. Oxford University Press, Oxford, pp. 97–130.
14. Steptoe A, Feldman PJ, Kunz S, Owen N, Willemsen G, Marmot M (2002). Stress responsivity and socioeconomic status. A mechanism for increased cardiovascular risk? *European Heart Journal* 23, 1757–1763.
15. Siegrist J, Klein D, Voigt KH (1997). Linking sociological with physiological data: the model of effort–reward imbalance at work. *Acta Physiologica Scandinavica* 161, Suppl 640, 112–116.
16. Brunner E, Marmot M (2005). Social organisation, stress and health. In: Marmot M, Wilkinson RG, ed. *Social determinants of health*, 2nd edn. Oxford University Press, Oxford, pp. 6–30.

17. Stansfeld SA (2006). Social support and social cohesion. In: Marmot M, Wilkinson RG, ed. *Social determinants of health*, 2nd edn. Oxford, Oxford University Press, pp. 148–171.

18. Lawlor DA, Ben Shlomo Y, Leon DA (2004). Pre-adult influences on cardiovascular disease. In: Kuh D, Ben Shlomo Y, ed. *A life course approach to chronic disease epidemiology*, 2nd edn. pp. 41–76. Oxford University Press, Oxford.

19. Bartley MJ, Plewis I (2002). Accumulated labour market disadvantage and limiting long-term illness. *International Journal of Epidemiology* 31, 336–341.

20. Power C, Hertzman C (1999). Health, well-being and coping skills. In: Keating D, Hertzman C, ed. *Developmental health and the wealth of nations*. Guilford Press, New York, pp. 41–54.

21. Blane D (2006). The life course, the social gradient, and health. In: Marmot M, Wilkinson RG, ed. *Social determinants of health*, 2nd edn. Oxford University Press, Oxford, pp. 54–77.

22. Maynard M, Gunnell D, Abraham L, Ness A, Bates C, Blane D (2004). What influences diet in early old age? *European Journal of Public Health* 16, 316–324.

23. Rutter M, the ERA research team (1998). Developmental catch-up and deficit following adoption after severe global early privation. *Journal of Child Psychology and Psychiatry,* 39, 465–476.

24. Lin N, Ye X, Ensel W (1999). Social support and depressed mood. *Journal of Health and Social Behaviour* 40, 344–359.

25. Kawachi I, Berkman LF (2001). Social ties and mental health. *Journal of Urban Health* 78, 458–467.

26. Weiss LH, Schwartz JC (1996). The relationship between parenting types and older adolescents' personality, academic achievement, adjustment and substance abuse. *Child Development* 67, 2101–2114.

27. Paz I, Jones D, Byrne G (2005). Child maltreatment, child protection and mental health. *Current Opinion in Psychiatry* 18, 411–421.

28. Champagne FA, Curley JP (2005). How social experiences influence the brain. *Current Opinion in Neurobiology* 15, 704–709.

29. Ryff CD, Singer BH (2005). Social environments and the genetics of aging: advancing knowledge of protective health mechanisms. *Journals of Gerontology* 60B, 12–23.

30. Caspi A, McClay J, Moffitt TE, Mill J, Martin J, Craig IW, *et al.* (2002). Role of genotype in the cycle of violence in maltreated children. *Science* 297, 851–854.

31. Marmot MG, Theorell T, Siegrist J (2002). Work and coronary heart disease. In: Stansfeld SA, Marmot MG, ed. *Stress and the heart*. BMJ Books, London, pp. 50–71.

32. Huppert F (2004). A population approach to positive psychology. In: Linley PA, Joseph S, ed. *Positive psychology in practice*. John Wiley, New Jersey, pp. 693–709.

33. Ryff CD, Singer BH, Love GD (2004). Positive health: connecting well-being with biology. *Philosophical Transactions of the Royal Society B: Biological Science* 359, 1381–1394.

34. Giddens A (1984). *The constitution of society: outline of the theory of structuration*. University of California Press, Berkeley.

35. Schooling MJ (2001). *Health behaviour in a social and temporal context*. PhD thesis, University of London.

36. Doyal L, Gough I (1991). *A theory of human need*. Macmillan, London.

37. McMunn A, Bartley M, Kuh D (2006). Life course roles and women's health in mid-life. *Journal of Epidemiology and Community Health* 60, 484–489.

38. McMunn A, Bartley M, Kuh D (2006). Women's health in mid-life: life course social roles and agency as quality. *Social Science and Medicine* 63, 1561–1572.

39. Wakschlag LS, Pickett KE, Cook E, Benowitz NL, Leventhal BL (2002). Maternal smoking during pregnancy and severe antisocial behavior in offspring: a review. *American Journal of Public Health* 92, 966–974.

40. Conger RD, Ge XJ, Elder GH, Lorenz FO, Simons RL (1994). Economic-stress, coercive family process, and developmental problems of adolescents. *Child Development* 65, 541–561.

41. Plomin R, Defries JC, Loehlin JC (1977). Genotype–environment interaction and correlation in analysis of human-behavior. *Psychological Bulletin* 84, 309–322.

42. Caspi A, Moffitt TE, Morgan J, Rutter M, Taylor A, Arseneault L, *et al.* (2004). Maternal expressed emotion predicts children's antisocial behavior problems: uising monozygotic-twin differences to identify environmental effects on behavioral development. *Developmental Psychology* 40, 149–161.

43. Kim-Cohen J, Moffitt TE, Taylor A, Pawlby SJ, Caspi A (2005). Maternal depression and children's antisocial behavior—nature and nurture effects. *Archives of General Psychiatry* 62, 173–181.

44. Jaffee SR, Caspi A, Moffitt TE, Polo-Tomas M, Price TS, Taylor A (2004). The limits of child effects: evidence for genetically mediated child effects on corporal punishment but not on physical maltreatment. *Developmental Psychology* 40, 1047–1058.

45. Freedman D, Thornton A, Camburn D, Alwin D, Young de ML (1988). The life history calendar: a technique for collecting retrospective data. *Sociological Methodology* 18, 37–68.

46. Blane D, Berney L, Davey Smith G, Gunnell D, Holland P (1999). Reconstructing the life course; a 60 year follow-up study based on the Boyd Orr cohort. *Public Health* 113, 117–124.

47. Makepeace G, Dolton P, Woods L, Joshi H, Galinda-Rueda F (2003). From school to the labour market. In: Ferri E, Bynner J, Wadsworth MEJ, ed. *Changing Britain, changing lives.* Institute of Education Press, London, pp. 29–70.

48. Hardt J, Rutter M (2004). Validity of adult retrospective reports of adverse childhood experiences: review of the evidence. *Journal of Child Psychology and Psychiatry* 45, 260–273.

49. Barker DJP (1992). *Fetal and infant origins of adult disease.* BMJ Press, London.

50. Forsdahl A (1977). Are living conditions in childhood and adolescence an important risk factor for arteriosclerotic heart disease? *British Journal of Social and Preventive Medicine* 31, 91–95.

51. Berkman LF, Glass T, Brissette I, Seeman TE (2000). From social integration to health: Durkheim in the new millennium. *Social Science and Medicine* 51, 843–857.

52. Siegrist J, Marmot M (2004). Health inequalities and the psychosocial environment. *Social Science and Medicine* 58, 1463–1473.

53. Steptoe A, Feldman PJ, Kunz S, Owen N, Willemsen G, Marmot M (2002). Stress responsivity and socioeoconomic status. A mechanism for increased cardiovascular risk? *European Heart Journal* 23, 1757–1763.

54. Suomi SJ (1997). Early determinants of behaviour: evidence from primate studies. *British Medical Bulletin* 53, 170–184

55. Wilkinson RG (1996). *Unhealthy societies.* Routledge, London.

56. Bruhn JG, Wolf S (1979). *The Roseto story.* University of Oklahoma Press, Oklahoma.

57. Dalgard OS, Tambs K (1997). Urban environment and mental health: a longitudinal study. *British Journal of Psychiatry* 171, 530–536.

58. World Bank (2003). *World development indicators.* World Bank, Washington.

59. United Nations (2003). *Human development report 2003.* United Nations, New York.

60. Makinen IH (2000). East European transition and suicide mortality. *Social Science and Medicine* 51, 1405–1420.

61. Shkolnikov V, Cornia GA (2000). Population crisis and rising mortality in transitional Russia. In: Cornia GA, Paniccia R, ed. *The mortality crisis in transitional economies.* Oxford University Press, Oxford, pp. 253–279.

62. Esping-Andersen G (1999). *Social foundations of post-industrial economies.* Oxford University Press, Oxford.

63. Korpi W, Palme J (1998). The paradox of redistribution and strategies of equality—welfare state institutions, inequality and poverty in the Western countries. *American Sociological Review* 63, 661–687.

64. Navarro V, Shi L (2000). The political context of social inequalities and health. *Social Science and Medicine* 52, 481–491.

65. Coburn D (2000). Income inequality, social cohesion and the health status of populations. *Social Science and Medicine* 51, 135–146.

66. Coburn D (2004). Beyond the income inequality hypothesis. *Social Science and Medicine* 58, 41–56.

67. Bartley MJ (2003). Health inequality and societal institutions. *Social Theory and Health* 1, 108–129.

68. Wadsworth MEJ, Bartley MJ (2006). Social inequality, family structure and health in the life course. *Koelner Zeitschrift für Soziologie und Sozialpsychologie* 46, 125–143.

69. Roseboom TJ, van der Meulen JH, Michels, RP, Osmond C, Barker DJP, Ravelli ACJ, *et al.* (2001). Adult survival after prenatal exposure to the Dutch famine 1944–45. *Paediatric and Perinatal Epidemiology* 15, 220–225.

70. Rutter M, Kreppner J, O'Connor T (2001). Specificity and heterogeneity in children's responses to profound institutional privation. *British Journal of Psychiatry* 179, 97–103.

71. Marmot MG, Syme SL, Kagan A (1975). Epidemiologic studies of CHD and stroke in Japanese men living in Japan, Hawaii and California: prevalence of coronary and hypertensive heart disease and associated risk factors. *American Journal of Epidemiology* 102, 514–525.

72. Salmond CE, Joseph JG, Prior IAM, Stanley, DG, Wessen AF (1985). Longitudinal analysis of the relationship between blood pressure and migration: the Tokelau Island migrant study. *American Journal of Epidemiology,* 122, 291–301.

73. Montgomery SM, Bartley MJ, Cook DG, Wadsworth MEJ (1996). Health and social precursors of unemployment in young men in Great Britain. *Journal of Epidemiology and Community Health* 50, 415–422.

74. Elder GH (1974). *Children of the great depression.* University of Chicago Press, Chicago.

75. Costello EJ, Compton SN, Keeler G, Angold A (2003). Relationships between poverty and psychopathology—a natural experiment. *Journal of the American Medical Association* 290, 2023–2029.

76. Pembrey ME, Bygren LO, Kaati G, Edvinsson S, Northstone K, Sjostrom M, *et al.* (2006). Sex-specific, male-line transgenerational responses in humans. *European Journal of Human Genetics* 14, 159–166.

77. Shanahan MJ, Hofer SM (2005). Social context in gene–environment interactions: retrospect and prospect. *Journals of Gerontology* 60B, 65–76.

78. Finch CE, Crimmins E (2004). Inflammatory exposure and historical changes in human life-spans. *Science* 17, 1736–1739.

79. Ferri E, Bynner J, Wadsworth MEJ (2003). *Changing Britain, changing lives: three generations at the turn of the century.* University of London, Institute of Education, London.

80. Rutter M, Smith DJ, ed. (1995). *Psychosocial disorders in young people.* John Wiley, Chichester.

81. Siegrist J, Marmot M, ed. (2006). *Social inequalities in health.* Oxford University Press, Oxford.

82. Halsey AH, Webb J, ed. (2000). *Twentieth century British social trends.* Macmillan, London.

83. Young M, Willmott P (1962). *Family and kinship in East London.* Pelican, London.

84. Wadsworth MEJ (1991). *The imprint of time.* Clarendon Press, Oxford.

85. Ely M, Richards MPM, Wadsworth MEJ, Elliott BJ (1999). Secular changes in the association of parental divorce and children's educational attainment: evidence from three British birth cohorts. *Journal of Social Policy* 28, 437–455.

86. Roche AF (1992). *Growth, maturation and body composition: the Fels longitudinal study 1929–1991.* Cambridge University Press, Cambridge.

Chapter 4

Designs for large life course studies of genetic effects

Camilla Stoltenberg and Andrew Pickles

Abstract

The need to investigate genetic aetiology has led to studies of an unprecedented size and cost. We review designs, methods of genetic analysis and some current major studies including case–control, cohort and collaborative studies. We assess critically the potential of these major data sources for life course research.

4.1 Introduction

Over the last 10 years, there has been an increasing interest in large population-based studies of genes, environment and health, mainly springing out of scientific discoveries in genetics, but also as a result of the development of molecular biology in general, information technology and life course epidemiology. Many experts agree that by merging genetics and epidemiology it may be possible to overcome major limitations of the classic approaches in both disciplines, and answer important scientific questions about causes of disease.

This chapter will review the reasons why scientific thinking has now concluded that large-scale population studies of genetic and environmental effects are necessary, summarize the background and methods of genetic analysis, and consider some of the strengths and weaknesses of different designs for life course research. The focus will be on large population-based studies, and in particular prospective cohorts, where both data and biological material are included. *Large* will in this context mean studies where there are, or will be, more than 100 000 participants.[1] However, examples will also be drawn from smaller projects, simply because most studies that have been used to explore genes, environment and health *are* smaller. Studies where analysis of biological material, and in particular genetic analysis, is or will be included are primary in this review, while purely quantitative genetic studies will be secondary to those involving 'wet' laboratories in one way or another. Thus, for simplicity, the term *population biobanks* will be used to describe the kind of studies that are the core topic of this chapter. Establishment of new population biobanks, conversion of existing epidemiological studies into population biobanks by adding collections of biological material, pooling of data and samples from existing population biobanks in national and international collaborations, and meta-analysis of such studies are the main approaches towards the establishment of large population studies of genetic and environmental effects.[1] These approaches, and the possible design options for such studies, will be reviewed and discussed.

Issues regarding access to samples and data, ethical, legal and societal aspects, funding, management and governance of population biobanks have been prominent in the published literature about large population-based studies of genes, environment and health. In comparison, systematic published literature on the scientific rationale and objectives, and of the actual outcomes of such initiatives after about 10 years of attention and intense activity, is surprisingly scarce. In this context, the focus will be solely on the latter aspects of population biobanks. It is also important to note that this review will not provide a comprehensive description of all population biobank projects, but rather use a selection as examples to illustrate the main types of projects.

4.2 What is a population biobank?

Strictly, a biobank is a collection of biological material. Biobanks are not much worth without information on demographic variables, environmental exposures and/or diseases or other phenotypes. However, because the use of really large biological collections in genetic research is relatively new and requires considerable resources, the emphasis on the biobanks that are part of such large studies may be appropriate, at least for a period of time. Also, the biobank concept has attracted more public attention lately than the more precise concepts of cohorts and case–control studies.

Collections of biological material from humans can be categorized according to the aim of the biobank, for example as clinical biobanks such as archival collections in pathological departments, therapeutic biobanks such as blood banks, research biobanks such as those collected in drug trials or health surveys, or judicial biobanks such as DNA collections from criminals. Alternatively, biobanks can be categorized according to whether they are patient based or population based.[2] Also, some require that the material is collected with the intention of being stored for a long period of time before it is categorized as a biobank, while others consider the information derived from analysis of the biological sample as part of the biobank, which means that the biobank will exist even when all the material has been consumed. Lastly, the term biobank often includes the organizational structure managing the biological samples, such as in UK Biobank. In this context, the term will be used in an unspecific way, as a description of studies that include biological material from individuals.

The term *population biobank* will be used to describe population-based studies where information on health and biological material from the participants is available. Population biobanks can have many different sources of data and biological material. There are at least five principal sources. (1) They can be part of large disease oriented population-based case control studies as in deCode genetics in Iceland (www.decode.com) or the Wellcome Trust Case Control Consortium (www.wtccc.org.uk). (2) They can be opportunistic nested case–control or case–cohort studies based on non-scientific 'natural' experiments. (3) They can use national screening programmes where biological material is collected routinely from all newborn children, as in the PKU-biobanks in Sweden and Denmark.[3,4] (4) They can be part of old or new prospective pregnancy, birth or adult cohorts as in the Danish (www.ssi.dk/sw9314.asp) and Norwegian pregnancy cohorts (www.fhi.no/morogbarn) or UK Biobank (www.ukbiobank.ac.uk/). (5) They can be national or international collaborations between established epidemiological cohorts such as in the European Prospective Investigation into Cancer and Nutrition (EPIC) (www.iarc.fr/epic/intro.html) and GenomEUtwin (www.genomeutwin.org).

Although not by definition, the perception of a biobank is more closely associated with DNA banking and genetics than with measurements of environmental factors, and it seems to be only loosely linked up with the vernacular of life course epidemiology.[5] Several of the new large population biobank initiatives reviewed in this chapter have been established with a limited interest in environmental factors and little attention directed to life course perspectives, while others have these interests as explicit aims. It may seem that although the original initiatives towards conversion of epidemiological studies into DNA banks were driven by the prospects of gene identification, the potential for exploiting information on environmental exposures and longitudinal follow-up is becoming clearer over time, as epidemiologists and geneticists are learning from each other. The focus has been on conversion of epidemiological studies into infrastructures for genetics, but along the road it is becoming clear that regardless of what the origin was, large studies with information on both genes and environment at different stages in life will eventually become valuable resources for aetiological research, provided that they are managed well. In many ways, population biobanks are old phenomena with a new name. However, the size, and, in the case of cohorts, the very long-term perspective, of these enterprises raises a whole range of new issues about funding, access to data and samples, management and governance that represent new challenges both to the research community and to the community at large.

4.3 Methods of genetic analysis and the rationale for population biobanks

Before proceeding to consider why biobanks might be necessary, it is helpful to consider the other common designs that have been used for genetic analysis and the kinds of analyses that we should be looking for them to support in the future.

4.3.1 Biometrical genetics

The simplest biometrical genetic models treat the genetic and environmental effects as 'anonymous', merely contributing to components of phenotypic variation that may be differentially shared by relatives of varying degrees of relatedness. As described in Chapter 2, twin and adoption studies have been the principal study designs for this approach in humans. The extension of the analysis methodology to multivariate outcomes has allowed an elegant array of sophisticated analyses to be undertaken that, for example, can distinguish an individual's impact on their environmental exposure from its impact on them (see Chapter 3), or identify that different genes influence blood pressure at rest and at exercise[6] or physical growth in childhood and adolescence. The models and designs thus lend themselves to addressing many questions of interest to life course researchers. It is likely that twin studies, in particular the large collaborative studies such as GenomEUtwin, will continue to deliver much of interest. Nonetheless, many remain sceptical of assumptions required for variance decomposition, and anyway wish to progress beyond anonymous genes to identifying specific genes and biosocial processes.

4.3.2 Linkage and pedigrees

For diseases predominantly determined by the inheritance of a single gene, considerable power is available from the analysis of extended families with multiple affected relatives using parametric linkage analysis. However, it is likely that we have exhausted the diseases easily amenable to this kind of analysis. Where the genetic aetiology of the disease is more complex and the genetic model correspondingly more uncertain, non-parametric or model-free methods are preferred. For these, large numbers of smaller pedigrees are generally preferred, both for their computational simplicity and for the greater generalizability expected from avoiding reliance upon a small number of (possibly just one) idiosyncratic families. Whether using parametric or non-parametric approaches, linkage does not directly identify the causal gene but instead uses markers (heritable functional or non-functional genetic variation at various positions along the genome) to localize fairly large regions as containing a potentially causal gene. In so doing, since linkage could do this with the use of a comparatively modest number of markers (hundreds), it provided a feasible means of screening the whole genome for regions of potential interest. Initially restricted to binary phenotypes, the method has now been widely applied to quantitative 'disease' traits, such as language and literacy scores, with further extension to multivariate score profiles, notionally allowing increased power and the localization of genes with specific effects. Do any of these linkage methods have any specific relevance to life course epidemiology? In principle, searches for specificity of effect for early versus late onset disease, or some life course-defined outcome such as a trajectory class (see Chapter 8) would be possible, but few such applications appear to have been undertaken.

4.3.3 Association methods

When genotyping was costly and the density of available markers limited, linkage was the sensible starting point on the path to identifying genes. Neither of these applies any longer. Moreover, there are enough examples of disease genes being located without prior localization by linkage analysis, such as the IF1H1 region for type 1 diabetes,[7] that many no longer consider it a necessary preliminary step.

Instead, researchers are now much more keen to test for direct association between a gene and disease. Genotypes may be included in epidemiological life course analyses alongside traditional environmental covariates. For example, Payton *et al.*[8] show an association in a growth curve context (see Chapter 8) in which the serotonin transporter gene was tested for association with both the initial level and the decline of cognitive performance that occurs in older age. Such analyses can include interactions between genotype and environment.

Examples include the finding of Caspi *et al.*[9] where the effects of the 5HT transporter gene on depression appears to be modified by life events and the finding that increased endotoxin exposure is protective against respiratory allergic disease but only for the CC form of the CD14 gene.[10] Association methods therefore lend themselves readily as the means to include genetics in a life course approach, in particular where there is a restricted set of candidate/hypothetical causal genes.

4.3.4 Confounding in genetics

Just as in identifying environmental aetiology, identifying genetic aetiology can be complicated by the existence of confounding. The confounders can be environmental or genetic. An example of the latter is where both a genotype and the disease are more common in a subpopulation. Such confounding can be approached via stratification by potential confounder, be that environmental or genetic. In addition, elegant methods specific to genetics have been proposed, such as the transmission disequilibrium method in which affectedness is examined conditional upon the set of alleles available to be inherited from a set of parents. Such an approach requires genotypic data from child and parent trios. However, parent data are often unavailable, particularly for studies of diseases of older age, and experience suggested that the risks of genetic confounding were lower than we had once feared (we later discuss a resurgent concern that this may reflect premature complacency). As a consequence, increasing attention is being paid to simple designs that involve unrelated individuals.

4.3.5 Multiple testing

However, although association methods do not require prior specification of the causal gene, the genetic marker typically has to be very close to it. This makes any proposed screening for contributory genes by associational methods much more speculative than via linkage, simply because so many markers must be tested to cover the whole genome that the multiple testing problem becomes very severe. How do we detect the true effect signal above the clamour of false-positive associations? The severity of this problem has placed great emphasis on the importance of statistical power, in turn leading to the conclusion that studies need to be of a very considerable size indeed.

4.3.6 Mendelian randomization

This concern with size and statistical power has been reinforced more recently from an unexpected source, namely researchers primarily interested in non-genetic effects. Their concern has been focused upon the difficulties in obtaining estimates of the causal effects of a risk factor when there are ongoing concerns about potential bias from residual confounding. As explained in Chapter 8, under certain assumptions it is possible to obtain bias free estimates, even in circumstances where the confounders are unmeasured or unknown, by the use of an instrumental variable. It turns out that there are some instances where genes can act as instrumental variables.[11] What is required is that a gene influences the outcome of interest, but solely through the risk exposure of interest. Davey Smith and Ebrahim[11] give an example of the gene for the alcohol dehydrogenase enzyme, which acts as a source of variation in alcohol consumption that is uncorrelated with smoking and other common confounding risks. The impact of this variation in alcohol consumption on, for example, high-density lipoprotein (HDL) cholesterol or blood pressure, offers scope for estimating the confounder-free effect of alcohol consumption. There are, of course, many potential pitfalls that must be guarded against, but one of the sources of concern is the low power of this approach when the available contender instrumental variable genes have only modest impact on the risk exposure, which is the common situation. Application of such weak instruments, as they are called, requires large samples.

4.3.7 Epigenetics

The analysis methods that we have described for the most part examine the relationship between genotype and phenotype as a black box. However, the mechanisms that regulate gene expression are coming to be seen as of increasing importance, especially in relation to life course epidemiology.[12] Often gene expression is regulated by other genes, but it is also regulated by environmental exposure, both contemporaneous exposure and historic. The latter can include exposures early in development, such as in the example described in Chapter 5 of the early maternal care received by rat pups influencing lifelong cortisol levels through methylation of the DNA during the immediate post-natal period.[13] This provides a mechanism by which programming, in the Barkerian sense, may come about. However, it also seems that some aspects of gene regulation are themselves heritable, and not just through inheritance of regulatory genes. By means of a mechanism that is termed imprinting, some aspects of the gene regulation induced by an environmental exposure in one generation can be passed on to another, as described in Chapter 3. This provides an explanation of how famine in one generation can influence both the child and grandchild.[14]

The extent to which methylation, histone acetylation, RNA-mediated silencing pathways and other regulatory mechanisms[15] operate only in the early stages of development or in response to extreme environmental stress such as famine is unclear. Studies of identical twins have suggested progressive phenotypic divergence throughout the life course, with parallel divergence in the genomic distribution of 5-methylcytosine DNA and histone methylation.[16] Such instability would suggest regulatory processes as key targets for life course research, and the potential for reversibility would suggest them as targets for therapy, pharmaceutical or otherwise. However, other DNA methylation profiling studies find no relationship with age,[17] suggesting greater stability and a more limited potential role in life course research.

These processes present a number of major challenges to routine genetic analysis. First, phenotypic associations with genotype will be at best attenuated due to the variable expression of that genotype between individuals and within individuals over time. Secondly, in addition to needing to know the regulatory status of a gene, we must contend with the fact that this can be expected to be tissue specific. Knowledge gained from saliva or blood will commonly not be sufficient. Thirdly, since regulatory status can change, repeated measurement may be necessary. Fourthly, as elaborated in Chapter 8, synergism may be expected between genes and an exposure potentially distant in the past or even between gene and past exposure that together set up a condition of vulnerability for a current precipitating exposure. Fifthly, epigenetic processes again emphasize the importance as to the timing of the exposure process with respect to development.

Thus, while knowledge of gene regulation processes may offer much in respect of understanding aetiology, prevention and therapy, particularly from a life course perspective, they present an enormous challenge for measurement and analysis. Where biobanks are presented as a long-term scientific resource, we will also need to assess their usefulness from such an epigenetic perspective.

4.4 Aims of biobanks

So what are biobanks intended to deliver? In the wake of the sequencing of the human genome, attention has turned towards the relationships between identifiable genes, environment and complex disease. It is believed that most, if not all, common human diseases, such as hypertension, coronary artery disease and psychiatric disorders, develop through interactions between our genome and the environment from conception to death. Many have pointed out that a particularly valuable strategy to dissect the relationship between genetic factors and complex disease is to utilize large epidemiological studies with biological samples from different populations.[18,19]

Most of the large biobank initiatives have declared grand ambitions. Box 4.1 displays a selection of the aims that the population biobank initiatives have stated in publications

---

Box 4.1 Aims of selected population biobanks

Case–control studies

deCODE genetics (www.decode.com accessed 9 August 2006): using our population approach and resources, we can efficiently conduct population- and genome-wide scans to home in on the key genetic factors involved in any common disease in a virtually hypothesis-free manner. We have been able to do this through the analysis of genotypic and medical data from over 100 000 volunteers in our gene research in Iceland—more than 50 per cent of the adult population—in tandem with our genealogical data linking together the entire present-day population and stretching back over 1100 years. By mining these data sets, we can effectively trace the inherited components of a given disease, pinpointing the key disease genes as well as the specific markers or haplotypes within these genes that correlate with the disease.

The Wellcome Trust Case Control Consortium (WTCCC): WTCCC is a collaboration of 24 leading geneticists, who will analyse thousands of DNA samples from patients suffering with different diseases to identify common genetic variations for each condition. It is hoped that by identifying these genetic signposts, researchers will be able to understand which people are the most at risk, and also produce more effective treatments (http://www.wtccc.org.uk/ accessed 9 August 2006).

Box 4.1 Aims of selected population biobanks *(continued)*

Cohorts

UK Biobank: the main aim of the study is to investigate the separate and combined effects of genetic and environmental factors (including lifestyle, physiological and environmental exposures) on the risk of common multifactorial diseases of adult life (UK BioBank 2002).

The Kadoorie Study of Chronic Disease in China (KSCDC): a blood-based prospective study of environmental and genetic causes of premature death in 500 000 Chinese adults: The Kadoorie Study of Chronic Disease in China (KSCDC) is an open-ended prospective study with very broad research aims.[20] This study will help sort out the complementary roles of genetic factors and of environmental factors such as tobacco, infections and diet as causes of premature deaths in China, and could have important implications for disease control worldwide (http://www.ctsu.ox.ac.uk/%7Ekadoorie/ public/).

Potential large US cohort for the study of genes, environment and health: to ascertain and quantify all of the major environmental and genetic causes of common illnesses, setting the stage for a future of better preventive medicine and more effective therapy. Such a study could examine the environmental exposures, genetic risk factors, lifestyle and medical experiences of a cross-section of America of unprecedented size and scope (http://www.genome.gov/Pages/About/ OD/ ReportsPublications/ PotentialUSCohort.pdf website accessed 11 August 2006).

The Danish National Birth Cohort (DNBC): we wanted to study pregnancy complications and diseases in offspring as a function of factors operating in early life, fetal growth and its determinants. We aimed especially at studying side effects of medications and infections. We focused not only on diseases in the period from conception to early childhood, but also on all diseases with a possible origin in the fetal time period.[21]

The Norwegian Mother and Child Cohort Study (MoBa): the objective of MoBa is to test specific etiologic hypotheses by estimating the association between exposures (including genetic factors) and diseases, aiming at prevention.[22]

Collaborations—pooling of cohorts

The European Prospective Investigation into Cancer and Nutrition (EPIC): the European Prospective Investigation into Cancer and Nutrition (EPIC) was designed to investigate the relationships between nutritional status, lifestyle and environmental factors a incidence of cancer and other chronic diseases (http://www.iarc.fr/epic/intro.html accessed 9 August 2006).

GenomEUtwin: To develop novel strategies to utilize maximally the unique features of twin cohorts, including the availability of longitudinal data and ample information about lifestyle and environmental factors, in the characterization of complex traits.

To utilize the synergy between the twin cohorts and the representative population cohorts (MORGAM) from the same countries, in studies of genetic and environmental predictors of traits (www.genomeutwin.org, accessed 10 August 2006).

or at websites. All of them are aiming at discovering the causes of common, complex diseases, but the emphasis on genetic rather than environmental factors, or on understanding how disease develops through the life course versus identifying drug targets, differs.

Box 4.2 summarizes the arguments put forward by UK Biobank as to why large population-based longitudinal cohorts are necessary.[23] These reasons are simply the arguments for cohort studies overall, but with particular attention to genetics and the use of biological samples. The arguments for population cohorts have been repeated and reformulated in many other biobank projects, such as the NIHGR 2005 initiative.

Box 4.2 Reasons why large prospective population cohorts with biobanks are needed

Prospective cohort design

- Investigation of a large number of conditions/end-points, including all-cause mortality
- Provides information on exposure prior to development of disease, thus avoiding recall bias and allowing accurate measurement of variables
- Allows measurement of blood-based molecular and proteomic factors using samples collected prior to the development of disease
- Provides prospectively collected blood samples, with genetic information from all cases in the cohort regardless of the severity
- Allows investigation of conditions that cannot generally be investigated retrospectively, (e.g. fatal conditions, dementia), and inclusion of all cases of disease where there is high case fatality rate (e.g. myocardial infarction)
- Provides data allowing the broader consideration of both the risks and benefits associated with a specific genotype and/or exposure, through the inclusion of multiple end-points
- Provides a straightforward source of comparable controls
- Minimizes the assumptions made regarding the underlying relationships between genotypes, exposure and outcome (in contrast to designs such as those employed in case-only studies, which assume independence between genotype and exposure)
- Allows the investigation of continuous outcomes
- Provides a framework for a variety of studies to be conducted within the cohort
- Provides a resource for the future, where investigation of outcomes and relationships unforeseen at the time of commencing the study is possible
- Provides a research resource which grows in value as time passes and more health events arise

> **Box 4.2 Reasons why large prospective population cohorts with biobanks are needed** (continued)
>
> ## Large-scale
>
> - Yields statistically reliable results
> - Provides appropriate information on a range of important health outcomes
> - Yields accurate information on moderate effects, which are of clinical and public health relevance
> - Provides an accurate and comprehensive quantification of combined genetic and environmental effects
>
> ## Population-based recruitment
>
> - Allows acquisition of information of direct relevance to health in the general population
> - Provides a heterogeneous population, with a range of relevant exposures
> - Provides direct information on rates of disease
> - Allows inclusion of large numbers of participants
> - Encourages a sense of public ownership and inclusivity
>
> Adapted from UK Biobank Protocol (2002, pp. 10–11).[23]

Box 4.3 outlines the uses of cohorts, including the secondary uses which are not sufficient reasons for investing in population biobanks, but are scientifically valuable and cost-efficient applications of them.

In summary, population cohorts with biobanks are perceived as necessary for discovering the aetiology of complex diseases because of their size, because of their combined information on genetic and environmental factors and phenotypes, and, in the case of longitudinal cohorts, for their ability to overcome certain methodological problems and for life course studies.

4.5 Design options for population biobanks

Although there are divergent opinions on what types of population biobanks are worthy of the necessary investments, there seems to be consensus about the need for population biobanks to drive forward research on genes, environment and complex diseases.

The three main design options for large population-based studies on genes and environment are (1) case–control studies, (2) cohorts and (3) harmonization and pooling of existing studies. There are already a number of initiatives using each of these strategies, and considerable debate about what the most efficient and appropriate design might be. One major debate is about the choice between series of case–control studies versus a limited number of large prospective cohorts. Another debate is about the usefulness of very large

Box 4.3 Uses of prospective cohorts in studies of genes, environment and health

Primary uses

- Studies of joint effects of genes and environment
- Genotype-based studies
- Genetics of disease progression

Secondary uses

- Direct association of genes with disease
- Genotype-based studies
- Environmental exposure-based studies
- Universal controls
- Family-based studies
- Replication of associations found in smaller studies in selected populations (patients, multiplex families)

Additional features under optimal circumstances

- Linkage with routine registries covering the total population for collection of outcomes and adjustment for attrition and biases in recruitment
- Linkage with routine clinical biobanks

Adapted from presentation by Paul Burton, May 2006[24]

---

sample sizes versus the need for in-depth and high quality data collections, particularly regarding environmental exposures and phenotypes. The former debate focuses specifically on designs that allow investigation of gene–environment interaction, while the latter focuses on what has been labelled 'thick versus thin' longitudinal studies.[25]

4.6 Case–control studies

Clayton and McKeigue[26] have argued strongly against the use of cohort studies as a basis for examination of gene–environment interactions. They have promoted case–control studies as the design of choice for studies of gene–environment interaction because such studies are less expensive and time consuming, can include the necessary number of cases without the great risk of attrition involved in longitudinal follow-up, and can achieve more precise measurements of outcomes. Supporters of large population-based cohorts have disputed their views, and claim a number of advantages of cohort studies.[27,28] The cohort defenders say that population biobanks with a cohort design will be a foundation for medical research for the next 20–30 years or longer, allow for studies of multiple end-points in the same base population, represent an investment that is profitable over time compared with series of case–control studies, and provide a basis for nested case–control and case–cohort studies, and for good control samples. In addition, prospective cohorts allow for assessment of both the risks and benefits of specific genotypes and environmental exposures. Lastly, effects on all-cause and specific mortality, genetic and exposure data are available regardless of disease outcome and severity.[29] If the opportunity for life course studies is added, this list summarizes the additional advantages of cohorts compared with case–control studies for a series of purposes. However, a review of results so far seems to support the view that case–control studies are, at least currently, better suited for discovery of genetic variants and mechanisms. DeCode genetics in Iceland and the Wellcome Trust Case Control Consortium can illustrate this point.

4.6.1 deCODE genetics

deCODE genetics in Iceland has effectively employed a variety of case–control approaches to identify genetic loci and specific alleles conferring increased risk of a series of diseases, and for studies of basic genetic mechanisms and methods. The original aims of deCODE were both to identify genes and to study the interaction between genes and environment. However, identification of genes and genetic mechanisms, validation and replication is still a daunting task, and deCODE has focused on identification of genes and drug development, while they have not collected or utilized environmental information. The company is organized as a private enterprise, and has collected informed consent, blood samples and phenotypic information from more than 100 000 Icelanders, of which about 50 per cent are 40 years or older, and about 60 000 individuals from countries outside Iceland. According to their web-page, deCODE is working on gene discovery in about 50 common diseases, and has isolated 15 genes and drug targets in 12 common diseases, and mapped genes in some 16 more.

   In the first years after the establishment of the company in 1996, both patients and all their first-degree relatives were invited to donate blood. The relatives were used as family controls and also provided information on broader, subclinical phenotypes or endophenotypes. Later, a more traditional case–control approach has been used with a standard set of about 1800 controls for whom as much as possible has been genotyped (Augustin Kong, personal communication, June 2006).

   Genealogical information has provided additional efficiency to the basic case–control approach. Famously, the genealogical database in Iceland covers the total population alive today and includes about 726 000 individuals throughout the history of human settlement in Iceland. The basic idea is that common diseases do not show Mendelian inheritance patterns. Affected siblings are therefore not frequent in common diseases, but many patients have more distant relatives with the same (or related) diseases (see Table 4.1). Scientifically, however, information on biological relatedness has proven to be useful for three to four generations, while more distant relations have not been used as much in scientific studies.[30,31] Table 4.1 demonstrates a clear relationship between

Table 4.1 Use of genealogies in studies of common complex diseases. Risk ratio in relatives of patients with atrial fibrillation by degree of relationship

Degree of relatives	Risk ratio (95 per cent CI)
1	1.77 (1.67–1.88)
2	1.36 (1.27–1.44)
3	1.18 (1.14–1.23)
4	1.10 (1.06–1.13)
5	1.05 (1.02–1.07)

CI = confidence interval.

All *P*-values are >0.001.

Adapted from Arnar *et al.*[32]

degree of relatedness and risk of atrial fibrillation in a recent study using the Icelandic genealogical database.

Very few countries have genealogical information of this kind. In Sweden, there is a multigeneration register covering about three generations of all residents born in Sweden,[33] and a few other total populations are or can be included in similar databases.

The combination of genealogical information and a traditional case–control approach has been efficient in directing the research towards chromosomal loci that contain highly penetrant alleles in families with a high aggregation of disease, as in traditional linkage analysis. Such linkage peaks are probably caused by rare variants with high penetrance, and are used as guides to where the common variants with variable penetrance and small to moderate linkage peaks are located. Thus, even smaller linkage peaks may be of interest if they occur in locations where the rarer variants have been observed.

The genealogical database is a basis for family studies, and is also helpful in studies of fertility, longevity and genetic history.[34–38] deCODEs population-based resources include a large proportion of the population in Iceland, and some individuals have been part of many different studies as cases, controls or both. This allows for studies of more than one disease or trait simultaneously, just as in cohort studies. Clearly, when a series of population-based case–control studies are as comprehensive and intertwined as the Icelandic one, it acquires some of the features of a longitudinal cohort and can easily be transformed into a cohort study. Life course studies have never been part of deCODE's strategy. Still, it seems that the biobank with clinical information that deCODE has established, in combination with linkage to existing health registries, demographic information and environmental information, could potentially be transformed into a resource for life course studies.

deCODE is currently performing genome-wide scans with 317 000 TagSNPs (Illumina) on the 100 000 Icelandic samples in the biobank, which will yield a unique resource internationally for genome-wide association studies.

Originally, much attention was directed towards the genealogical database, a proposed national healthcare database which has never materialized, and the homogeneity of the

Icelandic population. However, these features may not be absolutely necessary for genetic research of the kind that deCODE has devoted itself to, and deCODE's main advantage may therefore be their efficiency and capacity for doing genetic research on common and complex diseases rather than the population structure of Iceland.

4.6.2 **The Wellcome Trust Case Control Consortium (WTCCC)**

Pooling and harmonization of projects is ongoing for both case–control and cohort studies. A good example of pooling of case–control studies is the Wellcome Trust Case Control Consortium (WTCCC), although it does not qualify as a population biobank according to the cut-off at 100 000 participants which is employed here regardless of whether these are participants from the general population waiting for cases to accrue, or already phenotyped cases. The Consortium is funded by the Wellcome Trust and was established in 2005 as a collaborative project between 24 British geneticists who are responsible for a series of disease-based case–control studies (http://www.wtccc.org.uk/). The aim is to use existing biological samples and ascertained phenotype information, in combination with new genetic technologies, to acquire genome-wide association data rapidly. The declared objectives of WTCCC are to analyse these genome-wide association data in order to identify genetic variants displaying evidence of disease association. In addition, further rounds of genotyping and functional studies will be needed to obtain assessments of the contribution each variant makes to disease pathogenesis, but these rounds are not part of the current project plan. Also, the Consortium aims to develop insights into technical, analytical, methodological and biological aspects of genome-wide association analysis.

In 2005–2006, the WTCCC genotyped up to 675 000 single nucleotide polymorphisms (SNPs) on 2000 samples from each of seven diseases; type 1 diabetes, type 2 diabetes, coronary heart disease, hypertension, bipolar disorder, rheumatoid arthritis and inflammatory bowel disease. There will be a common set of 3000 controls from England, Scotland and Wales. The 1958 British Birth Cohort provides a representative sample of 1500 controls, while the rest will be blood donors recruited from the National Blood Service. Interestingly, according to the WTCCC website, one of the questions that the Consortium intends to address is the *relative merits of these alternative strategies for the generation of representative population controls*. A possible interpretation of this is that if blood donors are as representative genetically as the 1958 cohort, it may not be necessary to use costly and precious population cohorts as sources of common controls.

In addition to the core genome-wide association studies, three additional studies have been established: the first on host resistance to infectious diseases in African populations; the second on autoimmune thyroid disease, breast cancer, ankylosing spondylitis and multiple sclerosis; and the third on a number of other diseases including obesity. Common to all WTCCC projects are the clear aims of identifying genetic variants and mechanisms, using cutting edge genetic technologies and methods, and employing recent discoveries such as those derived from the International HapMap Consortium.[39] There is no intention of studying environmental factors or joint effects of genes and environment, not to mention gene–environment interaction.

Although the organization and history are different, the genetic focus and the aims of the WTCCC have many similarities with deCODE's research aims. DeCODE's advantages are the genealogical data on the total population, the total size of the biobank and a streamlined work process. However, the WTCCC is based on established British studies where access to a much larger number of patients within each disease category is possible due to the size of the population, allowing for detection of smaller effects and for analysis within subgroups. Both projects focus strictly on genetic discovery and are currently performing genome-wide screening with a high number of SNPs on large and thoroughly phenotyped populations, preparing for the next generation of genome-wide association studies.[40]

4.7 Cohorts

The main aim of a prototypical cohort study is to establish causal relationships between exposures, be it environmental or genetic, and health outcomes.[41] Prospective population-based cohorts are essential for life course studies of genetic and environmental exposures. In a prototypical cohort, the participants are recruited from the general population, not based on diseases or exposures. Data and biological samples for determining both genetic and environmental exposures should be collected prior to the development of disease or death, and ideally one should include multiple data collections so that trajectories of disease can be described, allowing for evaluation of normal variation, subclinical forms of the disease in question and so-called endophenotypes. The cohort design reduces the uncertainty about the temporal order of exposure and disease; it avoids recall bias, and allows investigation of continuous traits and conditions with high fatality or reduced ability to participate in research (Box 4.2).[42] Cohorts can normally not answer questions about the causes of secular trends.[43] Because investment in cohorts is expensive and long term, it can be very difficult to use cohorts to study rare diseases, or exposures that show little variation in a given population. However, once a cohort is established and the population has been followed for a sufficiently long time, cohorts may also prove superior for rare diseases and small to moderate exposure variance. Also, in registry-based cohorts with continuous recruitment of participants from total populations, even causes of secular trends can be addressed.

In general, the arguments for establishing large prospective cohorts differ from those for establishing large population-based case–control studies. Mostly, the perspective of cohort enthusiasts is broader, very long term and open regarding research questions. The aims listed in Box 4.1 are a reflection of this difference. The large case–control initiatives are primarily directed towards gene discovery, while the aims of prospective cohorts overlap with these aims; this is not where cohorts are competitive, at least not in the short term.

UK Biobank published a protocol in 2002 where the scientific rationale and the plans for the study were outlined. After that, both the detailed plans and organizational structure of UK Biobank have been altered. However, the aims and basic ideas seem not to have changed.

The National Human Genome Research Institute (NHGRI), in collaboration with several other NIH institutes, commissioned a group of experts to examine the scientific foundations and broad logistical outlines of a hypothetical US cohort for genes, environment and health. The recommendations of the expert panel were published in 2005 on the NIH website (http://www.nature.com/nrg/journal/v7/n10/full/nrg1919.html.).

Other similar protocols are available on the websites of the different biobank projects and initiatives, but the UK Biobank protocol and the NHGRI report provide detailed presentations of the reasons for initiating cohort-based biobanks and have been used as the main sources here.

4.7.1 New prospective cohorts

The delineation between new prospective cohorts and old ones is blurred. Two examples of new cohorts that are in very different phases will be reviewed, UK Biobank and the 'potential US cohort'.

4.7.1.1 UK Biobank

UK Biobank was conceived in the late 1990s and funded in 2000 by the Wellcome Trust, the Medical Research Council and the Department of Health. UK Biobank has gone through a long period of scientific planning, community consent and organizational development. It is now (November 2006) set up as a centrally managed charitable company, UK Biobank Limited, which coordinates six regional collaborating centres across Britain. It is a prospective population-based cohort study that will recruit 500 000 adult (40–69 years) volunteers. Recruitment is not based on disease or exposure. A pilot was conducted in 2005, and the main study began early 2007. Invitees are identified from central registries. However, the UK Biobank web-pages do not provide information on what the exact selection criteria are. Social, demographic and health data will be obtained via questionnaires and a physical examination. Blood and urine will be taken and stored as a source of DNA, and for assessment of environmental exposures and phenotypes. Follow-up for at least 20–30 years is indicated in the invitation. Monitoring of outcomes will mainly be through routine medical and other records, but also through renewed contact with selected participants for additional data collections in subcohorts or nested case–control studies. Information on a range of diseases will be collected, and the number of expected incident cases has been estimated for diseases such as common cancers, heart disease, diabetes, chronic obstructive pulmonary disease and rheumatoid arthritis (Tables 2–5 from Davey Smith et al.[1]).

4.7.1.2 A potential US prospective cohort (NHGRI)

A potential US prospective cohort has been described in a series of papers,[19,42,44] and in the NIHGR recommendations.[45] For simplicity, the proposal will be referred to as the 'US cohort' although it is not yet clear whether it will be established or not. The US cohort is clearly inspired by UK Biobank and shares many of its features. The report considers the usefulness of existing cohorts versus a new cohort, and concludes that a new cohort would serve the purpose better. However, partial recruitment from existing cohorts is recommended. Sample sizes of 200 000, 500 000 and 1 000 000 are considered, but for practical purposes the plan describes a cohort of 500 000 individuals. Data collection is meant to be population based but, contrary to UK Biobank, the report proposes to recruit a *representative* sample selected to match the most recent decennial US Census population on six stratifying variables: age, sex, race/ethnicity, geographic region, education and urban/rural residence. The importance of a high response rate is emphasized.

A household sampling frame is recommended, although only 30 per cent of the cohort is proposed to consist of related individuals. Biological specimens, including DNA and cells for possible transformation, should be collected, and the 'most extensive genotyping possible at the time the cohort is collected' should be performed. A rather intensive scheme for follow-up and monitoring of end-points is suggested. Public consultation is ongoing, and development of technology to collect and analyse phenotypic data and environmental exposure data is recommended as part of the project.

4.7.2 Existing prospective cohorts

Naturally, existing cohorts with biobanks are more varied, and often less explicit in their aims than new very large cohorts seeking considerable funding and legitimacy in the population. Many existing population-based cohorts are now being used for genetic studies or studies of joint effects of genes and environment. Few are large enough to qualify as population biobanks in this context; however, because many of them already have many years of follow-up, repeated measurements, good information on exposures and phenotypes, they are and will be of great value for those very large cohorts that will be realized. The birth cohort ALSPAC in Bristol, for example, already serves as a source for knowledge on how to run a longitudinal cohort, and of scientific hypotheses that can be tested or replicated in larger birth cohorts such as the Danish and Norwegian cohorts.

Some of the best existing population-based biobanks for studies of genes, environment and health have not been categorized as such until recently. The use of natural experiments and of routine population-based biobanks can be more efficient and a lot cheaper than the establishment of new cohorts.

4.7.2.1 Kadoorie study

The Kadoorie Study of Chronic Disease in China (KSCDC)[20] is a large population-based cohort currently recruiting 500 000 adults aged 35–74 from 10 regions in China. Recruitment started in 2004 and will be completed in 2008. According to Chen *et al.*,[20] it is an open-ended prospective study with very broad research aims. The study aims to investigate the effects of both established and emerging risk factors for many different diseases, including the growing tobacco epidemic. Participants undergo a face-to-face interview and clinical measurements, and donate blood. Both plasma and buffy coat samples are stored. Every fifth year, a sample of about 10 000 surviving participants will be invited for re-survey, and end-points will be identified through mortality and morbidity registries and medical records. Nested case–control studies will be one of the main designs used to select samples for assessment of genetic and other factors determining disease. The KSCDC will be among the largest population biobank studies ever conducted.

4.7.2.2 **Cohort of Norway**

Cohort of Norway (CONOR) is a national collaboration between regional cohorts in Norway (www.fhi.no/artikler/?id=28138). The four medical faculties and the Norwegian Institute of Health are partners in the collaboration which already includes close to 200 000 adults (18 years or older) that have provided health data and blood samples since 1994. Recruitment is ongoing, and the health studies in the county of North Trøndelag (HUNT 3) and the city of Tromsø are conducting new circles of recruitment. There is an identical CONOR core questionnaire included in all the regional health studies, and through the individual regional health studies access can be gained to an additional wealth of questionnaire data and clinical data going back to the 1970s for subsets of the population. End-points are identified through linkage to national health registries, the cause of death registry, hospital and primary health care records, and intensive clinical nested case–control studies. A national biobank for the DNA from CONOR samples has been established at the HUNT biobank. Together with the Norwegian mother and child cohort study, CONOR is part of a more comprehensive national collaborative project called Biobanks for Health in Norway (Biohealth) (www.fhi.no/artikler/?id=56737). Biohealth aims at extracting DNA from about 460 000 individuals of all ages in Norway by the end of 2008, and at strengthening national organization and scientific use of Norwegian population biobanks.

4.7.3 **'Natural' experiments**

In most cases, natural (or rather man-made and politically induced) experiments occur in populations where there has been no prior collection of biological material. However, provided that there is sufficient information on environmental risk factors prior to the development of the outcomes, biological samples for assessment of the genetic factors involved could be collected at a later stage on a case–control basis.

An increased risk for schizophrenia has been demonstrated among children who were exposed to famine *in utero* in The Netherlands under the Nazi occupation in 1944–1945,[46] and in China in 1959–1961 following the failure of the Great Leap Forward.[47] In both of these epidemiological studies, one could envisage collection of DNA from cases and controls retrospectively for analysis of genotypes that may be particularly vulnerable to the development of schizophrenia as a result of famine, or of *de novo* mutations that may have arisen more frequently among cases than controls as a result of the famine.[48]

4.7.4 **'When an entire country is a cohort'**

'When an entire country is a cohort'[49] was a title used to describe the advantages of Danish epidemiology. It is applicable to the situation in Denmark, and a few other countries and regions in the world, characterized by populations where all inhabitants have *personal identification numbers* following them from birth or immigration until death or emigration, and where there are routine health registries recording births, deaths, exposures and diseases on all inhabitants without individual informed consent.

In many ways, one can say that the ideal prospective population-based cohort is a very large cohort established in a society with this kind of infrastructure, where the participants are recruited at conception, and followed through fetal life, birth and onwards. The routine PKU-biobanks in Sweden and Denmark, and the Danish and Norwegian pregnancy cohorts may be the infrastructures that come closest to this ideal.

4.7.4.1 Routine population biobanks

The PKU-biobanks in Denmark and Sweden are good examples of routine collections of biological samples from the total population providing these countries with complete birth cohorts with biobanks.[4,50] In combination with national registries, this has proven to be an extremely valuable source of high quality aetiological research. These filter paper biobanks with minimal amounts of blood (blood spots) were originally established for the purpose of newborn screening, but have recently been used to show that there is an increased prevalence of enteroviral RNA in blood spots from newborn children who later developed type 1 diabetes, supporting the hypothesis that early enteroviral infections may play a role in the pathogenesis of type 1 diabetes,[4] that there is a low incidence of toxoplasma infection during pregnancy and in newborns in Sweden[51] and that clone-specific markers are present at birth in children with acute lymphoblastic leukaemia (ALL), a finding with important implications for the understanding of the causes of ALL.[3] The completeness of these population-wide biobanks and their potential for assessment of both environmental (infections) and genetic early determinants of disease make them particularly valuable as sources for future life course studies.

4.7.5 Pregnancy and birth cohorts

Birth cohorts are regarded as one of the best sources for life course studies. There are a number of established pregnancy and birth cohorts internationally, and an unknown number of efforts to establish such cohorts are ongoing (European Birth Cohorts www.birthcohorts.net).[52] In pregnancy cohorts, information and samples are collected from fetal life onwards, while in birth cohorts the children are recruited at birth. For simplicity, the term birth cohort is commonly used to describe both pregnancy and birth cohorts. Most of the existing birth cohorts are small (10 000 participants or less) and have not collected biological samples at recruitment. However, many have obtained blood samples recently or are in the process of doing so, allowing for genetic studies, and assessment of environmental exposures prospectively, although not from pregnancy onwards.

What are the advantages of pregnancy cohorts? In addition to the general advantages of cohorts, information is collected ideally from conception, and follow-up is indefinite, and preferably through generations. Thus, pregnancy cohorts are better suited for aetiological studies than birth cohorts. A series of subdesigns are possible in pregnancy cohorts. Obvious important subdesigns are the nested case–control study, allowing for cost-efficient use of the advantages of both the case–control design, and the cohort design.[46] Magnus et al.[22] has described additional valuable subdesigns that are possible within pregnancy cohorts that include biological samples from parents and women who contribute more than one pregnancy during the course of the study. One is the case–parent design, which opens the possibility of detecting effects of maternal genes, fetal genes and their interaction.[53] In triad designs, one can estimate the main effects of genotypes, gene–gene interactions and gene–environment interactions.[54] Case–parents triads can also be stratified by environmental exposures to detect gene–environment interactions. Another subdesign is the repeated pregnancy design, in which the maternal genome is unchanged, the fetal genotype is in each pregnancy a random sample from the parental genotypes, and the environment may change.[22] By modelling this design, the interaction between the maternal genotype and the environment can be partitioned out as can also the interaction between the fetal genotype and the environmental exposure. Other possibilities are the use of generation databases linked to the cohorts for studies of trans-generational effects, or studies of siblings or twins within the cohorts.[55] Pembrey[56] argues that unselected birth cohorts, where DNA is available from parents, have at least three special advantages. The first is in their potential for studying whether or not there is a distortion of the expected Mendelian transmission of alleles from parents to children, indicating differential loss of embryos of one genotype. The second is that such birth cohorts can be used to study the possible advantage or disadvantage of heterozygotes compared with homozygotes at any given loci. The third is the use of cohorts as a screen for genetic effects on phenotypes. Provided that the population is intensively phenotyped, one may investigate the effect of a certain genotype on a whole range of outcomes. Provided that we manage to describe phenotypes sufficiently well, and that genotyping of individual whole human genomes will be possible in the future, this is clearly an advantage of pregnancy cohorts.[57]

4.7.5.1 The Danish and Norwegian birth cohorts

The two largest birth cohorts in the world are the Danish National Birth Cohort (DNBC) www.ssi.dk/sw9314.asp) and the Norwegian mother and The Norwegian Mother and Child Cohort Study (MoBa) (www.fhi.no/morogbarn). Both are pregnancy cohorts with blood samples and health information collected from the mother (Denmark and Norway) and the father (Norway only) early in pregnancy, and cord blood collected from the child at birth. The two studies were originally planned together and will include 100 000 pregnancies each. Due to difficulties with funding and recruitment through general practitioners, the Norwegian study did not start until 1999, while the Danish study collected data from 1996.[21,22] The Danish study has completed recruitment, while the Norwegian will complete recruitment in late 2007 or early 2008. Both studies aim to investigate aetiology of diseases in the children throughout their life course, as well as parental diseases. They were inspired by hypotheses on early origins of adult disease and the fetal programming hypothesis,[58] and could more appropriately have been called life course cohorts. The design of the cohorts is not guided by specific hypotheses, although subpro-jects influence priorities in data collection. In the Norwegian cohort, DNA is extracted from fresh whole blood on all samples. In addition, urine is collected from all mothers during pregnancy, RNA is extracted from cord blood on the last 50 000 newborns, and samples are frozen as whole blood, plasma and serum, allowing for a range of future environmental exposure assessments.[59]

Denmark and Norway are relatively homogenous regarding certain environmental exposures such as diet, breastfeeding and vaccination coverage. Large variability in environmental exposures strengthens a cohort study, and the long recruitment period of the Norwegian study may have an advantage in covering periods with, for example, different epidemic infections.

The Danish and Norwegian pregnancy cohorts have schemes for follow-up that are relatively thin, compared for example with ALSPAC, a UK pregnancy cohort of about 14 000 children born in 1992,[60] or the plans indicated for the National Children's Study (http://nationalchildrensstudy.gov) which aim to develop a combined thick and very large study. However, both Denmark and Norway have a wealth of health registries and socio-demographic registries with which the pregnancy cohorts can be linked to obtain both additional exposure and end-point information. Collaborations with ALSPAC can provide opportunities for testing hypotheses derived from a 'thicker' cohort such as ALSPAC, in the 'thinner' but larger Scandinavian cohorts. Also, ALSPAC may serve as validation of instruments used in the larger cohorts.

4.7.6 Cohort collaborations

In order to increase sample sizes and environmental exposure variability, some large collaborative cohorts have been established. To date, EPIC (European Prospective Investigation on Cancer, Chronic Diseases and nutrition) and GenomEUtwin are the largest. EPIC is still probably the largest existing prospective cohort study with already collected biological material worldwide. EPIC was originally designed to study nutrition and cancer, but has recently been transformed to investigate the relationships between a series of environmental exposures, genetic factors and cancer, coronary heart disease and stroke. The total EPIC cohort from 26 regional centres in 10 European countries has 521 400 participants.[61] Enrolment in the cohort took place between 1993 and 1999. Blood samples were collected from about 400 000 subjects and DNA has been extracted from about 50 000. In addition, plasma, serum, leukocytes and erythrocytes have been stored. EPIC's original emphasis was on collection of blood samples for assessment of environmental exposures, and diet in particular. In recent years, a number of studies including genetic analyses have been published based on EPIC.

GenomEUtwin is a collaborative project funded by the EU fifth framework programme, and led from Finland (www.genomeutwin.org).[62] It has collected data from 1.6 million participants from already existing twin studies in eight countries, and from the MORGAM collaboration (www.ktl.fi/morgam/) including cardiovascular risk factor studies in 11 countries.[63] The first stage in GenomEUtwin consists of genotyping 10 000 samples with genome-wide markers and specific target SNPs in relation to stature, obesity, migraine, coronary heart disease, stroke and longevity. Analyses of the first 6000 completed genome scans are ongoing, according to the P3G observatory (last updated 23 October 2006). The project started in 2002 and runs to 2007. To date, publications from the GenomEUtwin project have demonstrated both the formidable wealth of data in the collaboration and the complexities of merging cohorts from many different countries and of many different kinds.[64]

4.8 **Harmonization of cohorts**

Numerous meetings, consortia and projects such as the Human Genome Epidemiology Network, the Public Population Project in Genomics (P3G) (www.p3gconsortium.org) and Population Biobanks (PHOEBE) a coordination action funded by EU framework programme 6 (www.populationbiobanks.org or www.phoebe-eu.org), have been created in order to harmonize and standardize population biobanks, and develop guidelines for access, governance and reporting of genetic association studies in particular.[65–67] Ioannidis and colleagues recently described how networks of investigators have begun sharing best practices, tools and methods for analysis of associations between genetic variation and common diseases.[65] Their plan is to integrate published literature databases, and unpublished data, including 'negative' studies, and capture these by online journals and through investigator networks.

The Population Biobanks (PHOEBE) coordinated action aims to harmonize population-based biobanks and cohort studies to strengthen the foundation of European biomedical science. The idea is to establish a collaborative research network to ensure that Europe makes best use of its rich array of population-based biobanks and longitudinal cohort studies. These include major cohorts that already exist and new initiatives that are starting up. P3G has similar ambitions on an international scale and has developed an observatory describing population-based biobanks from all over the world.

Currently, harmonization efforts are moving towards more concrete harmonization of biobanks and collaborative use of more than one large population-based biobank. The next few years will show whether the ambitious aims for harmonization and standardization can be met, and lead to important results in the field of genetic epidemiology.

In many instances, particularly in relation to existing studies, harmonization of measures will not be possible. How can we combine studies when each uses, for example, their own measure of exposure? One approach is to exploit or collect additional samples of subjects where each participant has been assessed using two or more of the alternative measures. Under certain assumptions, instruments can be calibrated against each other, allowing scores on one measure to be translated into scores from another. In practice, this should be done using a method such as multiple imputation that preserves the uncertainty in this translation process, illustrated by Collishaw *et al.*[68] in their comparison of adolescent behavioural and emotional problems from three major UK studies that spanned more than 25 years.

Even the same measures cannot always be assumed to perform in the same way in different samples. Here tools such as anchoring vignettes may be useful. Originally introduced in political research by Gary King, these allow basic self-rated survey data to be complemented by ratings of very short descriptions (vignettes). These provide a common anchor point to the scale that helps calibrate the same measure across cultures, respondent groups and studies. There use in health studies is still at an early stage.[69]

4.9 Biobanks and life course epidemiology

4.9.1 'Small is beautiful, but size matters'

As we have seen, sample size dominates the case for biobanks and is relevant both for case–control studies and for prospective cohorts. According to Burton and Hansell's estimates,[70] it takes 36 and 22 years, respectively, to get 5000 incident cases of rheumatoid arthritis and lung cancer (Table 4.2), while obviously these are diseases where one can recruit incident cases that are not from cohorts much faster than that. The sample sizes needed in genetic epidemiology vary with the research questions. However, one of the main purposes of establishing population biobanks is to achieve large sample sizes in order to be able to detect moderate and perhaps small effects, and to investigate gene–environment interaction. Power calculations have been undertaken for UK Biobank[70] and for the National Genome Institute initiative,[45] demonstrating the large size and long-term perspectives of the cohort approach. According to Collins,[19] a minimum of 5000 cases, and preferably 10 000 cases, is required to provide 80 per cent power to detect a moderately sized interaction effect, which means for example an interaction odds ratio of around 1.5–2.0 between two binary exposures each with a population prevalence between 10 and 25 per cent.

However, as we target increasingly small genetic effects, so the issue of confounding becomes more important. Quite small degrees of confounding can, in these very large studies, lead to significant false association. In addition to natural population structure,[71] genotyping errors, even of quite a modest scale, have been identified as another source of confounding,[72] particularly where genotyping of cases and controls has not been balanced across laboratories and undertaken without blinding as to caseness. This suggests that designs with internal genetic control, such as parent–child trios, may continue to be valuable and that much greater attention needs to be paid to what are routine methods for ensuring validity in experimental studies—notably blindness, randomization and designed test–re-test of measurement.

Table 4.2 The expected rate of accrual of incident cases of selected complex diseases in UK Biobank[70]

	Years to achieve cases numbering				
	1000	2500	5000	10 000	20 000
Myocardial infarction and coronary death	2	4	5	8	14
Diabetes mellitus	2	3	5	7	11
Chronic obstructive pulmonary disease	4	6	9	14	27
Rheumatoid arthritis	7	15	36		
Breast cancer	4	7	11	19	
Colorectal cancer	6	10	15	25	
Lung cancer	7	13	22		
Stomach cancer	17	36			

4.9.2 **Thick versus thin measurement**

What about 'small is beautiful'? One aspect of that beauty is the quality of measurement, and it does seem as if most of these studies, even the most expensive, have gained their massive sample sizes at the expense of the quality and richness of the measurement.

While the cohort studies can claim the apparent advantage of prospective measurement (i.e. prior to disease onset[11,19,23,42]), their enormous size can imply that even the baseline measures of the physical and psychosocial environment are extremely limited. The problem is made more severe by the additional demands of life course epidemiology. First, for many diseases, we would want that baseline to be very early in childhood, if not pre-natal. A significant part of the advantage of prospective measurement error is non-differential measurement error—that error in exposure measurement is not correlated with disease outcome. For studies that start in middle-age, this advantage is limited to those diseases with no expression prior to the middle-age baseline, and thus rarely applicable to, for example, any psychiatric disorder. Secondly, life course analysis often demands repeated measurement, something obviously expensive in a large study.

4.9.3 **Resolving the problem: exploiting existing infrastructure and elaborating the design of the measurement protocol**

In short, the 'dumb' biobank is thus not the obvious study design for life course researchers. There would seem to be two main strategies to overcoming its shortcomings.

First we should build on data and systems that already exist and those systems should be large enough such that the great bulk of the study sample will remain within their scope for the whole of their lives. Centralized, organized and research-engaged health services clearly offer such a capability. In such contexts, study design issues are then judged through the lens of marginal rather than average costs, which may deliver quite different decisions in relation to optimal design.

Secondly, we must further elaborate the design and analysis of studies where the data are thicker in parts. Perhaps the most familiar of these designs in epidemiology is the nested case–control design (where, as they occur, onset cases are matched to controls on certain variables). However, power can also be increased by increasing the variability in the exposure and disease of interest, an approach taken by Langholz and Clayton[73] when they introduced the idea of counter-matching. Counter-matching is particularly valuable when either disease or exposure, or both, are rare. The advantage of these nested designs is that an extended range of expensive and possibly invasive measures needs be acquired only for the selected cases and controls. Stored biological material clearly lends itself to this approach, and indeed it has been taken for granted that biobank cohorts would undertake this routinely. However, it would also be possible to apply this approach to some measures of the environment and behaviour, such as the coding of stored video-tape of behaviour (e.g. Walker *et al.*[74]) or other archival data. The other related common design is the two-phase (often called two-stage) design in which a subsample is drawn that is stratified on the basis of some screening, surrogate or auxiliary measures. A much more in-depth assessment is then made of this subsample. Analyses involving these more detailed measures can be undertaken using weights (see Chapter 8) or in various other ways.[75,76] The stratification on screening variables applies not just to factors related to the outcome (as in the nested case–control design) but to risk factors (as in the usual high risk design), and to sampling by strata defined on screens for both. The efficiency of the design depends strongly on the strength of relationship between the screen variables and the disease and exposure measures.[77]

Such designs can be helpfully viewed from the perspective of data missing by design. Such designs offer potential not just to reduce cost but also to reduce participant burden. The measurement protocol is divided up into a core section (commonly containing screen measures) and optional sections. Participants would be assessed on the core section and a subset of the optional sections, the subset depending upon a fractional sampling design and perhaps some of the responses obtained as part of the core section. This approach can sometimes also be used in circumstances where asking or undertaking one assessment risks contaminating or biasing another assessment. However, considerable further work is required to ensure that these complex, and thus in practice high risk designs, can yield the data we need and that our analysis tools are flexible enough to yield the answers we need for life course research.

4.10 Conclusions

Large-scale biobank studies will undoubtedly become of increasing importance. Like other epidemiological researchers, life course researchers can appreciate the value of sample size and power. Nonetheless, the measurement requirements of life course researchers are complex and justify a greater degree of scepticism as to the value of a number of these studies to life course research. Standard case–control studies may in general offer rather modest possibilities from this perspective, but occasionally can offer critical insight, for example when coupled with unusual historic exposures arising from natural experiments, and deliver results in a short time frame. However, life course researchers generally have a predilection for birth cohorts. The enormous long-term cost of large cohort studies requires the most careful and imaginative thought to build on freely available data and infrastructure, sample archiving and designed selective processing of archived material and in-depth assessment of subsamples. Further methodological work in this area, to suggest designs that are efficient without being unduly cumbersome for researchers and participants, should be a priority. Cohort studies starting later in life obviously shorten the waiting time for findings for many diseases, and may offer scope for prospective measurement of contemporaneous precipitant exposures but, unless linked to measurement of rich historic administrative data or to current measures that appropriately integrate prior exposure over time (see Chapter 8), these often may be unsuited to answer developmental questions. Whatever the individual design, constructive collaboration is clearly going to be essential. While current emphasis may be on harmonization of parallel studies with a view to a larger pooled sample size, there may be greater scope in collaboration among studies of quite different but complementary designs. In any event, the variations between countries in data availability, cost of collection, and public understanding and acceptance of science are such that the marginal costs of different study designs vary hugely. Fortunately, this is likely to ensure that we will have a portfolio of biobanks of varied designs.

Further reading

Davey Smith G, Ebrahim S, Lewis S, Hansell AL, Palmer LJ, Burton PR (2005). Genetic epidemiology and public health: hope, hype and future prospects. *Lancet* 366, 1484–1498.

Manolio TA, Bailey-Wilson JE, Collins FS (2006). Genes, environment and the value of prospective cohort studies. *Nature Reviews Genetics* 7, 812–820.

Susser E, Schwartz S (2006). Prototypical cohort study. In: Susser E, Schwartz S, Morabia A, Bromet EJ, ed. *Psychiatric epidemiology*. Oxford University Press, Oxford, pp. 91–107.

Hjalgrim LL, Madsen HO, Melbye M, Jorgensen P, Christiansen M, Andersen MT, *et al.* (2002). Presence of clone-specific markers at birth in children with acute lymphoblastic leukaemia. *British Journal of Cancer* 87, 994–99.

Kong A, Barnard J, Gudbjartsson DF, Thorlieffson G, Jonsdottir G, Sigurardottir S, *et al.* (2004). Recombination rate and reproductive success in humans. *Nature Genetics* 36, 1203–1206.

References

1. Davey Smith G, Ebrahim S, Lewis S, Hansell AL, Palmer LJ, Burton PR (2005). Genetic epidemiology and public health: hope, hype and future prospects. *Lancet* 366, 1484–1498.
2. Husebekk A, Iversen O-J, Langmark F, Laerum OD, Ottersen OP, Stoltenberg C (2003). *Biobanks for health—Report and recommendations from an EU workshop*. Technical report to EU Commission, Oslo.
3. Hjalgrim LL, Madsen HO, Melbye M, Jorgensen P, Christiansen M, Andersen MT, *et al.* (2002). Presence of clone-specific markers at birth in children with acute lymphoblastic leukaemia. *British Journal of Cancer* 87, 994–999.
4. Dahlquist GG, Forsberg J, Hagenfeldt L, Boman J, Juto P (2004). Increased prevalence of enteroviral RNA in blood spots from newborn children who later developed type 1 diabetes. *Diabetes Care* 27, 285–286.
5. Kuh D, Ben-Shlomo Y, Lynch J, Hallquist J, Power C (2003). Life course epidemiology. *Journal of Epidemiology and Community Health* 57, 778–783.
6. Van den Bree MB, Schieken RM, Moskowitz WB, Eaves LJ (1996). Genetic regulation of hemodynamic variables during dynamic exercise. The MCV twin study. *Circulation* 94, 1864–1869.
7. Smyth DJ, Cooper JD, Bailey R, Field S, Burren O, Smink LJ, *et al.* (2006). A genome-wide association study of nonsynonymous SNPs identifies a type 1 diabetes locus in the interferon-induced helicase (IFIF1) region. *Nature Genetics* 38, 617–619.
8. Payton A, Gibbons L, Davidson Y, Ollier W, Rabbit P, Worthington J, *et al.* (2005). Influence of serotonin transporter gene polymorphisms on cognitive decline and cognitive abilities in a non-demented elderly population. *Molecular Psychiatry* 10, 1133–1139.
9. Caspi A, Sugden K, Moffitt TE, Taylor A, Craig IW, Harrington H, *et al.* (2003). Influence of life stress on depression: moderation by a polymorphism in the 5-HTT gene. *Science* 301, 386–389.
10. Simpson A, John SL, Jury F, Niven R, Woodcock A, Ollier WE, *et al.* (2006). Endotoxin exposure, CD14, and allergic disease: an interaction between genes and the environment. *American Journal of Respiratory and Critical Care Medicine* 174, 365–366.
11. Davey Smith G, Ebrahim S (2005). What can Mendelian randomisation tell us about modifiable behavioural and environmental exposures? *British Medical Journal* 330, 1076–1079.

12. Goldsmith HH, Gottesman, II, Lemery KS (1997). Epigenetic approaches to developmental psychopathology. *Developmental Psychopathology* 9, 365–387.

13. Meaney MJ (2001). Maternal care, gene expression, and the transmission of individual differences in stress reactivity across generations. *Annual Review of Neuroscience* 24, 1161–1192.

14. Pembrey ME, Bygren LO, Kaati G, Edvinsson S, Northstone K, Sjostrom M, *et al.* (2006). Sex-specifc, male-line transgenerational responses in humans. *European Journal of Human Genetics* 14, 159–166.

15. Santos-Reboucas CB, Pimentel MM (2007). Implication of abnormal epigenetic patterns for human diseases. *European Journal of Human Genetics* 15, 10–17.

16. Fraga MF, Ballestar E, Paz MF, Ropero S, Sentien F, Ballestar ML, *et al.* (2005). Epigenetic differences arise during the lifetime of monozygotic twins. *Proceedings of the National Academy of Sciences, USA* 102, 10604–10609.

17. Eckhardt F, Lewin J, Cortese R, Rakyan VK, Attwood A, Burger M, *et al.* (2006). DNA methylation profiling of human chromosomes 6, 20 and 22. *Nature Genetics* 38, 1378–1385.

18. Peltonen L, Mc Kusick VA (2001). Genomics and medicine. Dissecting human disease in the postgenomic era. *Science* 291, 1224–1229.

19. Collins FS (2004). The case for a US prospective cohort study of genes and environment. *Nature* 429, 475–477.

20. Chen Z, Lee L, Chen J, Collins R, Wu F, Guo Y, *et al.* (2005). Cohort profile: the Kadoorie Study of Chronic Disease in China (KSCDC). *International Journal of Epidemiology* 34, 1243–1249.

21. Olsen J, Melbye M, Olsen S, Sorensen TI, Aaby P, Andersen AM, *et al.* (2001). The Danish National Birth Cohort—its background, structure and aim. *Scandinavian Journal of Public Health* 29, 300–307.

22. Magnus P, Irgens LM, Haug K, Nystad W, Skjærven R, Stoltenberg C, the MoBa Study Group (2006). Cohort profile: the Norwegian Mother and Child Cohort Study (MoBa). *International Journal of Epidemiology* 35, 1146–1150.

23. UK BioBank UK (2002). *A study of genes, environment and health*. 14 February 2002. The Wellcome Trust, Medical Research Council, Department of Health.

24. Burton P (2006). Personal Communication.

25. Kramer M (2006). Personal Communication.

26. Clayton D, McKeigue PM (2001). Epidemiological methods for studying genes and environmental factors in complex diseases. *Lancet* 358, 1356–1360.

27. Wacholder S, Garcia-Closas M, Rothman N (2002). Study of genes and environmental factors in complex diseases. *Lancet* 359, 1155.

28. Burton PR, Tobin MD, Hopper JL (2005). Key concepts in genetic epidemiology. *Lancet* 366, 941–951.

29. Banks E, Meade T (2002). Study of genes and environmental factors in complex diseases. *Lancet*, 359, 1156–1157.

30. Sveinbjornsdottir S, Hicks AA, Jonsson T, Petursson H, Gugmundsson G, Frigge ML, *et al.* (2000). Familial aggregation of Parkinson's disease in Iceland. *New England Journal of Medicine* 343, 1765–1770.

31. Kong A (2006). Personal Communication.

32. Arnar DO, Thorvaldsson S, Manolio TA, Thorgeirsson G, Kristjansson K, Hakonarson H, *et al.* (2006). Familial aggregation of atrial fibrillation in Iceland. *European Heart Journal* 27, 708–712.

33. Statistics Sweden (2001). *Bakgrundsfakta till befolknings-och välfärdsstatistik* (The Multi-Generation Registry). Statistiska Centralbyrån, Örebro.

34. Gudmundsson H, Gudbjartsson DF, Frigge M, Gulcher JR, Steffanson K (2000). Inheritance of human longevity in Iceland. *European Journal of Human Genetics* 8, 743–749.

35. Helgason A, Hickey E, Goodacre S, Bosnes V, Steffanson K, Ward R, *et al.* (2001). mtDNA and the islands of the North Atlantic. Estimating the proportions of Norse and Gaelic ancestry. *American Journal of Human Genetics* 68, 723–737.

36. Helgason A, Sigurdardottir S, Gulcher JR, Ward R, Stefansson K (2000). mtDNA and the origin of Icelanders. Deciphering signals of recent population history. *American Journal of Human Genetics* 66, 999–1016.

37. Helgason A, Sigurdardottir S, Nicholson J, Sykes B, Hill EW, Bradley DG, *et al.* (2000). Estimating Scandinavian and Gaelic ancestry in the male settlers of Iceland. *American Journal of Human Genetics* 67, 697–717.

38. Kong A, Barnard J, Gudbjartsson DF, Thorlieffson G, Jonsdottir G, Sigurardottir S, *et al.* (2004). Recombination rate and reproductive success in humans. *Nature Genetics* 36, 1203–1206.

39. The International HapMap Consortium (2005). A haplotype map of the human genome. *Nature* 437, 1299–1320.

40. Barrett JC, Cardon L (2006). Evaluating coverage of genome-wide association studies. *Nature Genetics*, 38, 659–662.

41. Susser E, Schwartz S (2006). Prototypical cohort study. In: Susser E, Schwartz S, Morabia A, Bromet EJ, ed. *Psychiatric epidemiology*. Oxford University Press, Oxford, pp. 91–107.

42. Manolio TA, Bailey-Wilson JE, Collins FS (2006). Genes, environment and the value of prospective cohort studies. *Nature Reviews Genetics* 7, 812–820.

43. Rose G (1985). Sick individuals and sick populations. *International Journal of Epidemiology* 14, 32–38.

44. Collins FS, Green ED, Guttmacher AE, Guyer MS on behalf of the US National Human Genome Research Institute (2003). A vision for the future of genomics research. A blueprint for the genomic era. *Nature*, 422, 1–13.

45. NIHGR initiative (2005). Recommendations for a populationbased cohort. http://www.nature.com/nrg/journal/v7/n10/full/nrg1919.html.

46. Susser E, Neugebauer R, Hoek HW, Brown AS, Lin S, Labovitz D, *et al.* (1996). Schizophrenia after prenatal famine. *Archives of General Psychiatry* 53, 25–31.

47. St Clair D, Xu M, Wang P, Yu Y, Fang Y, Zhang F, *et al.* (2005). Rates of adult schizophrenia following prenatal exposure to the Chinese famine 1959–1961. *Journal of the American Medical Association* 294, 557–562.

48. McClellan JM, Susser E, King MC (2006). Maternal famine, *de novo* mutations and schizophrenia. *Journal of the American Medical Association* 296, 582–584.

49. Frank L (2000). When an entire country is a cohort. *Science* 287, 2398–2399.

50. Norgaard-Pedersen B (1998).[The PKU registry and biobank at the National Serum Institute. Rules and applications]. *Ugeskr Laeger* 160, 2266–2267. Danish.

51. Evengard B, Petersson K, Engman ML, Wiklund S, Ivarsson SA, Tear-Fahnehjelm K, *et al.* (2001). Low incidence of toxoplasma infection during pregnancy and in newborns in Sweden. *Epidemiology and Infection* 127, 121–127.

52. Landrigan PJ, Trasande L, Thorpe LE, Gwynn C, Lioy PJ, D'Alton ME, *et al.* (2006). The National Children's study: a 21-year prospective study of 100,000 American children. *Pediatrics* 118, 2173–2186.

53. Gjessing H, Lie RT (2006). Case–parent triads: estimating single- and double-dose effects of fetal and maternal disease gene haplotypes. *Annals of Human Genetics* 70, 382–396.

54. Umbach DM, Weinberg CR (2000). The use of case–parent triads to study joint effects of genotype and exposure. *American Journal of Human Genetics* 66, 251–261.

55. Hopper JL, Bishop DT, Easton DF (2005). Population-based family studies in genetic epidemiology. Genetic epidemiology 6. *Lancet* 366, 1397–1406.

56. Pembrey M (2004). Genetic epidemiology: some special contributions of birth cohorts. *Paediatric and Perinatal Epidemiology* 18, 3–7.

57. Freimer N, Sabatti C (2004). The use of pedigree, sib-pair and association studies of common diseases for genetic mapping and epidemiology. *Nature Genetics* 36, 1045–1051.

58. Barker DJ (1997). Fetal nutrition and cardiovascular disease in later life. *British Medical Bulletin* 53, 96–108.

59. Rønningen KS, Paltiel L, Meltzer HM, Nordhagen R, Lie KK, Hovengen R, *et al.* (2006). The biobank of the Norwegian mother and child cohort study. *European Journal of Epidemiology* 21, 619–625.

60. Golding J, Pembrey M, Jones R, the ALSPAC study team (2001). ALSPAC—The Avon longitudinal study of parents and children. I. Study methodology. *Paediatric and Perinatal Epidemiology* 15, 74–87.

61. Riboli E, Hunt KJ, Slimani N, Ferrari P, Norat T, Fahey M, *et al.* (2002). European Prospective Investigation into Cancer and Nutrition (EPIC): study populations and data collection. *Public Health Nutrition* 5, 1113–1124.

62. Peltonen L (2003). GenomEUtwin: a strategy to identify genetic influences on health and disease. *Twin Research* 6, 354–360.

63. Evans A, Salomaa V, Kulathinal S, Asplund K, Cambien F, Ferrario M, *et al.* (2005). MORGAM (an international pooling of cardiovascular cohorts). *International Journal of Epidemiology* 34, 21–27.

64. Silventoinen K, Zdravkovic S, Skytthe A, McCarron P, Herskind AM, Koskenvuo M, *et al.* (2006). Association between height and coronary heart disease mortality: a prospective study of 35,000 twin pairs. *American Journal of Epidemiology* 163, 615–621.

65. Ioannidis JPA, Gwinn M, Little J, Higgins JP, Bernstein JL, Boffetta P, *et al.* (2006). A road map for efficient and reliable human genome epidemiology. *Nature Genetics*, 38, 3–5.

66. Khoury MJ, Millikan R, Little J, Gwinn M (2004). The emergence of epidemiology in the genomics age. *International Journal of Epidemiology* 33, 936–944.

67. Lowrance WW (2006). *Access to collections of data and materials for health research.* The Wellcome Trust, London.

68. Collishaw S, Maughan B, Goodman R, Pickles A (2004). Time trends in adolescent mental health. *Journal of Child Psychology and Psychiatry* 45, 1350–1362.

69. Salomon JA, Tandon A, Murray CJL, World Health Survey Pilot Collaborating Group (2004). Comparability of self rated health: cross sectional multi-country survey using anchoring vignettes. *British Medical Journal*, 328, 258–260.

70. Burton PR, Hansell A. (2005). *UK Biobank: the expected distribution of incident and prevalent cases of chronic disease and the statistical power of nested case control studies.* UK Biobank Technical Reports. Manchester.

71. Seldlin MF, Shigeta R, Villoslada P, Selmi C, Toumilehto J, Silva G, *et al.* (2006). European population substructure: clustering of northern and southern populations. *PloS Genetics* 2, e143.

72. Clayton DG, Walker NM, Smyth DJ, Pask R, Cooper D, Maier LM, *et al.* (2005). Population structure, differential bias and genomic control in a large-scale, case–control association study. *Nature Genetics* 37, 1243–1246.

73. Langholz B, Clayton D (1994). Sampling strategies in nested case–control studies. *Environmental Health Perspectives* 102 (Suppl 8), 47–51.

74. Walker EF, Savoie T, Davis D (1994). Neuromotor precursors of schizophrenia. *Schizophrenia Bulletin* 20, 441–451.

75. Clayton DG, Dunn G, Pickles A, Spiegelhalter D (1998). Analysis of binary longitudinal data from multiphase samples (with discussion). *Journal of the Royal Statistical Society, Series B* 60, 71–102.

76. Breslow NE, Chatterjee N (1999). Design and analysis of two-phase studies with binary outcome applied to Wilms tumour prognosis. *Applied Statistics* 48, 457–468.

77. Cologne J, Langholz B (2003). Selecting controls for assessing interaction in nested case–control studies. *Journal of Epidemiology* 13, 193–202.

Chapter 5

Human development, life course, intervention and health

Clyde Hertzman

Abstract

This chapter proposes three generic models of life course trajectories in health, well-being, and behaviour and learning skills, starting from the essential early life processes of physical growth and development in socio-emotional, and language and cognition terms. For the adult period, models are proposed of how life course experience affects human biology. These principles are then reviewed in terms of how they can be implemented in intervention study designs, and criteria are outlined for a new generation of intervention studies.

5.1 The life course as a basis for intervention

5.1.1 The scientific case for the life course as a basis for intervention

There are many diseases that affect the young, such as depression and asthma, which are serious and very costly. Yet, in wealthy societies, adult chronic disease predominates when it comes to the overall societal burden of morbidity and mortality. Much less well understood is the fact that many of the illnesses and disabilities that emerge in adult life, and the patterns of behaviour and lifestyle that serve as proximate risk factors for them, have roots in childhood and back further to the fetal period. The health status of populations cannot, therefore, be adequately understood without recognizing health-determining influences across the life course. Life course factors affect a diverse range of outcomes, from general well-being to physical functioning and chronic disease in mid to late life.[1–3] Accordingly, this chapter makes two arguments:

1. That our understanding of life course contributions to adult disease demands an understanding of human development and the adoption of models of life course observation and intervention that involve decades, rather than just months and years, of follow-up.

2. Without careful attention to existing life course research and a long-term investment in the follow-up of birth cohorts, it is unlikely that we will be able to understand the underlying mechanisms of adult disease adequately and design effective health-improving social or healthcare policies.

From a life course perspective, many determinants of health are 'quotidian' in the sense that they are properties of daily life, rather than discrete phenomena that are easily distinguishable from the experiences of daily life. For instance, it has long been understood that the conjunction of low birth weight (LBW) and small for gestational age (SGA) confers increased risk for a variety of developmental outcomes.[4–7] From the standpoint of influences on blood pressure and blood pressure-related disease in adulthood this becomes important because LBW/SGA may have its effects through early life course influences on cognitive development. Cognitive development is non-discrete and non-distinct in the sense described above. Its principal non-biological determinant is the richness and variety of language and cognitive stimulation occurring during the developing child's waking hours.[8] In theory, the association between LBW/SGA and adult blood pressure-related disease may be influenced by a variety of quotidian phenomena occurring during the intervening years and decades of life. Three examples include:

1. Shifts in the functioning of host defence mechanisms, such as the hypothalamic–pituitary–adrenal (HPA) axis, as a result of the same deprivation factors in the intra-uterine environment that lead to LBW/SGA. Changes in HPA axis function, in turn, will have life course influences on cortisol metabolism that, in turn, will increase the rate of ageing of several target organs and organ systems.[9]

2. Alterations in the function of pathways that mediate the relationship between the external environment and human biology as a result of the unusual post-natal experiences that many LBW/SGA children face. For instance, several weeks of neonatal intensive care may deny the child appropriate stimulation during the 'sensitive period' for developing attachment through eye contact with a consistent set of caregivers. The usual pattern of parent–child interaction, with the parent holding the child, provides a consistency of facial stimulation at the focal length of the developing eye, allowing experience-dependent development of central nervous system pathways linking face recognition to the experiences of social affiliation or sanction; emotional belonging or alienation. Absence of this consistency of faces, and facial expressions, at the child's focal length in the early post-natal period could result in fundamental alterations in visual–emotional pathways in the central nervous system, reducing the capacity of the developing child to access social and emotional support and feedback through the recognition of emotion on the faces of 'significant others'.

3. Early delays in cognitive development may, in turn, adversely affect the stimulant qualities of the environments where the child grows up; influence social mobility over time; and lead to compensatory coping styles that, in turn, have perverse cumulative effects on health and well-being.

Each of these examples raises the prospect that influences at an earlier stage of the life course, however small, may help initiate social and biological cascades over time that will be of significance to health at a later stage of life. Similarly, each case requires us to concentrate on three phenomena simultaneously: the state of the (nurturant) environment; the stage of the life course; and the role of unfolding time, measured in human experience. Here we have used examples of the relationship between post-natal and childhood environments/influences on adult health, but the same issues arise when mid-life factors influence health in later life. Two notable analogous examples are: the impact of mid-life circumstances on 'successful ageing',[10] and the role of psychosocial working conditions on heart disease mortality and morbidity.[11]

To understand the conjunction of environment, life course and outcome, we turn to the experiment of marbles in a bowl.[12] The experiment starts with two marbles in a bowl, one white and one black. Wearing a blindfold, one marble is removed from the bowl and replaced with two of the same colour. Now, with three marbles in the bowl, the process is repeated. However, at this point, two of three marbles are the colour of the first one removed, so the probability of removing that colour goes up. With repeated trials, it is most likely that the bowl will become disproportionately filled with marbles of the colour of the first one removed. In this experiment, the initial random selection is the most important one, and ends up having a profound and enduring influence over the long term. By the end of the experiment, three critical influences have emerged: an effect of the initial selection; an effect inherent in the principals of selection; and an effect based upon the relative prevalence of black versus white marbles in the bowl. Together, these three influences convert a small 'perturbation' of the system at its outset into a trajectory of change over the course of the experiment, resulting in a unique, and increasingly irreversible outcome state.

This is not just a thought experiment. It has practical consequences. For example, our recent research has suggested that the long-term consequences of gestational effects such as LBW are difficult to separate from early circumstances and cognitive trajectories.[13] Taking maths achievement in grade school as an example, we have shown that high socio-economic status (SES) children, on average, start school with above-average skills, and their advantage grows from age 7 to 16. LBW reduces, but does not eliminate, the advantage of growing up in a high SES family. Conversely, low SES children start school, on average, with below average maths skills, and this disadvantage increases from age 7 to 16. LBW among children growing up in a low SES family exacerbates this disadvantage. When these effects are combined, we have shown that LBW children from privileged backgrounds still have a developmental advantage over normal birth weight children from underprivileged backgrounds. Thus, socio-economic disadvantage and gestational factors have both declared their developmental impacts by early in the life course, and both go on to confer a risk of diabetes, high blood pressure and heart disease later in life. In this case, LBW or its absence are analogous to the colour of the marble selected first; SES is analogous to the choice of rules of selection throughout the experiment; and the maths trajectory is analogous to the increasing proportion of marbles in the bowl of the first colour removed from the bowl.

Can these principals be used to capture valid and reliable insights into how health status later in life may be determined by the quotidian experiences of daily living earlier in life? Building on the marbles in a bowl experiment, we have tried to simplify the problem by creating the following taxonomy of life course influences.[14]

Exposure to both beneficial and adverse circumstances over the life course will vary for each individual and will constitute a unique 'life exposure trajectory', which will manifest as different expressions of health, well-being, behaviour and learning skills. Studies that collect data from the earliest stages of life and follow individuals over time provide the best lens on the relative importance of, and interaction among, these exposure–expression relationships. The possible long-term exposure–expression relationships cluster into three generic models that we have labelled *latency, cumulative* and *pathway*. By *latency* we mean relationships between an 'exposure' at one point in the life course and the probability of health 'expressions' years or decades later, irrespective of intervening experience. (This is analogous to the influence of the initial random selection of a marble of a given colour.) A *non-quotidian* example of such a relationship is asbestos' elevation of the risk of various cancers decades after exposure to the substance has ceased. *Cumulative* refers to multiple exposures over the life course whose effects on health combine. (Analogous to the effect of the proportion of different coloured marbles in the bowl on each subsequent blinded selection.) These may either be multiple exposures to a single recurrent factor (e.g. chronic poverty or persistent smoking) or a series of exposures to different factors. A *non-quotidian* example of the latter would be the cumulative effects of exposure to respirable silica in the workplace with the tuberculosis bacillus, to produce the lethal silico-tuberculosis. Finally, the term *pathways* represents dependent sequences of exposures in which exposure at one stage of the life course influences the probability of other exposures later in the life course, as well as associated expressions. (Analogous to the principals of marble selection.) For example, the (non-quotidian) divorce of someone's parents in early childhood may reduce that child's readiness to learn at school entry, which may, in turn, affect school performance, which would affect later employment opportunities and the socio-economic trajectory throughout life.

By thinking in terms of latent, cumulative and pathway models, it is possible to open up the 'hypothesis space' much wider than is ordinarily the case. In particular, the models allow us to deal with the prospect that traditional approaches to the study of mortality and serious illness do not fully capture the potential of factors 'earlier' in life influencing outcomes 'later' in life. *Here we do not recommend creating 'best fit' models from amongst a jumble of variables collected at different stages of the life course. Nor is the emphasis on the statistical fine structure of the analysis (regression, structural equation modelling, hierarchical modelling, etc.). Instead, the priority is modelling latent, pathway and cumulative effects in a conceptually coherent manner.*[15] The most significant methodological challenge that needs to be overcome is not on the statistical side. As the examples in the above paragraph suggest, it is easy enough to recognize the influences of discrete and distinct phenomena, but the challenge is to find methods and approaches that allow researchers to recognize and distinguish latent, pathway and cumulative phenomena in the quotidian context of daily life. This is not just an intellectual exercise, but has implications for policy and intervention. In general terms, the implication of latent effects is to intervene early; of pathway effects is to intervene at strategic junctures in the life course; and of cumulative effects is to intervene consistently over time, building on models of social change.

5.1.2 Developmental health

In trying to understand latent, pathway and cumulative phenomena, the most useful insight of the last 15 years has been the importance of a human development perspective.

It begins with the premise that human development in general, and early child development in particular, are the principal 'agents' mediating the relationship between life course, human experience and health outcome.[1,16] The basic story line is as follows:

> Newborns' immediate postnatal social environment has profound, long-lasting influences on subsequent health and development. A prime example is infant attachment to a parental figure (usually, the mother) in both higher primates and humans. The parental figure's failure to provide the full set of necessary visual, tactile, and auditory—and, perhaps, olfactory—inputs during a 'critical early window' of infant development leads to profound developmental delay. Indeed, in cases of severe neglect, this deprivation can result in adult stunting or even death, despite the availability of theoretically adequate 'physical' nourishment, warmth, and other material necessities. Furthermore, there is much less effect of this form of psychosocial deprivation when it occurs at later ages, as if the infant is 'prewired' to require this input at precisely a certain developmental stage.[17]

Three broad domains of early child development (ECD) are of special relevance, and have a role to play in health across the life course: physical, social/emotional and language/cognitive. Social determinants play a crucial role in the early phases of conception, pregnancy and post-natal periods of children's development. Sensitive periods in brain and biological development start pre-natally and continue throughout childhood and adolescence. The brain continues to sculpt itself, albeit at a declining rate, such that it does not reach its 'adult' state until the end of the second or beginning of the third decade of life. For example, key executive functions, regarding how an individual responds to social and emotional stimuli, develop in the prefrontal cortex from approximately age 3 to 9. At the same time, there is evidence that neural connections to the prefrontal cortex, from centres in the midbrain that sense environmental threats, develop earlier. Thus, whereas the physiological sense of threat is developed at a very young age, the repertoire of responses to threatening circumstances may develop later. The extent to which these processes lead to successful development depends upon the qualities of stimulation, support and nurturance in the social environments in which children live, learn and grow.[18]

Socio-economic gradients in health across the life course begin as socio-economic gradients in physical, social/emotional and language/cognitive development.[19] Since these three broad domains are, in part, markers for brain development, early gradients have been interpreted as evidence of 'differential access' to environments that provide adequate attachment, support, nurturance and stimulation.[20] By school age, development has been influenced by factors at three levels of society: family, neighbourhood, and the broader society. At the most intimate level, the 'within-family' environmental attributes of stimulation, support and nurturance are of greatest significance. At the next level of social aggregation, 'neighbourhoods/communities' matter: safety, cohesion and the avoidance of ghettoization of poor and marginalized families. At the broadest level of aggregation, the socio-economic environment and provision of effective programmes and services makes a difference. When the child is very young, factors at the most intimate levels of social aggregation are most important, but as the child ages the role of factors in the neighbourhood and broader socio-economic environment become increasingly important.

Gradients become institutionally embedded when they translate into children's 'readiness for school', subsequent school performance [21] and, finally, into gradients in literacy and numeracy in young adulthood.[22] Literacy and numeracy are important determinants of adulthood socio-economic destinations that have well established relationships to health status. In adult life, gradients emerge as differential rates of death, illness and disability. Thus, the social environment is a fundamental determinant of child and human development and, in turn, development is a determinant of health, well-being and learning skills across the balance of the life course.

According to this perspective, three domains of development: physical, social/emotional and language/cognitive should be considered both outcomes of the quotidian processes of daily living and, in turn, determinants of subsequent health outcome.

5.1.3 The developmental biology of daily life

There is, of course, nothing to be gained by implying that life course research must study 'everything, all the time'. We already know that everything affects everything else but, as many before us have asserted, the key question is: 'how much?' One challenge posed by quotidian life course phenomena is how to choose efficiently where to look for the big pay-offs among all of human experience.

Here it is argued that the best place to start is at the level of the 'transduction' systems that allow human experience to get under the skin and affect human biology to an extent that will affect health across the life course. To be sure, there are many ways for experience to get under the skin. Inhalation of toxic fumes is one way. A massive transfer of kinetic energy from a moving automobile is another. However, these are processes that are either discrete and/or distinct from daily life. As the time of writing, there are several 'candidate systems' that meet four basic criteria for our purposes.

- The system develops according to quotidian life course experiences (often early in life), such that differential qualities of experience lead to a differently functioning system.
- The system responds to quotidian experiences throughout the life course.
- The system, if it dysfunctions, has the biological capacity to influence health status.
- Differential functioning of the system across the life course, to the extent that health status is affected, derives from the quotidian.

There are four 'candidate systems' that meet these criteria and are worthy of mention here: the HPA axis and its accompanying secretion of cortisol; the autonomic nervous system (ANS) in association with epinephrine and norepinephrine; the development of memory, attention and other executive functions in the prefrontal cortex; and the systems of social affiliation involving the primitive amygdala and locus coeruleus with accompanying higher order cerebral connections, mediated by serotonin and other hormones. Here we will highlight one, the HPA axis, as an exemplar of how experience may get under the skin.

5.1.4 The 'life course development' of the HPA axis in society

Here we describe an animal model of the life story of the HPA axis and consider how it might unfold across the life course in those with different social origins and destinations in human society. The HPA axis is highly relevant because of its role in our perception of, and response to, stressful circumstances. HPA stimulation leads to the secretion of the hormone cortisol, which, in turn, has widespread metabolic effects on various organ systems. These effects are adaptive in the acute stress response phase, focusing the body's energy on the immediate task at hand and reducing metabolic processes that do not contribute to the immediate response. However, over the long term, cortisol can damage these same organ systems as a result of a high level of exposure.[9]

Animal studies provide an intriguing model of the role the HPA axis may play in general vulnerability and resistance to disease. Three lines of evidence are particularly pertinent here. In rats, the apparently minimal intervention of removal from the cage in early life can bring about a cascade of events that permanently conditions the way the HPA axis functions over the remainder of the life course.[23] This conditioning effect can only be created by intervention during a limited and specific period in early life, which suggests that it depends on appropriate stimulation during a highly circumscribed window of opportunity in brain and biological development (i.e. a critical period). Most important, once the HPA axis has been conditioned, the effects appear to be lifelong. In the study conducted by Meaney, rat pup handling reduced total lifetime exposure of corticosterone (the rat equivalent of cortisol in humans) to the brain. Chronic overexposure to corticosterone, in turn, endangered selected neurons in the brain's hippocampus, such that the rate of loss of hippocampal neurons was reduced in the handled rats over their whole life span. Because of cognitive functions' sensitivity to relatively small degrees of hippocampal damage, the handled rats, by 24 months of age (elderly by rat standards), had been spared some of the cognitive deterioration typical of ageing. Rats not handled as pups showed a progressive deterioration in their memory, cognitive processing and learning performance with age; in contrast, much less deterioration occurred in aged rats handled in infancy.[24]

There is a fascinating subtext here. The apparently simple handling of the baby rats meant in practice that they were removed for half an hour per day from their cages, from week 3 to week 9 of their lives—a protocol that involved putting them on a sheet and gently agitating them. At the time, the researchers thought this was the main intervention. However, the *de facto* intervention turned out to be something different. When the researchers returned the baby rats to their cages, the mothers, who had been without them, then engaged in extra licking, grooming and other affectionate and stimulating behaviour that was not offered to the unhandled baby rats. Subsequent biochemical studies have shown that, after the intervention, the handled rats showed a more adaptive, or functional, corticosterone response pattern to stress: a low basal corticosterone level, an abrupt response to acutely stressful circumstances and an abrupt decline to baseline thereafter. Among the non-handled rats, there was a much broader range of responses, typified by higher baseline levels and a more blunted response to stressful circumstances. Thus, the cumulative lifetime exposure to the rat hormonal equivalent of cortisol was higher for the non-handled rats than for the handled rats, leading to a variety of ageing effects, including hippocampal neuronal damage documented by Sapolsky (1992)[23] after chronic stressor exposure. It is striking that when the researchers tried the handling protocol later in life, rather than during the critical window between 3 and 8 weeks of age, it had no biological effect, i.e. they did not detect the prolonged change in the corticosterone response pattern or the differential ageing of learning and memory functions. This research presents a model of a discrete stimulus occurring at a critical point in early development and affecting a basic biological function relevant to host stress response, defence, and organ system ageing—a latent effect that then had lifelong consequences for health, well-being and competence.

A second series of experiments adds important depth to this story. By comparing the development of rat pups that were frequently, versus infrequently, licked and suckled by their mothers, Meaney (2001) was able to elucidate a mechanism by which systematic differences in the function of the HPA axis emerge.[24] He showed that licking and suckling initiate a biochemical cascade that leads to long-term *alterations in the expression of genes* influencing the development, not only of response patterns in the HPA axis, but also of higher order executive functions in the brain.[25,26] In colloquial terms, Meaney speaks about a 'life is going to suck' pattern, wherein the less licked and less suckled rats end up with a more highly reactive HPA axis (good for fight or flight, but bad for sustaining learning and memory functions over time) and a reduction of neuron-to-neuron synapses in the cerebral cortex. It is a model wherein high quality early nurturance leads, *through mediation of gene expression*, to a more tranquil HPA axis, greater capacity for complex learning and reduced age-related declines in learning and memory capacity. In other words, the early nurturant environment has been 'biologically embedded'.[27]

This series of experiments has also shown that the benefits of licking and suckling can be transmitted from one generation to the next. It began with distinct subgroups of rats that had histories of either high or low licking and suckling. However, when female rat pups from the low licking and suckling group were 'cross-fostered' with high licking and suckling mothers, they experienced the same benefits as the natural offspring. Most importantly, these female offspring adopted the high licking and suckling behaviour when they became mothers. In other words, a pattern of intergenerational learning was taking place that transmitted the more adaptive nurturing pattern to those who had been 'predisposed' to the non-adaptive pattern. Taken as a whole, this research presents a complete working model of how experience can get under the skin and influence aspects of well-being across the life course and, also, from generation to generation.

Does the HPA axis truly have the same sort of life story in human society that it seems to have among rats? Evidence on this point has been much slower to accumulate. However, several lines of inquiry converge with the evidence just presented.

1. It has been shown that the quality of early maternal–child attachment affects both the HPA axis function and behaviour, such that poorly attached toddlers have both more reactive HPA axes and less adaptive behavioural responses in social conflict situations.[28] Early in infancy there are differences in cortisol reactivity that are associated, on the one hand, with differences in the level of attachment and, on the other, with infant behaviours that reflexively affect the social environment of the infant. There is an important interaction between the individual's behaviour and the qualities of his or her immediate environment. Attachment, for example, is under considerable social control, but failure of the environment properly to signal and set up the reactions of positive attachment in the HPA axis and brain of the child means that the

child will be at risk of missing significant social cues. This, in turn, can make the child less easy for caregivers and peers to relate to, which, in turn, can lead to deterioration of the child's immediate social environment, making it more stressful. This vicious cycle, in turn, can have significant consequences for his or her social, emotional and cognitive development. An extreme example of this is the plight of Romanian orphans studied by Gunnar et al.[29] After more than 8 months of neglect since birth in state-run orphanages, these children have tended to become high cortisol reactors and to suffer various behavioural disturbances—ranging to 'psychosocial dwarfism' in extreme cases who were never provided even minimal infant love and attention, to minor—and apparently often reversible—developmental delay in those only orphaned later.

2. There are systematic social class differences in basal cortisol levels among both primary and secondary school children.[30] Early morning, 'pre-peak' salivary cortisol levels vary widely among children from different social classes. These investigators found that in the elementary school population, the early morning cortisol levels were higher in children from families with low parental income, education and employment status, and higher levels of parental depression. This was especially so among the children who 'did not think that much was possible in their lives'; an attitude that was more common among lower than higher SES children.

3. Work comparing 50-year-old 'healthy' men from Sweden and Lithuania provides important insights.[31] In Eastern Europe during the last 20 years of the Soviet era, there was a mounting health crisis that was further exacerbated by the political, social and economic dislocations during the post-Soviet political and economic transition. Whereas heart disease mortality rates for middle-aged men were similar in Sweden and Lithuania in the mid-1960s, by the mid-1990s they were 4-fold higher in Lithuania than in Sweden. An early report on the East–West 'life expectancy gap' suggested that the difference between Eastern Europe and the West could be thought of as being analogous to SES differences.[32] In other words, the experience of life for people in Eastern Europe in recent decades was, in some respects, like that of low socio-economic groups in the West. Kristensen's work[31] was designed to test that idea. She studied 50-year-old men from one city in Lithuania and one city in Sweden, and examined their cortisol response pathways, using a challenge protocol. This involved three stress tests: psychosocial, mental–intellectual and straightforwardly physical (inserting the subjects' hands into cold water). She found that the pattern of salivary cortisol before, during and after these standardized stressors was such that the Lithuanian men had a higher baseline cortisol, and then a blunted response to the stressor (what she described as a 'burnout' pattern). The Swedish men had lower baseline levels, a sharp response to the stressor, regardless of which one, and then a quicker return to baseline levels; ultimately the Swedes' cortisol levels came down further.

Kristensen found that the Lithuanian pattern tended to be associated with low self-esteem, lower sense of coherence (i.e. a sense of conjunction between one's lived experience and one's sense of what life should bring),[33] and increased reported job strain, according to the Karasek model.[34] In general the Lithuanians showed decreased decision latitude in their jobs, increased 'vital exhaustion' and increased depression. This 'psychosocial risk factor complex' association with coronary heart disease risk was quite specific. Other biological variables known to predict coronary heart disease risk that were examined—such as serum cholesterol and blood pressure levels—could not in themselves explain the two populations' very different heart disease rates. The Swedish men's cortisol levels were reminiscent of the 'handled' rats, whereas the Lithuanian men tended to have cortisol profiles of non-handled rats and socially subordinate baboons.[35]

To conclude, the HPA axis fulfils the criteria for a candidate system identified at the beginning of this section. Less is known about the other candidate systems according to these criteria, and much work needs to be done, through birth cohort studies combined with developmental biology investigations, to work out the role of these systems. What is required here is an era of mixed methods research, bridging from developmental biology to life course epidemiology, that illuminates the most promising biological substrates for latent, pathway and cumulative effects, and improves the chances of identifying valid life course influences on health.

Life course intervention studies are an essential part of the mixed methods research programme. Methodologically they offer the opportunity to create an experimental design to test mediating processes in relation to specific outcomes in the context of many years of life, with prospectively designed means of controlling for the effects of the social environment.

5.2 Life course intervention studies

5.2.1 Strategic approaches to intervention

Ideally, a body of life course research would exist wherein human development interventions were implemented during one stage of the life course with the explicit purpose of altering health outcomes at a later stage of life. This author is not aware of any significant body of literature that meets this standard. At present, our level of understanding of the evidence regarding societal influences and transduction mechanisms strongly supports certain generic approaches to intervention. These can be best understood using the notions of primary, secondary and tertiary prevention. The reader from a public health background will find these terms familiar, since public health deals largely with the primary and secondary prevention of disease. Here, we apply these terms further 'upstream' to developmental trajectories that may confer differential risk of disease. Thus, from a public health standpoint, primary, secondary and tertiary prevention of adverse developmental trajectories are all forms of pre-primary, or primordial, prevention.

5.2.1.1 The nature of the interventions

The principal primary prevention strategy is to provide an 'experiential environment' during the child's waking hours, from as young as possible, that has stronger nurturant qualities than would otherwise be available. The rationale here is not to identify and intervene in relation to specific weaknesses, but rather to provide a generally stronger nurturant environment that will have positive influences on a wide range of brain and biological developmental parameters, behaviour and the development of basic competencies. This is the basic strategy taken by most of the successful early intervention programmes (see below). It is important to note, however, that most of the interventions studied to date focus directly on the child's daily experiences, and not on the socio-economic and institutional factors in society that influence them. Studies of state-level programmes, such as expanded family income support, parental leave, universal access to quality child care, neighbourhood renewal and flexible work-leave provisions, would all be considered primary prevention strategies.

Secondary prevention begins with a child showing delay or weakness in one or more domains of development (e.g. slow language acquisition; slow transition from physical aggression to verbal negotiation in situations of social conflict). Here, the principal strategy is to view the remainder of a sensitive period in brain development as a window of opportunity, and intervene by altering the child's experiential environment in ways that will strengthen the developmental domains showing vulnerability. For example, current studies applying functional magnetic resonance imaging (fMRI) to early language development in children across the socio-economic spectrum have shown that the vulnerability of low socio-economic children to language delay is largely confined to those with low levels of phonological awareness.[36] In other words, the 'developmental cost' to the child of low phonological awareness is greater in lower socio-economic contexts where the language environment may not be very rich, but in high socio-economic contexts the language environment tends to be rich enough to stimulate even those children who are relatively inattentive to spoken language. This observation implies an obvious form of developmental targeting that, if initiated early enough, can strengthen otherwise weak biological pathways, behaviour and basic competencies.

Tertiary prevention begins, by definition, after the primary windows of opportunity presented by sensitive periods in brain development have closed. Here the principal strategy is to open up alternative routes of perception and cognition that will pre-empt any weakness brought about by missing the original developmental opportunity. For instance, it is well known that second languages can be learned long after sensitive periods in language development have ended, but that this competency involves different synaptic pathways from original language learning. Increasingly, fMRI, magnetoencephalograph (MEG) and evoked response potential (ERP) techniques are being used to pinpoint the neurocognitive substrate of developmental weakness *post hoc*, in order to guide compensatory strategies for development. For example, MEG studies showing weak inter-hemispheric communication of receptive language among children with Down's syndrome has led to 'show and tell' methods of instruction wherein the showing component can 'speak to both hemispheres of the brain' simultaneously, and help weak inter-hemispheric communication.[37]

5.2.1.2 Strategic issues in sampling

The approaches to primary, secondary and tertiary prevention described above have unambiguous implications for intervention sampling strategies. Primary prevention depends upon an understanding that, *on average*, the room for improving the experiential environment through intervention gradually increases as one goes down the socio-economic spectrum. This is consistent with two types of sampling strategies: first, a population-based approach, that includes families across the full socio-economic spectrum, with the objective of 'flattening up' the socio-economic gradient in child development; and, secondly, an approach that targets low socio-economic families, neighbourhoods or ethnic enclaves in order to achieve improvements at the individual level. The former is both ambitious and complex in that it requires not only matching intervention and control communities across a range of socio-demographic characteristics but, also, sampling enough intervention and control communities to model the effects hierarchically. The latter is more straightforward in that it is only necessary to sample individually comparable control children from a comparable context. However, this approach has the limitation that it cannot address the question of how to 'scale intervention up' to the societal level.

Secondary prevention involves sampling children based upon early evidence of specific developmental vulnerabilities. This can be achieved in two ways. First, intervention could follow an early developmental screen, applied in the family, child-care or clinical context, allowing simultaneous identification of candidates for intervention and random assignment to intervention and control groups. Secondly, sampling could begin with a series of child-care environments where a high proportion of children have been shown, in the past, to face specific developmental vulnerabilities. Here, secondary prevention would take place across the whole group, regardless of their individual developmental status, with the objective of reducing vulnerability by shifting developmental norms. Like the population-based strategy described above, this would require sampling enough intervention and control environments for a hierarchical analysis of the outcomes.

Tertiary prevention, by definition, involves individual sampling; detailed knowledge of the developmental status of the individual; and careful matching of intervention and controls according to a full range of socio-demographic and individual capacity variables that would be likely to influence long-term outcomes.

5.2.1.3 Measuring the effect of interventions

The developmental science that underpins life course intervention suggests three special considerations in measuring outcomes. First, the influence of the intervention on 'phenotype' (i.e. physical, language/cognitive, social/emotional characteristics of the whole child) must be judged *separately from* changes detected by means of imaging or developmental biology tests. In other words, the working assumption must be that improvements in developmental trajectories can take place through biological mechanisms other than those that are currently recognized, without it being assumed that these improvements are ephemeral in nature. Secondly, successful interventions must be defined as those that strengthen one or more domains of development *without weakening the others*. There is much legitimate concern about strategies that 'teach to the test' and narrow the breadth of children's experience in order to help them achieve a specific competency. Thus, measurement of outcomes, especially over the life of the intervention, must tap each of the three broad domains of child development regardless of the focus of intervention.

Thirdly, outcome measurement must include a credible strategy to check whether or not short-term benefits of intervention are sustained over time. Ideally, outcomes would be measured over decades, and simple follow-up strategies can be put in place to track study subjects' residential moves so that this purpose is not defeated by loss to follow-up over time. However, in general, it is not practicable to judge effectiveness over decades of follow-up, since assessment of interventions, in order to be useful, must be timely.

A practical compromise is to insist that follow-up be taken to the next developmental transition point. For example, there is now an extensive body of research showing that well designed stimulation programmes in the pre-school period can improve the cognitive and social/emotional development of children. The focus on cognitive and social/emotional functioning is relevant because of its connection to school readiness. School readiness, in turn, is important because the complex web of early academic failure and early school misbehaviour is associated with lack of school readiness and, in turn, strongly predictive of school failure, employability, criminality and psychological morbidity in young adulthood.[38] Thus, we organize the following sections according to the age of intervention in the early life course.

5.2.2 Programmes beginning in infancy

Earliest in the life cycle are the 'parent/infant stimulation' programmes. These programmes usually start in the first few months, or years, of life. The specific details of the programmes vary, but they share certain common characteristics: the activities take place at home, with or without a separate learning centre focus; there is voluntary involvement of at least one parent; the role of the parent in the process of child development is actively reinforced and positive role models from the local community are promoted; contact with programme staff is frequent (i.e. at least twice monthly); and the programmes consciously focus on both cognitive and social/emotional factors. Examples of parent/infant stimulation programmes that have successfully altered developmental trajectories include the Parent Child Development Center,[39] project CARE[40] and the Family Rehabilitation Program.[41]

5.2.3 Programmes beginning in the pre-school period

The literature on school success following pre-school and school-age intervention is divided between those studies which seem to show improvements due, primarily, to gains in cognitive development and those which seem to suggest that the social/emotional effects may be more durable, and may have a longer lasting impact. Notwithstanding this dichotomy, most of the effective programmes attempt to intervene in both cognitive and social/emotional domains. In fact, gains may occur in the opposite domains from which they were intended. There is evidence that gains in cognitive development increase with increasing longevity of the programme. In one pre-school intervention programme for socio-economically disadvantaged children aged 4, gains in cognitive development increased with increased parental time commitment to the programme, and other measures of school readiness, such as task orientation, extraversion and verbal facility, increased with student participation time.[38]

In the Carolina Abecedarian Project,[42] socio-economically disadvantaged subjects were randomly assigned to the control or experimental group in two time periods: pre-school child care and school age. The first part of the programme was entirely based in a child-care environment, and did not have a home intervention component. This early intervention group made significant gains in cognitive development by 54 months of age, but by mid-primary school the pass rate was highest for those children who were part of both the day care and the school-aged educational intervention. Their success rate (84 per cent) was virtually the same as that of the local school system as a whole (87 per cent). The next most successful group were those who were given the pre-school but not the school-aged programme (71 per cent), followed by those given the school-aged programme only (62 per cent), and those given neither programme (50 per cent). By age 12, there was still a pre-school, but not a school age, treatment effect on IQ of approximately five points;[43] but the effects upon IQ distribution were impressive: 87.2 per cent of the pre-school group had IQs above 85, compared with 55.8 per cent of those in the school age and control groups. Figure 5.1 shows that the effects of the programme on reading skills were sustained until at least age 21.[44] Both the pre-school and the school-aged intervention had long-lasting benefits, but those children randomized to both programmes had the greatest benefit—0.8 of a standard deviation above controls on reading skills in young adulthood. The unanswered question is: will these gains in cognitive development translate into reduced risks for adult chronic disease? The answer to this question will have to await another 30 years of follow-up.

The Perry Preschool Study is perhaps the most significant because it was based upon one of the most comprehensive of the early stimulation programmes for underprivileged children (with both a centre-based and a home visiting/parental involvement component).[45–47] It was evaluated by comparing outcomes among children who were randomly assigned to 'preschool' and 'no pre-school' groups for approximately 18 months between

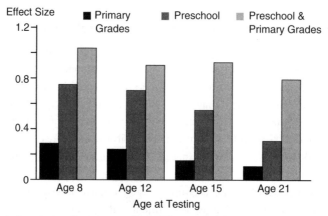

Fig. 5.1 Abecedarian study: effects on reading skills ages 8–21.
Note. From "Early childhood education; young adult outcomes from the Abecedarian project", by F.A. Campbell, C.T. Ramey, E. Pungello, J. Sparling, and S.Miller-Johnson, 2002, *Applied Developmental Science, 6*, p 50. Copyright 2002 by the American Psychological Association. Reprinted with permission.

age 3 and 5. Its special significance lies in the fact that it has been followed for the longest period of time. By age 19, the intervention group had higher rates of school graduation and college attendance, fewer arrests and teenage pregnancies, higher rates of employment, and lower proportions were on social assistance. By age 27, the intervention group were four times as likely to be earning US$2000 per month or more; three times as likely to own a home; one-fifth as likely to have been subject to multiple arrests; more likely to be in a stable marriage-like relationship; and 20 per cent less likely to have consumed social assistance as the controls.[46] By age 40, the advantages for earnings and for encounters with the justice system had persisted[47] and, by this age, it was estimated that US$17 had been saved over the previous 35 years on justice, special education, and social services costs for every dollar spent, even after discounting for 35 years of inflation.

Neither of these studies, nor any of the others, has been followed-up long enough to determine if the interventions will also have an effect on adult chronic disease. Most of the early intervention studies are relatively small, with sample sizes of a few hundred or less.[48] Thus, there is an urgent need for a coordinated effort to meta-analyse *interventions that were successful in altering developmental trajectories*, in order to assess their influence on adult chronic disease.

5.2.4 Life course and society

Life course relationships need to be considered in the context of broad societal influences, since the latter will determine the barriers and opportunities that individuals will confront at important stages in their lives. There is evidence that major social cataclysms: the Great Depression,[49] mass military mobilization[49,50] and the socio-economic and political transition in Central and Eastern Europe, for example, have had the capacity to change life course trajectories *en masse*. In these instances, everyone within society is affected by major societal changes that, in turn, have implications for human development and health. However, the relationship between life course and social context is not confined to social cataclysm. Less dramatic variations in the social environments that populations encounter over time could also be expected to influence life course trajectories and their healthfulness, albeit in ways more subtle, and more difficult to measure.

From the standpoint of understanding the societal factors that influence health, the most intuitively obvious and useful approach exploits the fact that they can be grouped, reasonably neatly, by 'levels of social aggregation'. At the macro level are such society-wide influences as levels and fluctuations of national income, and particularly patterns of distribution, and policies intended to affect these (e.g. income support, education, healthcare or employment policies). At an intermediate, or 'meso', level are the characteristics of one's neighbourhood, community or workplace. Influences here would include how people interact with each other; levels of social trust and community participation; working conditions in the local employment base; and the quality of local institutions such as schools, libraries, newspapers, policing and parks. At the most 'micro' level, there are the influences on health associated with private life, such as the nature and quality of personal social support: intimate relationships, friendships and the availability of personal help when needed. From the standpoint of child development, one is most interested in whether or not the intimate environments of childhood are stimulating, supportive and nurturing.

We have examined the life course in the context of broad social influences, by incorporating the concept of macro-/meso-/micro-levels of social aggregation to create the parsimonious predictive model of self-rated health at age 33 in the 1958 British birth cohort.[15] The model conceptualizes the life course development as an arrow, encompassing latent, pathway and cumulative effects, intersecting a bullseye that represents society at the micro-, meso- and macro-levels of aggregation. For the purposes of this discussion, the most important finding was the following: there were statistically significant effects of childhood factors—latent, pathway and cumulative—as well as factors operating at two of three levels of social aggregation (meso and macro), but the life course factors were not 'explained' statistically by the societal level factors, and conversely, society level effects were not 'explained' by life course factors. In other words, life course intervention research must take account not only of the individual life course and individual-level interventions. It must also take account of 'intervention' at different levels of social aggregation.

Recently, under the auspices of the WHO International Commission on the Social Determinants of Health, we have generalized this model to the global environment. In so doing, we have been much more precise about the different social environments that influence human development; the characterization of those environments; and the degree to which they overlap one another in different parts of the world. The result is the framework presented in Fig. 5.2.[51]

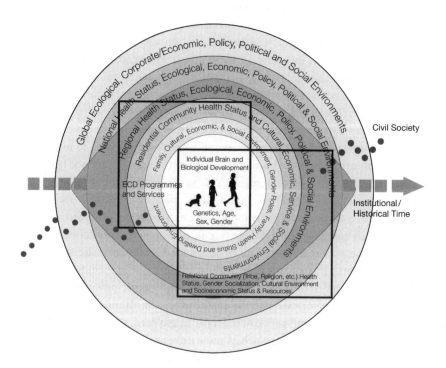

Fig. 5.2 Global model of the social determinants of human.

5.2.5 **Levels of intervention**

Life course interventions can take place at various levels of social aggregation: clinical, targeted, universal and civil society.

Civil society interventions are designed to make communities 'friendlier' to families and children. Examples of civil society interventions include socio-economically diverse neighbourhoods that reduce class, race and gender inequalities, access to parks and play spaces, strong inter-sectoral support for early child development, neighbourhood safety, and so on. Many of these interventions relate to town planning and access issues, as well as policies of senior levels of government. In the UK, the Sure Start programme is, in part, a programme of civil society intervention.[52] Civil society interventions are meant to influence the entire distribution of the developmental curve, so that if these programmes are successful, the entire curve will shift in a positive direction. If these interventions really 'bring a community together' to create family-friendly environments across class and ethnic divides, they should have disproportionate influence at the vulnerable end of the developmental distribution. In other words, the distribution should both improve and be compressed. As a result, the range, or inequality in distribution, should be reduced.

In theory, universal programmes are available for everyone to use (i.e. library story times, Family Resource Programmes, quality child care). However, a universally *available* programme is not the same as a universally *accessible one*, since there can be barriers for some groups of people that limit their access to these programmes. Universal interventions have the capacity to influence a large number of children and improve the distribution of development, *if* barriers of access can be addressed for children who are vulnerable. If barriers are not addressed, universal interventions will have a larger effect at the non-vulnerable end of the distribution. In other words, distribution will improve, but the range will *expand*, not compress.

Targeted programmes are designed for a subset of families and young children that are defined by some characteristic such as: income, geographic location, ethnicity, family risk (i.e. child protection issues) and biological risk (i.e. identified health problems). Most of the programmes that have been subject to evaluation to date (such as those described above) are targeted programmes. Targeted interventions, in principle, are meant to pick up a group of children who are likely to be vulnerable, and thus they can compress the distribution of development at the vulnerable end. The success of these kinds of programmes rests in part in correctly identifying vulnerable children so that interventions can have the greatest effect.

Clinical programmes are designed for treatment of a child and usually involve one-to-one treatment by a caregiver (i.e. speech and language services, physical therapy, etc.). They tend to affect a small percentage of children, who are identified individually as highly vulnerable.

5.3 **Evaluating human development as a societal objective: combining population-based and longitudinal data**

Child longitudinal studies in general, and birth cohort studies in particular, can provide an ongoing supply of information on developmental trajectories, and on the determinants of 'successful' and 'unsuccessful' developmental trajectories. However, just as they need to be complemented by studies of developmental biology and intervention, so too is there a need to complement them with population-based data collection. Here, two types of population-based studies are highlighted:

5.3.1 The early development indicator (EDI) as a population-based tool

The EDI was designed as a population-based tool for assessing the state of child development at school entry, useful for both communities and government in understanding ECD within their jurisdictions. It comes in the form of a checklist that can be filled out by teachers after they know a child for several months. The EDI takes approximately 20 min per child to fill out, such that an entire class can be assessed for the cost of a one-day teacher buy-out.[53]

A 5-year validation process took place during the late 1990s before the EDI was proposed for use in local communities. It was pilot tested on approximately 16 500 children in Toronto, North Bay, Baffin Island, Ottawa and New Brunswick, Canada. In this way, unreliable items and items that violated the UN Charter on the Rights of the Child were removed; scales were defined; and the range of utility of the tool was determined. The EDI is valid for interpretation at the level of the group, and can be analysed at the level of the individual, but it is not an individual *diagnostic* instrument. It is valid in the 4–6 year age range, and gives unbiased results by ethnicity and for children with English as a second language. Since implementation, further validation exercises have been undertaken in Australia and Canada. These exercises have been broadly consistent with the original validation. Most importantly, the EDI has been demonstrated to be predictive of individual student achievement on standardized tests of reading and mathematics at Grade 4.[54]

The EDI has five major scales: physical; social; emotional; language and cognitive; and communication skills and general knowledge. The five scales map directly onto the three broad domains of early child development: physical, social/emotional and language/cognitive that have lifelong influence on health, well-being, behaviour and learning skills. Thus, the EDI provides information that can be interpreted both backwards and forwards in time. The primary 'direction of interpretation' for the purposes of early child development is backwards in time, i.e. the results of the EDI, at the level of the group, can be construed to reflect the qualities of early experience that a particular group of young children have had up to that point in their lives. However, the EDI can also be interpreted prospectively, in that the results frame the challenge that families, schools and communities will have in supporting their children's development from kindergarten onward.

The principal parameter generated from each scale of the EDI is 'vulnerability', and for each scale there is a score that serves as a 'vulnerability threshold'. Children who fall below that score are said to be 'vulnerable' in that area of their development. The interpretation of vulnerability is that the child is, on average, more likely to be limited in their development in that area than children who fall above the cut-off. Because of the nature of the EDI, this is meant to be an interpretation at the level of the group. In other words, it is a meaningful use of the EDI to say something like '20 per cent of children in neighbourhood A are vulnerable in their physical development, whereas in neighbourhood B only 5 per cent are vulnerable' rather than comparing two individual children.

In British Columbia, we have mapped the 'proportion vulnerable' by geographic area for each scale of the EDI, and for one or more scales, for the whole province. Figure 5.3 shows the proportion of children who were vulnerable on one or more scale of the EDI according to the 59 school district areas of British Columbia, and Fig. 5.4 shows an individual school district broken down according to residential neighbourhood. This is the 'holistic' measure of ECD, covering all domains of development; in other words, they represent the 'differences that make a difference' for child development. It should be noted that the range of vulnerability by neighbourhood within the one small school district shown here is as large as across all 59 school districts in British Columbia.

The type of information that is generated through the use of the EDI shows how early development is distributed by neighbourhood and school, but does not directly provide strategic insight into the determinants of the differences. This latter is an important complementary role for child longitudinal/birth cohort studies, in particular for: demonstrating how the state of child development in a society can come to be an 'emergent property' of a complex of factors, many of them modifiable, at the intimate, civic and societal level; providing insights into the factors that underlie emerging gradients in the child; helping explain why the level of variation in 'vulnerability' is greater at the neighbourhood level

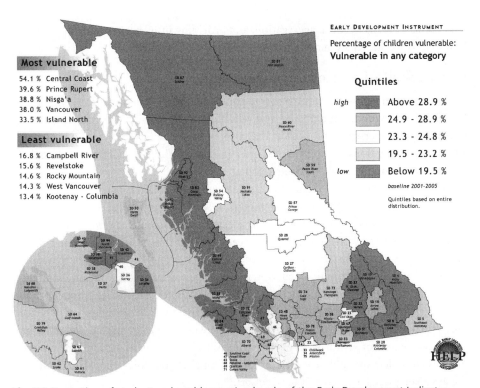

Fig. 5.3 Proportion of students vulnerable on ≤1 subscale of the Early Development Indicator.

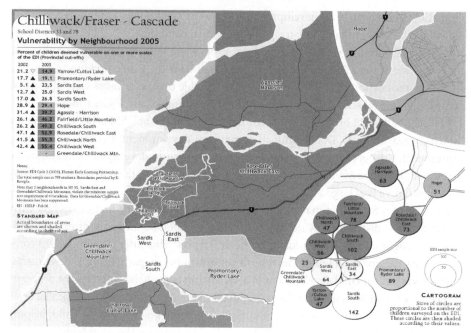

Fig. 5.4 Proportion of students vulnerable on ≥1 subscale of the EDI.

than at higher levels of social aggregation; and providing insights into where to look and how to look for strategies that might improve child development.

5.3.2 Portrait of a record linkage study

Over the long term, finding ways to merge population-based and life course methodologies should provide the most valid and reliable 'data system' for monitoring human development, experience and health, and, also, provide the most efficient platform for analysing interventions at any level of social aggregation. Here, we portray an example of the sort of output that could be contemplated.

A cohort of 28 794 British Columbian male sawmill workers was originally gathered to conduct a study of the effects of chlorophenol anti-sapstain exposure. Fourteen sawmills located in British Columbia, Canada were selected and personnel records were accessed for workers who had worked, for at least 1 year, in one of these mills at any time between 1950 and 1998. From the job history records, the number of episodes of unemployment, job mobility (classified as upward, downward or stable) and occupation (manager, skilled trades, machine operator or unskilled) were obtained. Historical estimates of job control, demands, noise and social support were obtained in two ways: from experienced job evaluators (two union and two management) who worked across the industry and, also, from panels of senior workers at each mill. These expert estimates for control, psychological demand, physical demand, social support and noise were then applied to the job history database in the fathers' cohort.[55]

The cohort of adult sawmill workers was linked to the British Columbia birth file from the provincial vital statistics registry in order to identify all of the children of these workers born in British Columbia between 1952 and 2000. There were 37 827 children in the cohort, of whom 19 833 satisfied the eligibility criterion that their father had at least 1 year of work in a study sawmill while the child or children were aged 0–16. Using probabilistic linkage techniques, the children's cohort was linked to the British Columbia Linked Health Database (BCLHDB), consisting of person-specific, longitudinal records on all British Columbians.[56] Eighty-eight per cent of the members of the children's cohort were linked to the BCLHDB in this way, allowing access to data on deaths, hospital discharges and other medical encounters for the years 1985–2001. Using ICD9 codes available in the hospital discharge database, it was possible to identify any suicide case (completed and attempted) that occurred between January 1985 and 31 March 2001. Children's exposure to adverse family socio-economic circumstances was assessed by applying the father's exposure (in terms of job mobility, unemployment experience and exposure to control, psychological demand, physical demand, social support and noise) during each year of the child's life from age zero to the end of the sixteenth year. Also available were father's marital status (married, divorced, widowed or single) and ethnicity (East-Indian, Chinese and other). Finally, from the BCLHDB it was determined whether a father had a completed or attempted suicide, a mental health diagnosis or an alcohol-related diagnosis prior to their child's attempted or completed suicide.

Of the 19 833 children in the cohort, 252 attempted or committed suicide between 1985 and 2001. After controlling for father's socio-demographic characteristics, occupation at the time prior to their child's suicide (attempted or completed), mental health diagnosis and alcohol-related mental health diagnosis prior to their child's suicide attempts or completion, it was found that:

◆ Male children of fathers with low duration of employment at a study sawmill while their child or children were less than age 16 had a greater odds of attempting suicide than children of fathers with high duration of employment.

◆ Female children of fathers who experienced low job control during the first 16 years of their child's life had significantly greater odds for attempting suicide.

◆ Male children of fathers employed in jobs with low psychological demand showed significantly greater odds for completing suicide.[57]

Although this example is somewhat circumscribed, it provides a glimpse of the power of record linkage technology in creating life course trajectories on large populations.

At the time of writing, we are working on a broader approach for studying life course intervention at the level of the population. The EDI records for British Columbia are being linked forwards in time to individual school records, and backwards in time to birth, medical, hospital and pharmaceutical records in order to create skeleton developmental trajectories for the whole population. Individual trajectories are then being re-aggregated by neighbourhood and/or school in order to 'nest' individuals properly within contexts of interest. At the time of writing, three significant advances have already been made in this regard. First, we have matched a Personal Education Number to 94 per cent of the EDI assessments carried out between 2000 and 2005, making it possible to relate EDI to school progress on an individual basis. Secondly, we have matched 97 per cent of the Personal Education Numbers to a Personal Health Number, allowing a cross-walk between education, health and development. Finally, we have established the physical infrastructure and ethical framework that will allow us to link birth, physician and hospital services, EDI and school records on a person-specific, population-based, but anonymous basis. Together, these advances mean that we will be able to create a developmental trajectory for each British Columbian child who has done the EDI, starting with birth experience (birth weight, small for gestational age, etc.), proceeding to early health status (inferred through medical and hospital services utilization), to state of development at school entry (using the EDI), to progress through school. From these data, we will be able to identify basic 'success' and 'failure' trajectories for British Columbian children in order to assist communities, schools, health authorities, local government and provincial policy-makers in understanding the determinants of development, and to serve as a platform for analysing life course interventions.

5.3.3 Design of a new generation of intervention studies

What, then, are the special issues that need to be considered when trying to achieve best practice in designing, conducting and analysing the data from a life course intervention study? The overarching consideration, of course, is the reality that life course intervention studies, with decades-long follow-up, must contend with determinants of health that are found in all aspects of daily life, such that potentially effective interventions can be concealed by an accumulation of adverse life experiences, and the reverse. From what has been described above, the following 13 criteria are proposed to reflect the special needs, and special circumstances, of this field:

1. Is the 'health status improving' rationale for the intervention meant to be an alteration in the developmental trajectory over time or a change in a discrete factor that is otherwise irrelevant to life course development?

2. Do the methods of data collection and analysis account for 'distinct and discrete' influences on health as well as the quotidian factors that are embedded in life course development?

3. Does the intervention take into account current knowledge in developmental biology, in terms of timing of developmental factors; inter-generational transmission; gestational influences; nature/nurture; and the development of biological transduction systems?

4. If the intervention is meant to alter developmental trajectories, have the special characteristics of life course development been considered? In particular, has the prospect been considered that effects may derive from some population subgroups being differentially sensitive to intervention than others, as opposed to the main effect being based upon dose–response? Has the role of stability versus residential transiency been considered? Has the intervention been designed/evaluated to take account of the interactive attributes of environment, not just the programmatic or static aspects?

Have slowly developing factors been considered (e.g. the development of a 'racialized' identity, the long-term consequences of stressful social comparisons)?

5. Has consideration been given to methods of analysis that are appropriate for developmental trajectories, including consideration of 'positive' and 'negative' developmental trajectories as both predictors of outcome and intermediate outcomes in their own right?

6. Do the data collection protocols and analytical methods take account of the fact that early language/cognitive, social/emotional and physical development can all influence health later in life?

7. Is the intervention appropriate to the stage of life course development for which it is proposed? What are the prospects that intervention at the proposed stage of development will, in fact, be long lasting?

8. Has consideration been given to the prospect that relationships between exposures and interventions, on the one hand, and outcome, on the other, may follow one or more of the latent, pathway or cumulative patterns?

9. Is there adequate accounting for determinants of health at the level of the family, community and broader environment? Has the intervention taken account of the ways in which slow-moving historical change might have affected the prospects for health across the population?

10. Has there been adequate accounting for the ways in which the factors that influence human development expand with age from strictly the family (when very young), to include an increasing range of aspects of the community environment, to finally including the broader societal/socio-economic environment?

11. Has consideration been given to the prospect that interventions may have different effects at different points along the socio-economic spectrum?

12. Have the problems of how selective participation and differential drop-out rates been considered, *especially with respect to long-term residential mobility*, and a plan put in place for minimizing loss to follow-up?

13. Have record linkage methodologies been considered, both for tracking individuals and for obtaining outcome information?

By careful design, using these criteria, intervention studies can have 'the major potential advantage of coming closest to true experimental design'.[57]

References

1. Keating D, Hertzman C, ed. (1999). *Developmental health and the wealth of nations*. Guilford Press, New York.

2. Kuh DL, Ben-Shlomo Y (1997). *A life course approach to chronic disease epidemiology: tracing the origins of ill health from early to adult life*. Oxford University Press, Oxford.

3. Marmot MG, Wadsworth MEJ, ed. (1997). Fetal and early childhood environment: long term health implications. *British Medical Bulletin* 53.

4. Shenkin SD, Starr JM, Pattie A, Rush MA, Whalley LJ, Deary IJ (2001). Birth weight and cognitive function at age 11 years: the Scottish Mental Survey 1932. *Archives of Diseases of Childhood* 85, 189–196.

5. Richards M, Hardy R, Kuh D, Wadsworth MEJ (2001). Birth weight and cognitive function in the British 1946 birth cohort: longitudinal population based study. *British Medical Journal* 322, 199–203.

6. Sorensen HT, Sabroe S, Olsen J, Rothman KJ, Gillman MW, Fischer P (1997). Birth weight and cognitive function in young adult life: historical cohort study. *British Medical Journal* 315, 401–403.

7. Matte TD, Bresnahan M, Begg MD, Susser E (2001). Influence of variation in birth weight within normal range and within sibships on IQ at age 7 years: cohort study. *British Medical Journal* 323,310–314.

8. Hart B, Risley TR (1995). *Meaningful differences in the everyday experience of young American children*. Paul H. Brookes Publishing, Baltimore.

9. McEwen B (1998). Protective and damaging effects of stress mediators. *New England Journal of Medicine* 338, 171–179.

10. Seeman TE, Crimmins E, Huang MH, Singer B, Bucur A, Gruenewald T, *et al.* (2004). Cumulative biological risk and socio-economic differences in mortaltiy: MacArthur studies of successful aging. *Social Science and Medicine* 58, 1985–1997.

11. Marmot M (2004). *The status syndrome*. Times Books, New York.

12. Pierson P (2003). Big, slow-moving, and … invisible: macrosocial processes in the study of comparative politics. In: Mahoney J, Reuschemeyer D, ed. *Comparative historical analysis in the social sciences*. Cambridge University Press, Cambrdge.

13. Jefferis B, Power C, Hertzman C (2002). Birth weight, childhood socio-economic environment and cognitive development in the 1958 birth cohort. *British Medical Journal* 325, 305–311.

14. Hertzman C, Power C (2006). A life course approach to health and human development. In: Heymann, J, Hertzman C, Barer ML, Evans RG, ed. *Healthier societies: from analysis to action*. Oxford University Press, New York.

15. Hertzman C, Power C, Matthews S, Manor O (2001). Using an interactive framework of society and life course to explain self-rated health in early adulthood. *Social Science and Medicine* 53, 1575–1585.

16. National Research Council Institute of Medicine (2000). *From neurons to neighbourhoods: the science of early childhood development*. National Academy Press, Washington, DC.

17. Cynader MS, Frost BJ (1999). Mechanisms of brain development: neuronal sculpting by the physical and social environment. In: Keating D, Hertzman C, ed. *Developmental health and the wealth of nations*. Guilford Press, New York.

18. Ramey CT, Ramey SL (1998). Prevention of intellectual disabilities: early interventions to improve cognitive development. *Preventive Medicine* 27, 224–232.

19. Ross DP, Roberts P (1999). *Income and child well-being: a new perspective on the poverty debate*. Canadian Council on Social Development, Ottawa.

20. McCain MN, Mustard JF (1999). *Reversing the real brain drain: Early Years Study final report*. Ontario Children's Secretariat, Toronto.

21. Human Resources Development Canada and Statistics Canada (1995). *Growing up in Canada: national longitudinal survey of children and youth*. Minister of Industry, Ottawa.

22. Statistics Canada and Organization for Economic Cooperation and Development (1995). *Literacy, economy and society*. OECD, Paris.

23. Sapolsky RM (1992). *Stress, the aging brain, and the mechanisms of neuron death*. MIT Press, Cambridge, MA.

24. Meaney MJ (2001). Maternal care, gene expression, and the transmission of individual differences in stress reactivity across generations. *Annual Review of Neuroscience* 24, 1161–1192.

25. Weaver ICG, Cervoni FA, Champagne FA, Alessio ACD, Sharma S, Seckl JR, *et al.* (2004). Epigenetic programming by maternal behavior. *Nature Neuroscience* 7, 847–854.

26. Szyf M (2003). *DNA methylation enzymology, encyclopedia of the human genome*. Macmillan Publishers, Nature Publishing Group, New York.

27. Hertzman C (2000). The biological embedding of early experience and its effects on health in adulthood. *Annals of the New York Academy of Sciences* 896, 85–95.

28. Gunnar MR, Nelson CA (1994). Event-related potentials in year-old infants: relations with emotionality and cortisol. *Child Development* 65, 80–94.

29. Gunnar MR, Morison SJ, Chisholm K, Schuder M (2001). Salivary cortisols in children adopted from Romanian orphanages. *Development and Psychopathology* 13, 611–628.

30. Lupien SJ, King S, Meaney MJ, McEwen BS (2001). Can poverty get under your skin? Basal cortisol levels and cognitive function in children from low and high socio-economic status. *Development and Psychopathology* 13, 653–676.

31. Kristenson M (1998). The LiVicordia study: possible causes for the differences in coronary heart disease mortality between Lithuania and Sweden. *Linkoping University Medical Dissertations No. 547*, Linkoping University.

32. Hertzman C (1995). *Environment and health in Central and Eastern Europe*. The World Bank, Washington, DC.

33. Antonovsky A (1993). The structure and properties of the sense of coherence scale. *Social Science and Medicine* 36, 725–733.

34. Karasek R, Theorell T (1990). *Healthy work: stress, productivity, and the reconstruction of working life*. Basic Books, New York.

35. Sapolsky RM (1995). Social subordinance as a marker of hypercortisolism: some unexpected subtleties. *Annals of the New York Academy of Sciences* 771, 626–639.

36. Noble KG, Wolmetx ME, Ochs LG, Farah MJ, McCandliss BD (2006). Brain–behavior relationships in reading acquisition are modulated by socioeconomic status factors. *Developmental Science* 9, 642–654.

37. Weeks DJ, Chua R, Weinberg H, Elliott D, Cheyne D (2002). A preliminary study using magnetoencephalography to examine brain function in Downs' syndrome. *Journal of Human Movement Studies* 42, 1–18.

38. Power C, Hertzman C (1999). Health, well-being and coping skills. In: Keating D, Hertzman C, ed. *Developmental health and the wealth of nations*. Guilford Press, New York.

39. Andrews SR, Blumenthal JB, Johnson DL, Kuhn AJ, Ferguson CJ, Lasater TM, *et al.* (1982). *The skills of mothering: a study of parent–child development centres*. Monographs of the Society for Research in Child Development 47.

40. Wasik BH, Ramey CT, Bryant DM, Sparling JJ (1990). A longitudinal study of two early intervention strategies: Project Care. *Child Development* 61, 1682–1696.

41. Garber HL, Heber R (1981). The efficacy of early intervention with family rehabilitation. In: Begab MJ, Haywood HC, Garber HL, ed. *Psychosocial influences in retarded performance: volume 2, strategies for improving competence*. University Park Press, Baltimore, MD.

42. Horacek HJ, Ramey CT, Campbell FA, Hoffman KP, Fletcher FH (1987). Predicting school failure and assessing early intervention with high-risk children. *American Academy of Child Adolescent Psychiatry* 26, 758–763.

43. Campbell FA, Ramey CT (1994). Effects of early intervention on intellectual and academic achievement: a follow-up study of children from low-income families. *Child Development* 65, 684–698.

44. Campbell FA, Ramey CT, Pungello E, Sparling J, Miller-Johnson S (2002). Early childhood education: young adult outcomes from the Abecedarian project. *Applied Developmental Science* 6, 42–57.

45. Weikart DP (1989). Early childhood education and primary prevention. *Prevention in Human Services* 6, 285–306.

46. Schweinhart LJ, Barnes HV, Weikart DP (1993). *Significant benefits: the High/Scope Perry Preschool Study through age 27*. Monographs of the High/Scope Educational Research Foundation 10.

47. Schweinhart LJ (2004). *The High/Scope Perry preschool study through age 40*. High/Scope Educational Research Foundation.

48. Karoly LA, Kilburn MR, Cannon JS, Bigelow JH, Christina R (2005). Many happy returns: early childhood programs entail costs, but the paybacks could be substantial. *Rand Review* 29, 10–17.

49. Elder GH (1986). Military times and turning points in men's lives. *Developmental Psychology* 22, 233–245.

50. Werner EE (1989). High-risk children in young adulthood: a longitudinal study from birth to 32 years. *American Journal of Orthopsychiatry* 59, 72–81.

51. Irwin LG, Siddiqi A, Hertzman C (2007). *Early child development: a powerful equalizer.* Final Report for the World Health Organization's Commission on the Social Determinants of Health. Human Early Learning Partnership, WHO, Geneva.

52. Belsky J, Melhuish E, Barnes J, Leyland AH, Romaniuk H (2006). Effects of Sure Start local programmes on children and families: early findings from a quasi-experimental, cross sectional study. *British Medical Journal* 332, 1476–1481.

53. Janus M, Offord DR (2000). Reporting on readiness to learn in Canada *ISUMA. Canadian Journal of Policy Research* 1, 71–75.

54. D'Anguilli A, Warburton W, Lloyd JEV, Kinar K, Irwin L, Dahinten S, Hertzman C (submitted). Grade-four basic skills are associated with pre-school vulnerability.

55. Ostry A, Marion SA, Green L, Demers PA, Hershler R, Kelly S, *et al.* (2000). Downsizing and industrial restructuring in relation to changes in psychosocial conditions of work in British Columbia sawmills. *Scandinavian Journal of Work, Environment and Health* 26, 273–278.

56. Chamberlayne B, Green B, Barer ML, Hertzman C, Lawrence WJ, Sheps SB (1998). Creating a population-based linked health database: a new resource for health services research. *Canadian Journal of Public Health* 89, 270–273.

57. Ostry A, Tansey J, Maggi S, Dunn J, Hershler R, Chen L, *et al.* (2006). The impact of father's physical and psychosocial work conditions on attempted and completed suicide among their children. *BMC Public Health* 6, 77.

58. Rutter M, Pickles A., Murray R, Eaves L (2001). Testing hypotheses on specific environmental causal effects on behaviour. *Psychological Bulletin* 127, 291–324.

Chapter 6

The life course plot in life course analysis

Tim Cole

Abstract

This chapter considers the life course in the context of an outcome in
later life as related to early growth status, where each subject is assumed
to have been measured as a child at two or more pre-specified ages.
The analysis is by multiple regression, with the outcome as the dependent
variable and the measurements at each age (expressed as z-scores) as the
independent variables. This analysis highlights measurements at any
particular age(s) that are predictive of outcome (size effects), and
simultaneously flags the predictive value of changes in the measurement
over different time intervals (i.e. growth effects). Size and growth are
intimately related, and the life course plot helps to interpret the results.

6.1 Introduction

6.1.1 Life course

Life course research involves the health and lifespan of individuals, and it arises in many
areas of research including psychology, sociology, demography, anthropology and biology.[1] It relates an outcome later in life, commonly health-related, to factors operating at
different stages earlier in life. In the context of chronic disease epidemiology, the life
course approach has been defined as

> the study of long-term effects on chronic disease risk of physical and social exposures during ges-
> tation, childhood, adolescence, young adulthood and later adult life. It includes studies of the bio-
> logical, behavioural and psychological pathways that operate across an individual's life course, as
> well as across generations, to influence the development of chronic diseases.[2]

One characteristic of life course chronic disease epidemiology is that while the outcome is health based, the earlier exposures are often social or behavioural, representing
say inequality measured by socio-economic status or lifestyle.

In contrast to this, one area of chronic disease epidemiology that has come to the fore
in the past two decades has an explicitly biological early exposure, the size and growth of
the individual in early life. The *fetal origins of adult disease* hypothesis originally focused
on birth weight as a proxy for fetal growth, aiming to explain its inverse association with

a variety of adverse adult outcomes in terms of biological programming.[3] More recent developments have extended the period of interest to include post-natal growth, but the approach is still firmly biological.

The pattern of growth is a particularly potent indicator of early life experience, as evidenced by serial measures of weight or height, or other anthropometry. Height and weight data are widely available and give a unique insight into the interaction of genes and environment in the development of the individual through time.

The aim of this chapter is to describe statistical methods to characterize growth patterns in such a way as to relate them to later outcome. The way that the *fetal origins* debate has proceeded over time has to some extent driven the forms of statistical analysis used, starting with simple correlation and proceeding to multiple regression. However, as later sections show, these relatively simple techniques can lead to results that are surprisingly complex to interpret, because of the duality between size and growth. It should be stressed that the more advanced statistical techniques discussed in later chapters do not necessarily help with the interpretation either.

Note that the term 'outcome' is used loosely here to indicate a health measure that occurs no earlier in time than the growth measures, so that any association between them is consistent—at least temporally—with a causal explanation.

6.1.2 Fetal origins of adult disease

The *fetal origins of adult disease* hypothesis (FOAD for short) is probably the best known example of a life course association. It states that poor fetal nutrition, as shown by small size at birth, leads to fetal adaptations that programme the propensity to adult disease.[3] The growth pattern is that seen during gestation, as summarized by birth weight, while the outcome is measured in adulthood and is a proxy for one of the chronic diseases of affluence such as heart disease, stroke, hypertension or type 2 diabetes. These adverse outcomes include all-cause or cause-specific mortality, blood pressure, serum cholesterol, plasma insulin and obesity (weight or body mass index).

The presence of obesity in this list is one of the intriguing aspects of life course research. Obesity has become a major public health concern worldwide in recent decades, its prevalence is rising steeply and it is in its own right a risk factor for adverse health outcome. Patients who are hypertensive, hypercholesterolaemic or hyperinsulinaemic are also likely to be overweight or obese. However, obesity reflects size, and adult size depends on the pattern of growth through childhood. So in epidemiological terms, later size is both an exposure and an outcome, and this dual role poses interesting questions of interpretation.

Evidence in favour of FOAD has steadily accumulated over the past two decades. Many studies have shown a negative correlation between birth weight and adult outcome, but latterly some of them have incorporated an adjustment, using multiple regression, for current (i.e. adult) weight or body mass index. This weight of evidence is summarized by two recent systematic reviews of birth weight related to later blood pressure.[4,5] The two reviews each covered the same 55 studies but came to rather different conclusions. Leon and Koupilova[4] distinguished between studies that adjusted blood pressure for current weight and those that did not. The latter group of 25 studies, unadjusted for current weight, included 20 with a negative birth weight association, of which seven (28 per cent) were significant. In the former group of 31 studies, where current weight *was* adjusted for, 29 showed a negative birth weight association of which 14 (45 per cent) were significant. So there was a higher rate of significance among the studies that adjusted for current weight.

In contrast, Huxley *et al.*[5] took the view that an adjustment for current weight was not appropriate, and they concluded that the birth weight associations, though present, were small and unimportant.

Irrespective of whether or not it can be justified epidemiologically or physiologically, adjusting for later weight does increase the inverse birth weight association. The multiple regression of blood pressure on birth weight and current weight depends on just three correlations: the two weights with blood pressure and one weight with the other. We know that birth weight has a small negative correlation with blood pressure while current weight has a large positive correlation, and birth weight and current weight are weakly positively correlated. So despite their positive correlation with each other, the two weights have opposite effects on blood pressure. This ensures that adjusting for current weight increases the strength of the inverse birth weight versus blood pressure association, though not necessarily making it significant.[6,7]

6.1.3 Use of multiple regression—outcomes and assumptions

Multiple linear regression analysis is a longstanding, powerful and flexible tool for relating the effects of correlated variables to some outcome. As such, it is well suited to life course analysis involving serial anthropometry, where the anthropometry is incorporated in the regression as a set of independent variables—two in the example above, early weight and current weight.

Statistically, the measurement scale of the outcome may be continuous (e.g. blood pressure), binary (presence/absence) or interval (survival), and the regression methodology extends naturally to include logistic regression (for binary outcomes), ordinal regression (ordered categorical outcomes) and Cox regression (for survival type outcomes).

6.2 An example

6.2.1 Split pro-insulin and weight patterns

To illustrate the value of regression analysis, and the difficulties of interpretation that come with it, take the life course example described by Lucas *et al.*[8] This was the first paper to point out the problem. The outcome was split pro-insulin concentration at age 10 years in 358 children born pre-term. Split pro-insulin is a precursor of insulin, and as such is a marker of insulin resistance and a risk factor for later type 2 diabetes. Weight was measured at birth and at several later ages, and its inverse correlation with split pro-insulin was found to be stronger at 18 months than at birth. So the focus here is the multiple regression of split pro-insulin at 10 years on weight at 18 months and 10 years.

The regression coefficients of the two weights are inversely proportional to the standard deviations (SD) of weight at the two ages. In general, weight SD increases with age, being 10 times larger at age 10 than at birth,[9] and this complicates the comparison of the coefficients. To compare like with like, the weights can be adjusted to a common SD, most simply by converting them to z-scores with a mean of zero and an SD of one. A z-score expresses the measurement in units of SDs relative to the median.[10]

So the two weights are converted to z-scores using the revised British growth reference,[9] which includes an adjustment for skewness,[11] and, to adjust for skewness in the outcome, split pro-insulin is 100 times natural log transformed to convert it to percentage units.[12] Table 6.1 model 1a gives the regression equation relating the two weights to outcome, including adjustments for sex and age at the later measurement. It shows the same pattern as for adult blood pressure discussed earlier, i.e. negative early weight and positive current weight effects, and both are highly significant (the ratio of coefficient to standard error is a t-value indicating the significance level, and both coefficients are highly significant with t-values exceeding 4). The current weight coefficient is almost three times that for early weight, +32 per cent compared with −12 per cent. The coefficients indicate the change in split pro-insulin associated with a unit change in weight z-score, i.e. a 1 SD change in weight.

Note the advantages of converting weight to z-scores: it standardizes the weight SDs to 1, which means that the weight regression coefficients are in the same units and can be directly compared with each other; it also adjusts for sex and age, and so compensates for slight variations in measurement timing.

6.3 Duality of size and growth

The weight coefficients in Table 6.1 model 1a are of opposite sign, so that the largest effects on split pro-insulin are seen in subjects whose weight z-score differs substantially at 18 months and 10 years. For example, a child with an early z-score of −1 (i.e. on the 16th centile) and later z-score of +1 (on the 84th centile) has an expected split pro-insulin that is (32 to −12) per cent or 44 per cent higher than for a child with weight z-score 0 (on the 50th centile) at

Table 6.1 Multiple regression analysis of split pro-insulin (percentage) on sex, age at measurement and: (1a) weight z-score at 18 months and 10 years; (1b) weight z-score at 10 years and z-score change from 18 months to 10 years; and (1c) weight z-score at 18 months and z-score change from 18 months to 10 years

Model	Variable	Coefficient	Standard error	t-value	Probability
	Constant	−58	39	−1.5	0.1
	Female sex	32	6.0	5.3	<0.0001
	Age at 10 years	20	3.4	5.7	<0.0001
1a	Weight z at 18 months	−12	2.6	−4.8	<0.0001
	Weight z at 10 years	32	2.7	11.7	<0.0001
1b	Weight z change	12	2.6	4.8	<0.0001
	Weight z at 10 years	20	2.8	7.0	<0.0001
1c	Weight z change	32	2.7	11.7	<0.0001
	Weight z at 18 months	20	2.8	7.0	<0.0001

The constant, sex and age terms are the same in all three models.

both ages. Conversely, a child with the opposite weight pattern of z-score, +1 changing to –1, is expected to have a 44 per cent lower split pro-insulin. So an important factor affecting the prediction is the *change* in weight z-score over time.

This can be seen algebraically. Omitting the sex and age terms, write the regression equation of Table 6.1 model 1a as

$$E(y) = \alpha + \beta_1 z_1 + \beta_2 z_2 \tag{6.1}$$

where y is the outcome, and z_i and β_i are the weight z-scores and their regression coefficients $(i = 1,2)$. The equation can re-arranged as

$$E(y) = \alpha + \beta_1(z_2 - z_1) + (\beta_1 + \beta_2)z_2 \tag{6.2}$$

where now the first term is the change in z-score from early to current, and the coefficient β_1 is the same as for early weight in equation 6.1 as shown in Table 6.1 model 1b. The second term is later weight, but with a numerically smaller coefficient than in equation 6.1 and Table 6.1 model 1a.

This is an important conclusion. Equation 6.1 illustrates the classic FOAD view, that early weight predicts later outcome. The public health implication is that early weight should be maintained where possible by focusing on maternal pregnancy nutrition. Conversely equation 6.2 shows the importance of weight change during childhood, and implies that the increase in weight should be minimized. This focuses the public health intervention in childhood. Yet both conclusions are based on the same data and the same analysis—so which is right?

The question relates to the duality of size and growth. Size here is weight at the two ages, while growth is the rate of change in size; here the change in weight z-score over time. However, these three pieces of information (two sizes and one growth increment) are based on only two measurements, so there is a redundancy—any one of the three can be calculated from the other two. This in turn means that the reparameterization of equation 6.1 in equation 6.2 is just one of an infinite number of reparameterizations.

Equation 6.3 is another parameterization involving weight change and early weight:

$$E(y) = \alpha + \beta_2(z_2 - z_1) + (\beta_1 + \beta_2)z_1 \tag{6.3}$$

Table 6.1 model 1c shows that here weight change is more significant than before $(t = 11.7$ versus 4.8), even though the information in the regression is unchanged. The unpalatable truth is that the three parameterizations in Table 6.1, and all the other possible reparameterizations, are as valid as each other.

It is important to understand how to interpret the parameterizations of size and growth in models 1b and 1c. Take the child shifting from the 16th centile at 18 months to the 84th centile at 10 years, a 2-unit increment in z-score. Each unit increase predicts a 12 per cent increment in split pro-insulin in model 1b and 32 per cent in model 1c, +24 and +64 per cent, respectively. These differ because they are conditioned differently—for later weight in model 1b and early weight in model 1c. If the weight adjustments are included, the two models are seen to be equivalent—add 20 per cent for later weight (z-score +1) in model 1b, and subtract 20 per cent for early weight (z-score -1) in model 1c. The net effect in both cases is $+44$ per cent, the same as for model 1a.

Equations 6.2 and 6.3 show that the regression coefficients for weight change in models 1b and 1c ($-\beta_1$ and β_2) are identical to those for early and later weight, respectively, in model 1a (apart from a sign change). Early and later weight can be viewed as weighted averages of the two weights, with weightings $(1, 0)$ and $(0, 1)$ respectively. In a model including weight change and the weighted average of the two weights, the significance of weight change alters as the weighting varies, while that for weighted average weight does not; note the constancy of the weight coefficients and standard errors in models 1b and 1c. It can be shown that models 1b and 1c are extreme cases—any other weighted average of the two weights gives an intermediate coefficient and standard error for weight change. This usefully demonstrates that however the model is parameterized, the significance of weight change is always within the range of significance seen for the two weights in model 1a.

6.4 Life course plot

The growth chart is used routinely to display the duality of size and growth. For a child weighed on two occasions, the weights are plotted against the ages of measurement, and the slope of the line joining the points is the weight velocity (the slope is the change in weight divided by the time interval between measurements). The chart shows the two weights (size) and also the weight velocity (growth).

As an aside, weight in the present context means weight z-score, so growth velocity is based on change in z-score not change in kg. This matches the clinical assessment of weight change on the growth chart, where relative growth is seen as centile crossing (i.e. z-score change). So growth here should be thought of as z-score change or centile crossing.

Just as size and growth are shown together in the growth chart, it is useful to display visually the results of the regression analysis in Table 6.1 in a form which exploits the size–growth duality. For want of a better name, the plot is called a *life course plot*, as described previously.[13] The two weight regression coefficients are plotted against the ages of measurement, and the line joining the two points added. This joining line summarizes the impact of growth, as opposed to the separate measures of size, on the outcome. The slope of the line is the difference between the two coefficients divided by the time interval between the measurements.

At first sight, this is perplexing, as the difference between the weight coefficients is $\beta_2 - \beta_1$, whereas the weight change coefficients in Equations 6.2 and 6.3 are $-\beta_1$ and β_2, respectively. However a third reparameterization of equation 6.1:

$$E(y) = \alpha + \left(\frac{\beta_2 - \beta_1}{2}\right)(z_2 - z_1) + (\beta_1 + \beta_2)\left(\frac{z_1 + z_2}{2}\right) \tag{6.4}$$

shows that conditioned on *mean* weight, the weight change coefficient is half the difference between the weight coefficients. So the difference between weight coefficients in the life course plot corresponds to twice the weight change coefficient conditioned on mean weight, as in equation 6.4. This symmetric parameterization of weight is a useful compromise over conditioning on one weight or the other. Note too that the weight coefficient in equation 1.4 is $\beta_1 + \beta_2$, the same as in equations 6.2 and 6.3.

Figure 6.1 shows the two weight regression coefficients from model 1a plotted against age, with the line joining them also shown. The fact that the coefficients are of opposite sign means that the points are far apart and the joining line has a steep slope, which highlights the importance of weight gain on the outcome.

6.5 Interactions

6.5.1 Single interactions

The regression models in Table 6.1 assume that the effect on split pro-insulin of weight at each age is the same whatever the child's other weight, i.e. that there is no interaction between early weight and later weight. However, the FOAD hypothesis implies that later weight may be important only or mainly in children who are relatively light early in life, and this needs testing by adding a suitable interaction to the model.

An interaction can be added in many different ways depending on the parameterization used, involving weight change as well as early or later weight, and these are discussed

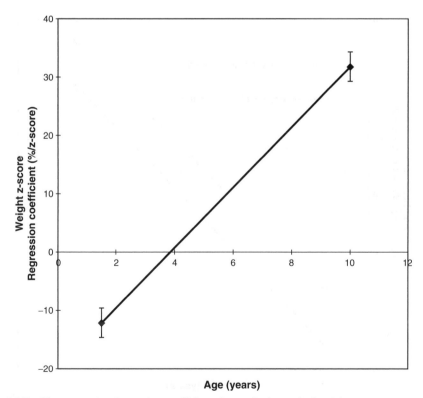

Fig. 6.1 The life course plot. Regression coefficients (± standard errors) of weight z-score at 18 months and 10 years on split pro-insulin at 10 years plotted against the age of measurement. The slope of the line joining the points indicates the importance of weight gain on later split pro-insulin.

in more detail below. However, the FOAD hypothesis focuses on differences in early weight, so a simple way to look for interactions is to divide the data into two equal groups according to their early weight. Figure 6.2 shows the life course plot for the data of Fig. 6.1 split into those whose early weight was on or above the median (upper points), and those with weights below the median (lower points).

Figure 6.2 shows that in the lighter infants, early weight is more important (the early coefficient is larger negative) and current weight less important (the current coefficient is smaller positive). Adding weight–group interactions to model 6.1 tests the significance of the group differences. The z_1 and z_2 coefficients turn out not to be significantly different between groups ($P = 0.13$) though they approach significance. In contrast, the slopes of the lines in Fig. 6.2, which represent the impact of growth on split pro-insulin, are very similar in the two groups, and the interaction term of group with $z_2 - z_1$ is far from significant ($P = 0.6$). This suggests, on the grounds of parsimony, that the important effect here may be growth rather than size, as the growth effect is the same in both light and heavy infants (though this is not particularly strong evidence in favour of the growth interpretation).

However, the growth interpretation also accords with the *growth acceleration* hypothesis recently put forward by Singhal and Lucas,[14] who argue that rapid acceleration soon after

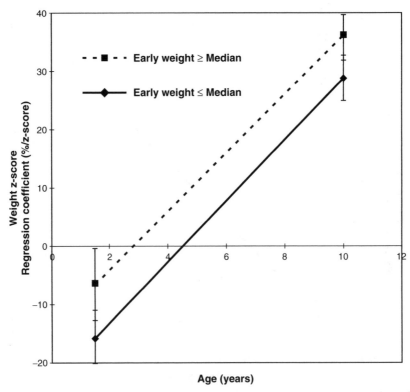

Fig. 6.2 The life course plot of Fig. 6.1 according to early weight status. Early weight has a larger inverse effect on later insulin, and later weight a smaller effect, among lighter infants, while the effect of weight gain (the slopes of the lines) is the same in the two groups.

birth (by which they mean upward weight centile crossing) leads to a poor outcome later. Their hypothesis includes the FOAD hypothesis as a special case, in that low birth weight infants tend to show post-natal catch-up growth. They argue that the risk factor in this group is not so much the low birth weight (as FOAD predicts) as the post-natal catch-up.

6.5.2 Many different interactions

As already shown, the regression model can be parameterized in many different ways and it has two distinct and contradictory interpretations. Extending the model to include an interaction between early weight and later weight introduces further ambiguity. Each parameterization of equation 6.1 has an associated interaction term but, unlike equations 6.1–6.4, the resulting models are distinct from each other. The four parameterizations lead to the following interactions:

◆ early weight with later weight, $z_1 \times z_2$

◆ weight change with later weight, $(z_2 - z_1) \times z_2 = z_2^2 - z_1 \times z_2$

◆ early weight with weight change, $z_1 \times (z_2 - z_1) = z_1 \times z_2 - z_1^2$

◆ mean weight with weight change, $\left(\dfrac{z_1 \times z_2}{2}\right) \times (z_2 - z_1) = \dfrac{z_2^2 - z_1^2}{2}$

Of the four interactions, three involve $z_1 \times z_2$ and three include quadratics in z_1 and/or z_2. In general, the interaction of weight change with a weighted average of the two weights involves the three terms z_1^2, $z_1 \times z_2$ and z_2^2.

The pro-insulin example, with separate models fitted to each half of the data ranked on z_1, corresponds to the interaction of z_1 with z_1 and z_2, i.e. z_1^2 and $z_1 \times z_2$. The quadratic term z_1^2 in the example simplifies to two regression lines of differing slope, one for each half of the z_1 distribution. The life course plot in Fig. 6.2 shows the values of the two corresponding z_1 coefficients, and also the two z_2 coefficients that correspond to the $z_1 \times z_2$ interaction.

However, quadratics in z_1 or z_2 do not represent interactions as such, and $z_1 \times z_2$ is the term to focus on. Adding this to the pro-insulin model 1a in Table 6.1 gives the results seen in Table 6.2 (model 2a), an interaction coefficient of +2.8 which is close to significance ($P = 0.06$).[8] This can be interpreted in either of two symmetric ways: among children with an early weight z-score of +1, the current weight coefficient is increased by this amount, i.e. from 32 to 34.8. Equally for children with a current weight z-score of +1, the earlier weight coefficient is larger by the same amount, increased from −12 to −9.2.

A more complete answer to the parameterization question is to include z_1^2 and z_2^2 in the model with $z_1 \times z_2$. Model 2b in Table 6.2 shows the effect of adding the quadratics, and now the interaction term is far from significant, having been displaced by z_2^2.

The take-home message is that interaction terms are tricky to interpret, but including the corresponding quadratic terms reduces the risk of making the wrong inference.

6.6 Extension to more than two occasions

6.6.1 Repeated measures

So far the discussion has focused on growth curves with measurements at just two ages. However, anthropometry is usually measured repeatedly, and the growth curve and its

Table 6.2 Multiple regression analysis of split pro-insulin (percentage) as in Table 6.1 with the interaction of weight z-score at 18 months and 10 years included; (2a) without and (2b) with quadratics in weight z-score at 18 months and 10 years

Model	Variable	Coefficient	Standard error	t-value	Probability
2a	Weight z at 18 months × weight z at10 years	2.8	1.5	1.9	0.06
2b	Weight z at 18 months × weight z at 10 years	−2.3	2.4	−1.0	0.3
	(Weight z at 18 months)^2	1.5	1.2	1.3	0.2
	(Weight z at 10 years)^2	4.6	1.8	2.5	0.01

The near significance of the interaction vanishes (and even the sign changes) once the 10 year quadratic is added.

associated life course plot can be generalized to multiple measurements. This also allows the effect on outcome of growth over different time periods to be compared. It is achieved by extending the basic model 6.1 to P measurements ($P > 2$):

$$E(y) = \alpha + \sum_{i=1}^{p} \beta_i z_i \qquad (6.5)$$

where z_i for $i = 1 \ldots p$ is the z-score for the ith measurement at age t_i, and β_i is the corresponding regression coefficient. So the outcome is predicted as a linear contrast of z-scores.

Equation 6.5 can be rearranged to focus on measurements at two particular ages:

$$E(y) = \alpha + \beta_1 z_1 + \beta_2 z_2 + \sum_{i=3}^{p} \beta_i z_i \qquad (6.6)$$

Here the ages are numbered 1 and 2 for convenience, but the principle applies to any pair of ages. The first three terms of equation 6.6 are the same as in equation 6.1 and so can be reparameterized as in equations 6.2, 6.3 or 6.4. The last term in equation 6.6 remains unchanged in these reparameterizations, and so makes no difference to the interpretation. This means that all the earlier inferences about a life course plot with two measurements apply equally to pairs of measurements in a life course plot with more than two measurements. It also applies to any other covariates that may be added to the model (e.g. age and sex in Table 6.1), which can be incorporated in the last term of equation 6.6.

6.6.2 Menarcheal age and earlier weight in the NSHD

The extended life course plot is demonstrated using data from the National Survey of Health and Development (NSHD),[15] a sample of British children born in March 1946 measured at 2, 4, 6, 7, 11 and 15 years for height and weight. Birth weight was also recorded, and at 15 years the girls reported their age at menarche. Weight and height at each age are expressed as internal z-scores, after log-transforming weight to account for skewness.

Table 6.3 shows a series of multiple regressions of menarcheal age on previous weight z-score in a sample of 1237 girls. For the 131 girls (11 per cent) still pre-menarcheal at 15, their age at menarche is taken here to be 16 years. The first model (a) includes all five ages

Table 6.3 Multiple regression analyses of age at menarche on weight z-score at earlier ages in 1237 girls from the National Survey of Health and Development: (a) ages 0, 2, 4, 6 and 7 years; (b) omitting 6 years; and (c) also omitting 4 years

Variable	Model a		Model b		Model c	
	Coefficient	t-value	Coefficient	t-value	Coefficient	t-value
Constant	13.2	362	13.2	362	13.2	362
Weight z-score at 0 years	0.126	3.1	0.126	3.1	0.127	3.1
Weight z-score at 2 years	0.128	2.8	0.130	2.8	0.141	3.2
Weight z-score at 4 years	0.040	0.6	0.047	0.8		
Weight z-score at 6 years	0.039	0.4				
Weight z-score at 7 years	−0.540	−6.2	−0.513	−8.9	−0.483	−11.3

from birth to 7 years, and Fig. 6.3 plots the weight z-score coefficients and standard errors in a life course plot. The first four coefficients are positive, of which the first two are significant, while the fifth, at 7 years, is highly significantly negative. From the previous discussion, this suggests that weight change from 6 to 7 years is important for predicting age at menarche, with the girls growing relatively slowly at this time tending to have a later menarche.

However, this interpretation ignores the fact that the 6 year coefficient is not significantly different from zero. It means that weight at 6 years is uninformative when the

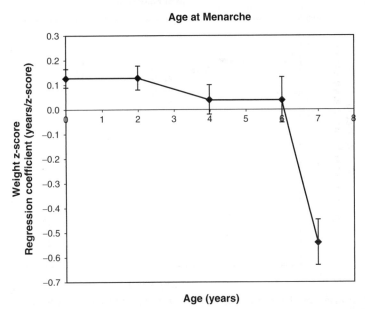

Fig. 6.3 Life course plot of age at menarche by previous weight status. Regression coefficients (± standard errors) of weight z-score at five ages. Age at menarche is later in girls who were relatively heavy at birth and 2 years, and relatively light at 7 years.

other weights are in the model, and therefore it ought not to appear in the plot as it is misleading. Put another way, we saw earlier that the significance of weight change from 6 to 7 years lay in between the significance of weight at 6 and weight at 7. Since weight at 6 is not significant, weight change 6–7 can also be insignificant depending on how weight is parameterized.

Figure 6.4 shows the effect of omitting weight at 6 years, and then subsequently omitting 4-year weight which is also not significant. The other three significant coefficients are little affected, and if anything become slightly more so. Overall there is a clear pattern of a small positive coefficient in the first two years switching to a much larger negative coefficient at 7 years, suggesting that growth from 2 to 7 years is important.

It is tempting to view this as a growth curve for a typical girl with a late menarche. However, this is not quite right—the coefficients at each age reflect the impact of a unit change in weight z-score on age at menarche, adjusted for the other weights in the plot. So the coefficients of +0.13 at birth and 2 years mean that a girl whose early weight z-score is +1 reaches menarche 0.13 years later than average, adjusted for weight at 7. Similarly, the coefficient of –0.5 at age 7 means that a girl with a weight z-score of +1 at age 7 reaches menarche half a year earlier on average, adjusted for her birth weight and weight at 2 years.

Biologically, the life course plot indicates two separate processes operating. Circumstances in early life mean that being above average weight at that age delays

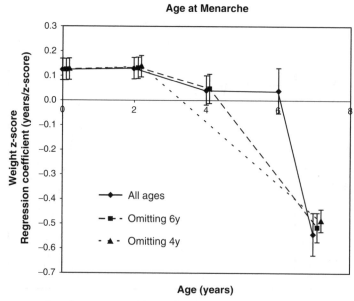

Fig. 6.4 Life course plot of age at menarche by previous weight status, sequentially omitting weights at 6 and 4 years which are conditionally uninformative. The ages are slightly offset for clarity. Age at menarche is later in girls who were relatively heavy at birth and 2 years, and relatively light at 7 years.

puberty, though why this should be is unclear. Then separately, girls with a slow rate of maturation become progressively lighter relative to their peers, so that weight at age 7 adjusted for earlier weight is a proxy for rate of maturation. However, late menarche also equates to a slow rate of maturation, and hence to a relatively low weight at age 7. The life course plot highlights this transition from being heavy in early life to being light at age 7 as a marker of delayed menarche. In this sense, low weight gain from 2 to 7 years predicts delayed menarche.

6.6.3 Height and earlier height in the NSHD

A second example is the outcome of height at 15 years in 1136 girls from the NSHD as predicted by height at the earlier ages of 2, 4, 6, 7 and 11 years. The heights are all converted to internal z-scores and adjusted for age of measurement. Figure 6.5 shows the life course plot based on the multiple regression of height z-score at 15 on height z-score at the five earlier ages. The pattern here is quite different from that in Figs 6.3 and 6.4, in that all the regression coefficients are both significant and positive (with t-values ranging from 2.6 to 10.8). Despite the high correlations between heights at the different ages past 2 years (0.66–0.88), they all contribute significantly to predicting height at age 15.

The size of effect increases roughly linearly with age, the coefficient at age 11 being six times that at age 2. The coefficient at age 11 is 0.33, indicating that a given height effect at this age predicts one-third of the effect at age 15. There also seems to be an important effect between 6 and 7 years, where the joining line is steeper than elsewhere (as seen in the previous example). The t-values for the coefficients at ages 6 and 7 are 3.6 and 7.0,

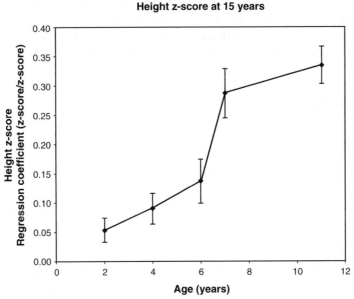

Height z-score at 15 years

Fig. 6.5 Life course plot of height z-score at 15 years by height status from 2 to 11 years. Being tall at any age, conditional on height at other ages, predicts tall stature at 15 years.

respectively, and, following the earlier discussion, this means that the t-value for height change from age 6 to 7 is between 3.6 and 7.0 depending on how the two heights are parameterized. So height gain over this 1 year period does seem to be biologically important, even though it is at a time in childhood when mean height velocity is low. Perhaps it presages the onset of puberty in the most advanced girls, when relatively rapid height gain is a marker of early maturation which predicts completed height growth by 15 years (and hence taller stature). In this sense, it is the reverse of the pattern in Fig. 6.3.

Had the outcome been height at say 20 years rather than 15, the plot would have looked rather different. Age 15 is towards the end of puberty in girls, so that the earlier heights are predicting two separate processes, stage of puberty and adult height. If the outcome had been at a later age, the stage of puberty would have been irrelevant, and height during the upheaval of puberty (e.g. at age 11) would have been less predictive than at earlier ages. As it is, height at age 11 predicts stage of puberty (as does height gain from ages 6 to 7) while the earlier heights predict adult height.

6.7 Disadvantages of the regression approach

The regression approach and its associated life course plot represent a simple tool for the analysis of life course data. However, it has three practical disadvantages: (1) each subject requires a full set of measurements to be included in the analysis; (2) the measurements need to be taken at the same age for each child; and (3) the regression coefficients at different ages are not constrained to vary smoothly across age.

6.7.1 Complete case analysis

The need to exclude from the analysis subjects with missing data is restrictive, and in a longitudinal study can appreciably reduce the sample size. In addition, it introduces bias, as the subjects with incomplete data may differ systematically from those with complete data. Various methods are available to impute the missing data, but using the incomplete data as they stand would be a simpler alternative if possible.

6.7.2 Fixed ages

The measurements through childhood have to be grouped by age to attach a regression coefficient to each corresponding age group. This is not ideal as children may be measured at any age, and indeed may not be measured at all for some periods of time. This is less of a problem in cohort studies where subjects tend to be measured at pre-specified ages, though with some variation around the nominal age, which can be handled in the regression by including the exact age of measurement as an additional covariate.

6.7.3 Collinearity effects

The regression coefficients in the life course plot are conditional on each other, but in general they do not change smoothly with age. This is a disadvantage of the method, since growth is intrinsically a smooth process, and changes in the coefficients over time ought to be smooth too. The example of menarcheal age in Fig. 6.3 shows what can happen, where two measurements are close together in time but very different in value, and the collinearity between them makes the interpretation difficult. Ideally there ought to be some form of constraint to ensure smooth changes in the coefficients over time.

6.8 Why not a regression solution?

These three disadvantages are all addressed by the powerful technique of functional data analysis, which is described in the next section. However, one might reasonably ask (as the editors have!) if there is not a simpler regression approach to achieve the same end.

The difficulty is that the regression coefficients of outcome on, for example, weight for the different ages, i.e. those appearing in the life course plot, cannot be summarized in a single model—each child contributes several measurements but has just one outcome. If it were otherwise, e.g. with each subject contributing several weight measurements and the same number of outcomes, then it would be straightforward to estimate regression coefficients for weight in different age groups. These regression slopes could be plotted against age, as in the life course plot, and the linear trend with age in the slopes could be modelled as a weight by age interaction. In practice, the trend might be more complex than linear, which could be estimated using Hastie and Tibshirani's varying coefficient model,[16] where the age-specific coefficients of outcome on weight are summarized as a cubic smoothing spline in age.

However, for the data structures under discussion here, i.e. a single outcome but multiple measurements, this approach does not work. Instead functional data analysis provides the way forward.

6.9 Functional data analysis

Functional data analysis is a recently developed method of analysing data consisting of serial measurements, where each data series, or growth curve in the present context, is termed functional data.[17] The principle behind functional data analysis is that each child's data series is summarized as a smooth curve, which allows it to be treated as a single entity in the analysis. Ramsay and Silverman describe in detail how to use functional data analysis,[18] providing a library of R functions applied to a wide variety of worked examples.

Regression analysis is feasible with functional data as the dependent or independent variable, and in the present case each child's growth curve is treated as an independent variable. This immediately addresses two of the problems of the regression approach, complete case analysis and fixed ages. Since each child's data are summarized as a curve, the number of measurements and the ages of measurement can vary from child to child. So as long as each child has at least two measurements in the target age range, they contribute to the analysis.

The output from the functional data analysis regression is a smooth regression function plotted against age. This addresses the third disadvantage of the regression approach, the age-specific regression coefficients not changing smoothly with age. For the special case of fixed measurement ages, the functional data analysis regression function is effectively a smooth curve summarizing the age-specific regression coefficients. However, in the general case, with random rather than fixed ages of measurement, age-specific coefficients cannot be calculated as such and the functional data analysis regression function provides a far more powerful and flexible summary of the impact of growth on outcome.

Here functional data analysis is used with the menarcheal age example of Figs 6.3 and 6.4. The data consist of 1810 girls with at least two weights (mean number 4.6), as against the 1237 with all five weights used in the earlier analysis. The results in Fig. 6.6 show four different life course plots, each with a functional data regression function summarizing the relationship between menarcheal age and weight over time. The five regression coefficients derived earlier are also shown. The shape of each regression function is specified by a cubic smoothing spline with the smoothing parameter (smoother) chosen by the user. Figure 6.6 shows smoothers of 0.5, 5, 50 and 500, and as the smoother increases the curve becomes progressively more smooth. The smoother can also be expressed in terms

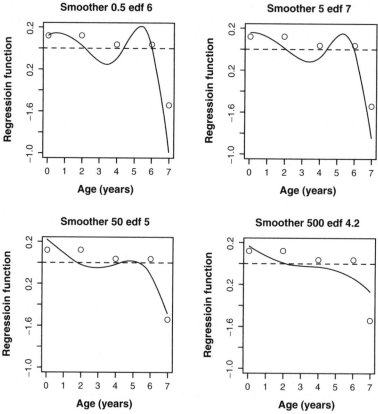

Fig. 6.6 Life course plot of age at menarche by earlier weight status, estimated using functional data analysis. Each plot contains a cubic spline regression function with different degrees of smoothing, indicated by the value of the smoother and its corresponding equivalent degrees of freedom (edf) above each plot. The regression coefficients from Fig. 6.3 are also shown, based on complete case analysis.

of equivalent degrees of freedom (edf), which correspond loosely to the degrees of freedom of a polynomial.

In Fig. 6.6a, the smoother is 0.5 and the edf is 6, corresponding to the five coefficients and intercept in the regression, so there is no smoothing as such. Here the regression function is an exaggerated version of the plot in Fig. 6.3. As the smoother increases, the curve becomes smoother and flatter, as indicated by the reduced edf, but the essential shape of the curve is retained. The optimal value for the smoother is around 50, which smoothes out the curve's peak at 5 years while retaining its cubic shape. In detail, the curve does not pass that close to the fixed-age coefficients. Despite this, the conclusion is broadly the same as for Fig. 6.3, that weight has a positive effect on menarcheal age in early life, followed by a neutral effect for a time, and then a strong negative effect leading up to age 7. In growth terms, the plot highlights the period from 5 to 7 years, where centile crossing downwards is a strong predictor of a later menarche.

6.10 Discussion

This chapter has shown how multiple regression can be used to gain insights into the relationship between, on the one hand, size and growth in childhood, and on the other, later outcome. The fundamental problem with analyses like this is the duality between size and growth, which makes their effects impossible to separate. If outcome is related both to early and later size, but the effects are in opposite directions, then a valid interpretation is that growth over the interval is itself predictive. Precisely this effect is seen in the pro-insulin and menarcheal age examples here, where the life course plot is useful for seeing both the size and growth effects in the same plot. The life course plot has also been applied in other life course analyses.[19,20]

The life course plot shows the size effects in terms of the mutually adjusted regression coefficients at the different ages. In addition, the difference between pairs of coefficients corresponds to the size of the regression coefficient for growth between the two corresponding ages. The significance of this growth effect is typically midway between the significance of the two size effects, depending on how size is parameterized in the regression. For life course plots with more than two points, these conclusions apply to any pair of ages.

Interactions between measures of size at different ages should be tested for but are hard to interpret, as they can also be parameterized in many different ways. In general, it is good practice to include quadratics in the regression when adding an interaction, i.e. for the interaction $z_1 \times z_2$ include the terms z_1^2 and z_2^2 as well.

Functional data analysis provides a powerful tool for extending the life course plot, in that it smoothes the regression coefficients across age while easing the requirement for complete data at specified ages. This is an area with considerable promise.

The biological conclusion from the pro-insulin example is that weight gain during childhood tends to increase pro-insulin at 10 years. Taken with the menarcheal age and height examples, this may reflect the impact of early maturation on outcome. The menarcheal age data have previously been analysed by dos Santos Silva et al.[21] using random coefficients models, and they reach broadly the same conclusions as here, that birth weight has a positive effect, but later growth a negative effect, on the timing of menarche. The sharp change in coefficient from 6 to 7 years seen in Figs 6.3 and 6.6 appears in their Figure 2 as a sudden increase in spacing of the menarche timing-specific curves of body mass index by age.

In conclusion, the relationship between size, growth and later outcome can usefully be investigated using multiple regression analysis. However, the interpretation of the results is not straightforward, and an understanding of the underlying biology is of critical importance to put the findings in context.

Acknowledgements

Data sources were MRC National Survey of Health and Development and MRC Childhood Nutrition Centre. I thank Professor Mike Wadsworth, Professor Di Kuh and Dr Mary Fewtrell for providing access to their data. I have also greatly benefited from discussions with Professor Dave Leon and Dr Bianca de Stavola. Comments on drafts of the paper by Professor Andrew Pickles and Dr de Stavola have been invaluable.

Further reading

Cole TJ (2004). Modeling postnatal exposures and their interactions with birth size. *Journal of Nutrition* 134, 201–204.

Huxley R, Neil A, Collins R (2002). Unravelling the fetal origins hypothesis: is there really an inverse association between birthweight and subsequent blood pressure? *Lancet* 360, 659–665.

Lucas A, Fewtrell M, Cole TJ (1999). Fetal origins of adult disease—the hypothesis revisited. *British Medical Journal* 319, 245–249.

Ramsay JO, Silverman BW (1997). *Functional data analysis*. Springer, New York.

Singhal A, Lucas A (2004). Early origins of cardiovascular disease: is there a unifying hypothesis? *Lancet* 363, 1642–1645.

References

1. Kuh D, Ben-Shlomo Y, Lynch J, Hallqvist J, Power C (2003). Life course epidemiology. *Journal of Epidemiology and Community Health* 57, 778–783.

2. Ben-Shlomo Y, Kuh D (2002). A life course approach to chronic disease epidemiology: conceptual models, empirical challenges and interdisciplinary perspectives. *International Journal of Epidemiology* 31, 285–293.

3. Barker DJP (1998). *Mothers, babies and health in later life*. Churchill Livingstone, Edinburgh.

4. Leon DA, Koupilova I (2000). Birth weight, blood pressure, and hypertension: epidemiological studies. In: Barker DJP, ed. *Fetal origins of cardiovascular and lung disease*. Marcel Dekker, New York.

5. Huxley R, Neil A, Collins R (2002). Unravelling the fetal origins hypothesis: is there really an inverse association between birthweight and subsequent blood pressure? *Lancet* 360, 659–665.

6. Tu YK, West R, Ellison GT, Gilthorpe MS (2005). Why evidence for the fetal origins of adult disease might be a statistical artifact: the 'reversal paradox' for the relation between birth weight and blood pressure in later life. *American Journal of Epidemiology* 161, 27–32.

7. Cole TJ (2005). Re: Why evidence for the fetal origins of adult disease might be a statistical artifact: the 'reversal paradox' for the relation between birth weight and blood pressure in later life [letter]. *American Journal of Epidemiology* 162, 394–395.

8. Lucas A, Fewtrell M, Cole TJ (1999). Fetal origins of adult disease—the hypothesis revisited. *British Medical Journal* 319, 245–249.

9. Freeman JV, Cole TJ, Chinn S, Jones PRM, White EM, Preece MA (1995). Cross sectional stature and weight reference curves for the UK, 1990. *Archives of Diseases in Childhood* 73, 17–24.

10. Cole TJ (1999). The importance of Z scores in growth reference standards. In: Johnston FE, Zemel B, Eveleth PB, ed. *Human growth in context*. Smith-Gordon, London, pp. 75–83.

11. Cole TJ, Green PJ (1992). Smoothing reference centile curves: the LMS method and penalized likelihood. *Statistics in Medicine* 11, 1305–19.

12. Cole TJ (2000). Sympercents: symmetric percentage differences on the 100 log$_e$ scale simplify the presentation of log transformed data. *Statistics in Medicine* 19, 3109–3125.

13. Cole TJ (2004). Modeling postnatal exposures and their interactions with birth size. *Journal of Nutrition* 134, 201–204.

14. Singhal A, Lucas A (2004). Early origins of cardiovascular disease: is there a unifying hypothesis? *Lancet* 363, 1642–1645.

15. Wadsworth MEJ (1991). *The imprint of time*. Clarendon Press, Oxford.

16. Hastie T, Tibshirani R (1993). Varying-coefficient models. *Journal of the Royal Statistical Society Series B* 55, 757–796.

17. Ramsay JO, Silverman BW (1997). *Functional data analysis*. Springer, New York.

18. Ramsay JO, Silverman BW (2002). *Applied functional data analysis*. Springer, New York.

19. Primatesta P, Falaschetti E, Poulter NR (2005). Birth weight and blood pressure in childhood—Results from the Health Survey for England. *Hypertension* 45, 75–79.

20. Stettler N, Stallings VA, Troxel AB, Zhao J, Schinnar R, Nelson SE, *et al.* (2005). Weight gain in the first week of life and overweight in adulthood—A cohort study of European American subjects fed infant formula. *Circulation* 111, 1897–1903.

21. dos Santos Silva I, De Stavola B, Mann V, Kuh D, Hardy H, Wadsworth M (2002). Prenatal factors, childhood growth trajectories and age at menarche. *International Journal of Epidemiology* 31, 405–412.

Chapter 7

Methods for handling missing data

Paul Clarke and Rebecca Hardy

Abstract

We begin by describing helpful typologies of missing data based on pattern and non-response mechanisms. We summarize a collection of commonly used but imperfect methods for dealing with missing data at the analysis stage. Three more rigorous methods, maximum likelihood, multiple imputation and weighting, are also considered.

7.1 The problem of missing data and the purpose of this chapter

Missing data are an almost unavoidable problem in experimental and observational research. There are many reasons for missing values in a data set, particularly when humans are the study unit of interest: cost considerations may have forced researchers to design a study in which complex physical measurements were taken only on a random subsample of study participants, rather than everyone in the study; it may have been impossible to contact everybody who was sampled; people may mistakenly have believed that some questions did not apply to them because they misread the questionnaire or misunderstood the interviewer; individuals may have refused to answer a sensitive question, such as one about their sexual behaviour, or refused to allow a physical measurement, such as a blood sample, to be taken.

While the missing data problem affects research in all areas, such as epidemiology, medicine and social science, the nature of life course research means that the problem may be particularly acute. Life course epidemiology concerns the analysis of how risk is accumulated during the different stages of individuals' lives, and the effect on these individuals of following different pathways through life. To address complex hypotheses concerning processes that develop over time, modelling techniques that incorporate a time dimension are required. Such techniques demand data from retrospective cross-sectional or prospective longitudinal studies, both of which are particularly prone to missing data. In the former case, it is usual for retrospective questions to have higher rates of non-response because individuals are unable to remember the relevant information in sufficient detail (or at all). In the latter case, the reasons for missing values listed above act on each wave of the study and the amount of incomplete data accumulates. While measurement error and response bias are also issues with retrospective data, they are taken to be beyond the scope of this chapter and the reader is referred elsewhere for further details (e.g. see Chapters 2, 8 and 9).

Why should we be worried about missing data? Most basic statistical routines require a complete data set with no missing values. So why not just discard the cases with missing values and just analyse the subsample of cases with complete data—a 'complete cases' analysis? Two important reasons are:

- High rates of missing data are often associated with poor study design, which can lead to low user confidence. Thus, the best studies use procedures to minimize the missing data rate.[1] However, even high-quality studies such as the National Survey of Health and Development that use such procedures still have appreciable rates of missing data.[2]

- Complete cases analyses can often yield biased estimates, of both the model parameters and their standard errors. Bias is a systematic error that can cause misleading conclusions to be drawn. Unlike random error (as quantified by significance tests or confidence intervals), bias does not decrease as the study size increases.

Complete cases analysis is just one of many approaches to handling missing data, but it is currently the most often used in life course epidemiology. There are a variety of other approaches, of varying complexity. No matter how complicated, each approach gives unbiased estimates only if certain assumptions (either explicit or implicit) about how the data came to be missing are true. The more sophisticated the method, the weaker these assumptions are (i.e. the more likely it is that they are true). If an inappropriate choice of approach is made, then misleading, biased estimates of the model parameters and their standard errors will result. It is therefore vital that analysts understand the assumptions made by each method, so that they can judge which method is the most appropriate for a particular application, and whether or not the results could be badly biased.

In this chapter, we do not set out to review the extensive literature in this area, as there are already a number of comprehensive reviews;[3–5] nor do we set out to provide a series of worked examples which researchers can follow to implement different methods. Instead, we aim to introduce a selection of methods for handling missing data, and outline some steps with which an appropriate one can be chosen. We focus on explaining the statistical reasoning behind each step, and the strengths and limitations of each method. These methods were chosen because: (1) they can be used for handling missing data in analyses based on statistical models for life course epidemiology, such as regression, proportional hazards (Cox) and structural equation models; and (2) they are relatively simple to implement, or are available as part of popular software packages.

7.2 Statistical models

The methods we consider are appropriate for handling missing data carried out using three types of statistical model suitable for life course research. Each method is described in terms of a generic epidemiological analysis that can be carried out using these models, which are:

1. *Regression models.* A regression model here refers to the appropriate generalized linear model for outcome Y. For example, if the error distribution is normal, then we refer to the normal linear regression model; if Y is dichotomous, then we refer to the logistic

regression model; and so on. The generic epidemiological analysis considers the effect of exposure E on outcome Y adjusted for confounding variable X; both covariates, X and E, may be multivariate.

2. *Cox models.* The outcome Y is a dichotomous event indicator. In addition to E and X, there is also censoring indicator C and follow-up time T at which time the follow-up was censored or the event occurred. Missing values on Y are naturally handled by censoring in Cox models under certain assumptions we will discuss further on. Thus we shall focus on missing data among covariates E and X.

3. *Structural equation models.* Structural equation models are an important generalization of regression models which can be used to specify growth curve models for analysing individual change using repeated measures data.[6] Whereas regression and multiple regression models classically allow for a single outcome variable and a number of covariates, the structural equation framework divides observed, or manifest, variables into endogenous variables determined by other variables in the system, and exogenous variables whose values are fixed. For growth curve models, the repeated outcomes Y are always endogenous, but covariates E and X can be a mixture of endogenous and exogenous variables. We consider missing data among the manifest (non-latent) variables.

7.3 Analysing the missing data

The first step in any analysis should involve becoming familiar with the characteristics of the data set being studied. This is also true when deciding on which method to use for handling missing data: an informed choice about how to handle missing data can only be made if the pattern of the missing values and the extent of missing data on each variable are known.

At this stage, we shall make a distinction between missing data in the study as a whole, and missing data in a particular analysis involving a subset of variables. For cross-sectional and longitudinal surveys, there are many variables measured on the study participants, possibly repeated measures over multiple waves. Hence, the 'study pattern' of missing data can be very complex. However, as it is likely that an analysis will involve a small subset of the study variables, the 'analysis pattern' will be less complex. For the present, we will refer only to the analysis pattern when referring to missing data, but the reader should be aware that there are occasions where the study pattern is also important. This issue will be referred to again further on.

The pattern of missing values is simply the arrangement of missing responses in the data set being studied. Missing values will often be denoted by special codes to avoid confusion with valid responses; for example, -9 is often used to denote a missing value in the British Household Panel Study. If there are multiple reasons for missing data, most software packages allow the user to specify different value codes for missing values, and to label these values. It is important at this stage to make a distinction between genuine missing values (i.e. those where a response was expected but none was obtained) and 'not applicable' values; for example, a man does not respond to a question about the number of times they themselves have been pregnant. If it is unnecessary to discriminate between different reasons for missing values, then most software packages allow 'system missing' values to be set.

The potential complexity of missing value patterns clearly increases in line with the number of variables. It is therefore useful to introduce a terminology which broadly speaking describes the main types of missing value patterns. Some examples of these types are shown in Table 7.1. The rows of the data set denote individuals/cases/participants, and the columns denote the three different variables in the generic epidemiological analysis.

- *Univariate.* The variables can be divided into two groups: (1) variables with no missing data (E, Y); and (2) a variable with some values observed and some missing (X).

- *Multivariate.* The same as a univariate pattern, except that group 2 can include more than one variable. Group 1 contains the variables that are always fully observed (Y), and group 2 contains the variables that are either fully observed or missing (E, X). Some authors also refer to this a univariate pattern, but we have decided to draw a distinction between them.

- *Monotone.* In general, the variables can be divided into G groups, where group 1 is fully observed and so 'more observed' than group 2, which in turn is more observed than group 3, and so on. A variable is more observed than another variable if (1) for all cases where it is observed, the other variable may be observed or unobserved, and (2) for all cases where it is missing, the other variable will also be missing. In this example, there are three groups, where Y is more observed than E, and E is more observed than X; notice that E is more observed than X because all cases with E observed either have X observed or missing, and all cases with E missing also have X missing.

- *Non-monotone.* Any pattern that is not univariate, multivariate or monotone.

Note that the variable ordering in Table 7.1 is not necessarily the natural ordering in the data set; it may be necessary for the analyst to rearrange the variables to show whether the missing value pattern is multivariate or monotone. The packages *SPSS*, *SAS* and *S-Plus* all have facilities to examine missing value patterns, as does the stand-alone specialist software for missing data *SOLAS* (http:\\www.statsol.ie\solas\solas.htm). As will become apparent further on, the pattern of missing values is important: simple patterns of missing data can make strong assumptions about the missing data more believable, and permit the use of simple methods.

7.4 Missing data assumptions

7.4.1 The non-response mechanism

It is rare for missing data to occur randomly. Generally, missing data are the result of a process (or processes) determined by unknown factors beyond the control of the study designers. This process is called the 'non-response mechanism'. Schafer and Graham[5] pointed out that this is a nebulous term, often used to describe one or more processes by which the data came to be missing. Some examples are given in the list below.

Table 7.1 Examples of univariate, multivariate, monotone and non-monotone missing value patterns for a three-variable analysis of Y, E, X

Cases	Univariate (a)			Multivariate (b)			Monontone (c)			Non-monotone (d)		
	Y	E	X	Y	E	X	Y	E	X	Y	E	X
1–25	O	O	O	O	O	O	O	O	O	O	O	O
26–50	O	O	O	O	O	O	O	O	?	?	O	O
51–75	O	O	?	O	?	?	O	O	?	O	?	O
76–100	O	O	?	O	?	?	O	?	?	?	?	O

The table contains four examples of missing value patterns for a study of 100 cases with measurements on Y, E, X. The first row denotes the missing value pattern for the first 25 individuals, the second row the for individuals 26–50, and so on. A column with O denotes that all the individuals within this group have the value corresponding to this variable observed; whereas a column with a ? denotes that the variable is missing for all individuals in this group.

Reasons for non-response in cross-sectional and longitudinal studies:

◆ *Unit non-response.* After sampling households or individuals using a random sampling design, it may not be possible to contact the selected individuals (by mail, telephone or interview), or the person may refuse to participate in the study.

◆ *Item non-response.* The questionnaire may be returned or the interview carried out, but the individual may refuse to answer certain questions, simply not know the answer to a question (particularly common for retrospective questions with long recall periods) or mistakenly fail to provide an answer (e.g. misreading the question or questionnaire routing).

Reasons for non-response in longitudinal studies only:

◆ *Attrition/drop-out.* After taking part in the first wave (or first few waves) of a study, an individual may: refuse to participate in any subsequent wave; die; be impossible to follow-up because they have moved house, emigrated, etc.

◆ *Wave non-response.* This is similar to attrition, but here the individual has been re-contacted and participates in further waves after previously not participating.

The factors causing the missing data are usually unknown. However, the possibility that these unknown factors will be associated with the variables in the analysis remains. In practice, this means that individuals with one missing value pattern may have very different epidemiological characteristics (health outcomes, exposures and confounders) from those individuals with another. Failure to account for these differences in the analysis will thus lead to non-response bias, i.e. biased model estimates caused by failure to handle the missing data properly. In sample surveys, it can be the case that missing data are caused by more than one non-response mechanism, each with very different causes; for example, non-contact and refusal in household interview surveys.[7] We will not pursue this issue further here and henceforth assume multiple processes to be strongly associated with each other.

Many (but not all) methods for handling missing data will give unbiased estimates of the analyst's model parameters provided that specific assumptions about the non-response mechanism hold. It is difficult to determine whether these assumptions are true or not because the factors causing missing data are rarely known. In addition, it is not guaranteed that any of the variables in an analysis will associate strongly with the factors causing non-response, which means that handling missing data is always an approximate exercise, with the aim being to minimize the bias given the available data. Given these qualifiers, we shall now consider the different types of missing data assumption.

7.4.2 Missing data assumptions

Assumptions about how the data came to be missing fall into three groups. Classification depends on which variables are believed to be most strongly associated with the factors causing missing data. These assumptions are:

* *MCAR: missing completely at random.* The missing values are distributed randomly across the data set.

* *MAR: missing at random.* For each individual, the probability of a missing value (or values) depends on the values of their observed variables.

* *MNAR: missing not at random.* For each individual, the probability of a missing value depends on the values of the missing variables and, possibly, the values of the observed variables.

Let us consider these assumptions in increasing order of complexity. If the data are assumed to be MCAR, then all occurrences of the missing values within an individual are random, i.e. each of the variables is equally likely to be missing. If we were able to be sure that the data were MCAR, then the problems associated with non-response are relatively simple, no matter what is being estimated or the extent and pattern of missing values in the data set. However, in practice, it should be remembered that MCAR is only an assumption, and a very strong one which does not often hold.

The next most complex assumption is MAR, an assumption widely made in practice, particularly as many methods are available for handling MAR data. It is thus pertinent to devote space here to a more careful consideration of what this assumption implies, which is less straightforward than is widely believed.

From the general definition given above, MAR data are the result of a non-response mechanism where the probability that an individual has a variable (or variables) missing depends on their observed variables. In multivariate problems, MAR thus defines a wide 'family' of different non-response mechanisms; depending on the data set, different individuals may have different variables observed and missing, and the true non-response mechanism may depend on some but not all of the observed variables. Given the nebulous nature of the MAR assumption, we shall now introduce two further definitions which are useful in practice.

* *Stratified-MCAR.* Conditionally on variables which are fully observed, the remaining variables are MCAR. For example, consider the variables Y, E, X in Table 7.1, where confounder X is completely observed but Y and E are incompletely observed, as in pattern d. If the data are stratified-MCAR then the probability that either Y or E or both are missing depends only on X. Stratified-MCAR is often called 'covariate-dependent drop-out' in longitudinal studies.

- *General-MAR.* Consider the following situation where there are four variables, Y is fasting blood glucose (FBG), E is body mass index (BMI) and X is age and sex. If we believe that the data are general-MAR but not stratified-MCAR, then for the individuals with FBG, BMI, age and sex all observed, the most complex non-response mechanism producing general-MAR data would have the following property: the probability that these values are missing depends on FBG, BMI, age and sex (and it follows therefore that the probability these variables are observed *also* depends on FBG, BMI, age and sex). For individuals with only BMI observed, the probability that other variables are missing depends on BMI, and so on.

In practice, the stratified-MCAR assumption is often used as a proxy for the MAR, when it is truer to say it is a member of the MAR family. Why is this distinction important? The answer is, the stratified-MCAR assumption can often be implausible (especially for non-monotone patterns), but the plausibility of mechanisms generating general-MAR data must also be pondered carefully.

First consider the situation for univariate, multivariate or monotone missing value patterns. The plausibility of the stratified-MCAR depends on the variables that are fully observed; if there are only a few such variables, and/or the fully observed variables are unlikely to be associated with the probability of non-response, the stratified-MCAR assumption is hard to sustain. However, a non-response mechanism that is general-MAR could still plausibly have generated the missing value pattern, because the non-response mechanism depends on a less limited set of variables.

Secondly, for non-monotone patterns, the same situation is also true, with the additional possibility that no variables are fully observed. In this case, the data *cannot* be stratified-MCAR, but they could be general-MAR. Robins and Gill[8] considered the types of non-response mechanism capable of producing MAR data with non-monotone missing value patterns, and named them 'random monotone missingness' (RMM) processes. The mechanisms for generating such data are necessarily complex, even convoluted, because the probability of missing values will vary between individuals depending on which variables were observed for each. RMM processes can also be shown to generate general-MAR data when the missing value pattern is univariate, multivariate or monotone, but the mechanisms are less complex and more plausible.

It is thus clear that when the stratified-MCAR assumption is implausible for a particular data set and the missing value pattern is non-monotone, careful thought must be paid to whether an RMM process is a plausible mechanism for generating the observed data. If it is not, then careful consideration must be given to whether the data can be assumed to be MAR at all. Moreover, as will be shown further on, while some methods are appropriate for stratified-MCAR data, they are not valid for general-MAR data.

The crucial distinction between non-response mechanisms causing MNAR data and those causing MCAR or MAR data is that the non-response probabilities depend on missing variable values. As will be discussed, this poses particular modelling problems that often require complex, computer-intensive solutions which are not available in standard software. As such, methods for MNAR data are not considered in this chapter. This does not mean that we consider the MNAR assumption to be unimportant (in many cases, it will be the only plausible choice), but the statistical and computational issues would require a further chapter to explain. Instead, the reader is referred to Little and Rubin[4] for an overview of methods for MNAR data.

7.4.3 Ignorable non-response

A concept closely related to MCAR and MAR is that of 'ignorable non-response'. Rubin[9] showed that to get unbiased estimates from an analysis of the incomplete data, it is generally necessary to model the data and the non-response mechanism; hence the expression 'non-ignorable'. However, under certain conditions, it is not necessary to model the non-response mechanism and so it is ignorable. When the data are MCAR, in almost every practical application the non-response mechanism is ignorable. Conversely, MNAR data are always the result of a non-ignorable non-response mechanism.

The situation for MAR data is less clear-cut. In Section 7.5, we shall divide methods for missing data into 'simple' and 'proper' methods. Broadly speaking, proper methods use information from both the complete and incomplete cases, usually through a likelihood function, to inform belief about the distribution of the missing values. Rubin[9] showed that the non-response mechanism is ignorable for MAR data provided that estimation is based on the likelihood function for the observed data, but in general requires that the data are MCAR. Simple methods are not based on observed data likelihoods, so the idea of ignorability is less useful.

7.5 Simple methods

7.5.1 How simple methods work

The methods we consider in this section are referred to as 'simple' because they are well known and relatively easy to implement without special software. This term is not to be taken too literally; as will become clear, some apparently simple methods become far from simple where standard error estimation or complex missing value patterns are concerned. As spelt out in Section 7.3, we focus on the pattern of missing values in one particular analysis, i.e. if our analytical data (sub-)set has three variables, we assume that we wish to make inferences about associations among these three variables, such as regression coefficients between an outcome and two covariates. We are also supposing that all the variables in our data set are associated with each other. Further on, we will show how independence or conditional independence between variables at the population level can often simplify things considerably.

We consider five simple methods in all: complete cases analysis, the indicator method, mean imputation, regression imputation and hot-deck imputation. The indicator and mean imputation methods are considered only as examples of methods that should *not* be used.

Simple methods such as complete cases analysis and hot-deck imputation use only information from the complete cases data to estimate the missing values. For individuals with a particular missing value pattern in which the missing variables are M and the observed variables O, it can be shown that the simple methods we consider require that the data are MCAR or MAR *and*

$$\Pr(M|O, \text{complete case}) = \Pr(M|O). \qquad (*)$$

holds, where $\Pr(M|O)$ represents the probability distribution of the missing variables given the observed variables for everyone in the population, and $\Pr(M|O, \text{complete case})$ represents this probability distribution among the complete cases. However, ($*$) does not hold in general. From the laws of probability, for any particular missing value pattern we can say only that

$$\Pr(M|O, \text{complete case}) = \frac{\Pr(\text{complete case}|O, M)\,\Pr(M|O)}{\sum_{\text{vals of } M} \Pr(\text{complete case}|O, M)\,\Pr(M|O)}$$

where $\Pr(\text{complete case}|O, M)$ is the probability of being a complete case given the observed and the missing variables, and the numerator involves summation over all possible values the missing variables could have taken.

To illustrate when ($*$) holds, consider again the example where outcome Y is FBG, exposure E is BMI, and X represents two confounders, age and sex. Then consider a data set with the following missing value patterns: as well as complete cases, the first involves individuals with age missing (M = age, O = FBG, BMI, sex), and the second has both FBG and age missing (M = FBG, age, O = BMI, sex). Now consider the situation under different assumptions about the missing data:

1. MCAR: for both patterns, $\Pr(\text{complete case}|O, M) = \Pr(\text{complete case})$ and the general expression simplifies to ($*$). This is true for individuals with any missing value pattern.

2. Stratified-MCAR: this assumption states that $\Pr(\text{complete case}|O, M) = \Pr(\text{complete cases}|S)$, where S is fully observed. In our example, only sex is fully observed and so S = sex, then ($*$) holds because sex is not in M for either pattern (Note that this depends on sex being associated with the non-sex mechanism.

3. General-MAR: recall that, under general-MAR, the probability a variable is missing depends on the values of the observed variables, i.e. in this example $\Pr(\text{complete case}|O, M) = \Pr(\text{complete case}|\text{FBG, BMI, age, sex})$, and so ($*$) cannot hold.

The example above makes clear the important distinction between stratified-MCAR and general-MAR when using simple methods. Even if the missing value pattern is a simple univariate or multivariate type, in order to apply the simple methods described below it is important to understand that the assumption being made is stratified-MCAR, and not general-MAR. A corollary of this is that for complex non-monotone patterns where there are no fully observed variables, or where the stratified-MCAR assumption is unreasonable, simple methods cannot be applied.

A brief summary of the simple methods is given below.

Complete cases analysis

Simply fit the analyst's model to the subsample of complete cases. This is called 'listwise deletion' in *SPSS*.

Indicator method

This is for covariates or exogenous variables only. Suppose that covariate X is incomplete. Replace X in the regression model with $OX = X$ if X was observed, and 0 otherwise; and $IX = 1$ if X is missing and 0 otherwise. Fit the regression model to the observed data.

Mean imputation

Imputation describes a large family of methods by which missing values are imputed, or 'filled-in', using some 'imputation model' for the values; the analyst's model is then fitted to the 'imputed data', namely the set of observed and imputed data. To describe mean imputation, consider the following simple example where only exposure E is incompletely observed. Mean imputation proceeds by replacing the missing values of E by the sample mean of E from the available cases. Using this approach, any set of incomplete variables can be imputed.

Regression imputation

Suppose again that only E is incomplete. Each missing value of E is replaced by a prediction of its expected value given the other variables that are observed. For example, if E were a continuous exposure, then

$$E^* = \hat{\alpha} + \hat{\beta}X + \hat{\gamma}Y,$$

could be used, where $\hat{\alpha}, \hat{\beta}, \hat{\gamma}$ are estimated by fitting the linear regression of E on X and Y to the complete cases. Recall that X and Y are observed for all individuals in this example; in general, if X was missing instead, then X^* could be estimated from the regression of X on E and Y. Variations on this basic method are possible by adding polynomial or piecewise-linear terms to the linear predictor, or using logistic, Poisson, etc. regression models if the missing variable is a count or categorical, or adding random noise to the expected value. See Little[10] and Little and Rubin[4] for details on regression imputation methods. Regression imputation is implemented in *SPSS*, and in *SAS* and *SOLAS* as 'predictive mean matching', together with an algorithm for calculating estimated standard errors.

Hot-deck imputation

Consider again an incomplete case with E missing but with X and Y fully observed. The complete cases are called 'donors', and imputation proceeds by taking a value of E from the donor with values E^*, X^*, Y^* such that

$$|(X - X^*, Y - Y^*)| = \min\nolimits_{\text{all } i \text{ in the complete cases}} |(X - X_i, Y - Y_i)|,$$

that is, the donor whose values of X and Y are closest to those of the incomplete case, where 'closeness' is assessed using the Euclidean distance defined by $|(A, B)| = \sqrt{A^2 + B_2}$.

If more than one case satisfies this equation, then the donor is drawn at random from the donors satisfying the equation. Similarly, for an incomplete case with both E and Y missing, imputation proceeds by taking the pair E and Y from the donor with values E^*, X^*, Y^* such that

$$|X - X^*| = \min_{\text{all } i \text{ in the complete cases}} |X - X_i|.$$

Further refinements to this basic rule are possible, depending on the measurement scales of the variables, e.g, using the Mahabalonis distance. Reilly[11], Relly and Pepe,[12] and Little and Rubin[4] consider the hot-deck method and its implementation in more detail.

Before proceeding further and showing how to choose which of these methods to use, we first remove indicator and mean imputation methods from consideration. Greenland and Finkle[13] showed that parameter estimates using the indicator method are generally biased, even when the data are MCAR. Statements such as 'this strategy continues to be employed in medical research ... the use of [this method] can improve the ability of a model to predict outcomes'[14] are often used to justify the indicator method, but we would not recommend its use at all. Likewise, mean imputation is the simplest imputation method, but this approach can never be recommended because its imputation model is wholly unrealistic. Even when the data are MCAR, the resulting estimates of the analyst's model will almost always be biased. Crawford et al.[15] illustrated this point nicely in their Figure 3, where a 'spike' corresponding to the imputed values on an incomplete variable can be seen to cause underestimation of the standard deviation in the imputed data. Moreover, associations between the variable being imputed and the other variables are not respected. We discuss the implications of the choice of imputation models further in Section 7.6.5.

7.5.2 Using simple methods

We now go through the situations in which one of the simple methods, complete cases analysis (CC), regression imputation (RI) and hot-deck imputation (HD), can be used. As we discussed in Section 7.2, the first step in choosing a method is to determine which variables are fully observed (and which are almost fully observed), which are incompletely observed and whether the missing value pattern is univariate, multivariate, monotone or non-monotone. We consider below the decisions on a pattern by pattern basis.

7.5.2.1 Univariate missing value patterns: outcome Y missing

Suppose that Y is incomplete but that E and X are fully observed. For example, suppose Y is birth weight, E is father's socio-economic status and X is year of birth. If the data are MCAR, then any one of CC, RI or HD can be applied. If the data are stratified-MCAR, then RI or HD can both be applied. The CC analysis will give estimates of the regression coefficients of Y on E and Y on X which are both unbiased, because the fully observed stratifying variable (or variables) are conditioned on in the analyst's model. (As an aside, note that the CC estimate of mean birth weight will be biased under stratified-MCAR in this case, but unbiased under MCAR.)

It is true that CC is an attractive prospect for univariate patterns with fully observed covariates, provided that the MCAR or stratified-MCAR assumptions are valid. In their

Table 2, Crawford *et al.*[15] showed CC to perform as well as one of the proper methods we consider in Section 7.6. However, it should be noted that they had a rich set of fully observed covariates available, which is of crucial importance to the stratified-MCAR assumption. Furthermore, the response rate was a relatively high (70 per cent) and so efficiency of the CC estimates is not unduly affected. When the response rate is low, then the efficiency (which can be interpreted as the power to detect exposure effects) is greatly reduced.

RI and HD are possible alternatives to CC when the number of complete cases is small. It is very important to note that both E and X should always be used when imputing values of Y (in the regression equation or choosing donors), even if only one of the covariates is believed to be a stratifying variable (recall we are assuming that all variables in the data set are associated with each other). It should also be noted that a naive application of the analyst's model to the imputed data under RI or HD will underestimate the standard errors. This is because the imputed values are treated as real observed values, and no account is taken of the uncertainty in the predictions made to obtain them. The RI implemented in *SAS* and *SOLAS* produces suitably adjusted standard errors, but neither method is particularly simple for obtaining standard errors.

HD is essentially a non-parametric method, and like all non-parametric methods it is affected by the 'curse of dimensionality'. In other words, if the number of variables used to choose donors is large, or there are a number of continuous variables, it may be that the 'best' donor is not 'close' to the incomplete case. This means that HD will work well for large studies with a few observed variables—where there are lots of 'good' donors—but HD may not always perform well. However, it makes minimal assumptions about the distribution of the missing variables and is easy to apply, although standard error calculation is complex.

7.5.2.2 Univariate missing value pattern: one covariate *X* or *E* missing

Now suppose instead that it is one of E or X that is incomplete, and that Y is completely observed. Many of the rules outlined above still hold, particularly with regard to CC. However, a naive implementation of RI is not possible when the covariates are missing. Suppose that E is incomplete, Y and X are fully observed, and RI is used to obtain E^*. The estimates obtained by using least-squares to fit the regression of Y on E and X to the imputed data set will be biased because RI introduces a correlation between exposure E and the regression error term through the dependence of E^* on Y. Weighted least-squares can be used to adjust for this bias when fitting the analyst's model, but calculation of the weights is complicated. An alternative approach is to exclude Y from the regression equation, but this undermines the stratified-MCAR assumption, and also requires weighted least-squares to adjust the estimates for underestimation of the residual variance. See Little[10] and Little and Rubin[4] for further details on these adjustments.

HD would appear to be a better option in this case. Provided that the curse of dimensionality does not result in too many bad donors, the method can be naively applied and will produce unbiased estimates of the analyst's model. Reilly and Pepe[12] developed a method of calculating standard errors which can be used when E and X have categorical outcomes.

7.5.2.3 Multivariate, monotone and non-monotone missing value patterns

Many of the comments from the preceding sections apply here. The general rule is that the number of fully observed covariates declines as the complexity of the missing value pattern increases, which in turn reduces the number of complete cases to small fractions of the sample size, and possibly weakens the plausibility of the stratified-MCAR assumption further.

Provided that the stratified-MCAR assumption is valid and the curse of dimensionality is not an issue, HD imputation is an attractive approach which can be applied naively to any missing value pattern (provided a set of fully observed variables exists), and the method developed by Reilly and Pepe[12] can be used to obtain standard errors if the variables are categorical. RI is implemented in *SOLAS* and *SAS* with correct standard error estimates for multivariate and monotone patterns, making use of available cases for each regression parameter; however, despite its apparent simplicity, the method is difficult to implement from scratch because standard error estimation is extremely complex.

7.5.3 Independence between variables

Throughout the preceding section, we have assumed that all variables in the data set being analysed are associated with each other. However, often it is the case that one or more variables may be independent or conditionally independent (i.e. independent given other variables in the data set). In such situations, the choice of variables used in the imputation (RI or HD) may not have to include the variable associated with non-response.

Take the following simple example where Y is FBG, E is BMI, and X is sex. In terms of missing data, suppose that FBG is incompletely observed, BMI and sex are fully observed and the non-response rate on FBG depends on sex. If there is no association between FBG and sex in the population (or no association for people with the same BMI), then it is unnecessary to include sex in the imputation model. In practice in such situations, including sex in the imputation model will not introduce bias, but is inefficient in terms of standard errors.

7.6 Proper methods

At this stage, we hope to have made the reader aware of the limitations of the simple methods considered, and understand the reasons why these methods cannot generally be used. In many non-trivial situations, the simplicity of regression and hot-deck imputation is lost because a naive application of the methods is not possible, particularly with regards to standard error estimation. Thus, we now consider four 'proper' methods. Schafer[16] notes that the term proper comes from Bayesian inference, but here it is used to denote missing data methods that can be used for MAR data, all missing value patterns, and give unbiased estimates of the analyst's model parameters and their standard errors. In other words, the analyst does not have to worry about missing data assumptions (stratified-MCAR versus MAR) or the missing value pattern. The proper methods we consider are likelihood-based, Bayesian, multiple imputation and inverse probability weighting. First, we describe each method in turn, and then we show that the choice between each method is about which makes the most realistic modelling assumptions.

7.6.1 Likelihood methods

7.6.1.1 Direct maximization

Suppose that there are no missing data and denote the analyst's model by $p(Y,E,X|\theta)$, where θ represents the 'interest' parameters (e.g. regression coefficients). Parameter estimation is often based on the unconditional likelihood function

$$L(\theta;Y,E,X) = \Pi_{\text{all cases}} \, p(Y,E,X|\theta).$$

The maximum likelihood estimate is the value of θ that maximizes the likelihood for a particular set of complete data. Estimates of standard errors are calculated using the expected information matrix $I(\theta)$, which is derived from the likelihood function.

When there are missing data, the log-likelihood becomes

$$L_{\text{obs}}(\theta) = \int_{\text{missing values}} L(\theta;Y,E,X),$$

that is, the average value of the likelihood function over all possible values that the missing variables could take. If the observed data likelihood is tractable, estimates can be obtained by maximizing $L_{\text{obs}}(\theta)$ and estimated standard errors using the observed data expected information matrix $I_{\text{obs}}(\theta)$. Structural equation models are based on a full likelihood for Y, E and X. Neither regression models nor Cox models are estimated using full likelihood functions: regression models are based on a conditional likelihood for Y given E and X (or the equivalent generalized least-squares minimization), and Cox models are based on the partial likelihood for Y given E, X, the follow-up time and the censoring indicator. Whereas full likelihood makes assumptions about $p(Y,E,X|\theta)$, conditional and partial likelihood make assumptions only about $p(Y|E,X;\theta)$.

The majority of software packages for structural equation modelling (e.g. AMOS by Arbuckle and Wothke[17]) can handle missing data in structural equation models by directly maximizing $L_{\text{obs}}(\theta)$, a method which it terms 'full information maximum likelihood' (FIML). The observed data likelihood is based on a multivariate normal model $p(Y,E,X|\theta)$. Structural equation models with normal latent variables can be specified, which means that missing data in normal linear regression models can also be handled by FIML.

For univariate or monotone missing value patterns, direct maximization is simplified in the following way. Consider a univariate missing value pattern with exposure covariate E incomplete but confounding covariate X and outcome Y complete. The likelihood factorises as

$$L_{\text{obs}}(\theta) = L(\theta_{YX}) \, L(\theta_{E|YX})$$

where θ_{YX} denotes the parameters of Y and X's joint distribution, and $\theta_{E|XY}$ the parameters of the conditional E given Y and X distribution. The two likelihood components are based on all available data on Y, X, and all the available data on E, Y, X—the complete cases; each likelihood component can be maximized separately using an appropriate method. The estimates can then be combined to give estimates of interest parameters θ. Little and Rubin[4] discuss the factorization method in more detail. Thus the impact of the missing value pattern can be seen to be on the ease of computation.

7.6.1.2 The EM algorithm

An approach more widely used in non-SEM frameworks than direct maximization is the 'EM algorithm'.[4,18] The general form of the EM algorithm is:

1. Choose starting value $\hat{\theta}^{(0)}$

2. Set $p = 1$

3. E-step: calculate $Q(q|\hat{\theta}^{(p-1)}) = E\{\log L_{obs}(\theta)|\text{observed data}, \hat{\theta}^{(p-1)}\}$

4. M-step: maximize $Q(\theta|\hat{\theta}^{(p-1)})$ to obtain $\hat{\theta}^{(p)}$

5. If $\hat{\theta}^{(p-1)} \approx \hat{\theta}^{(p)}$ then stop, else set $p = p + 1$ and repeat steps 2–4.

The beauty of the EM algorithm is that the M-step—maximizing the expected value of the full likelihood function given the observed data and the last parameter estimate—can be performed using a standard, complete data routine for $p(Y,E,X|\theta)$. In this case, the EM algorithm can be seen as a form of imputation; the difference between the EM algorithm and, say, regression imputation, is that the EM algorithm uses information from the complete and incomplete cases, no matter what the missing value pattern. An EM algorithm routine for multivariate normal missing data has been implemented in *SPSS*.

7.6.2 Bayesian full probability models

Bayesian estimation, now commonly undertaken using Monte-Carlo Markov chain methods, can be used as an alternative tool for estimating models that are for practical purposes standard likelihood models. In this approach, missing values are treated in much the same way as parameters, being quantities whose uncertainty is explicitly recognized.[19] However, Bayesian methods also offer the scope for being able to impose prior distributions on parameters, including those of missing data distributions and mechanisms. This offers a capability for exploring problems where either the extent of missing data, or where the weakness of the assumptions we are willing to make about the missing data mechanism, makes model identification difficult.

7.6.3 Multiple imputation

There are many good reviews of multiple imputation written for applied researchers, e.g. Schafer and Olsen,[20] Schafer,[21] Allison,[3] Faris *et al.*[14] and Patrician.[22] The basic idea behind multiple imputation is this: in simple, 'single' imputation methods, the imputed values were treated as the actual missing values, when they are predicted values based on some imputation model. Complicated adjustments must be made to reflect this uncertainty. Rubin[23] proposed multiple imputation as a generalization of simple imputation methods to allow for this uncertainty by simulating multiple missing values from a given imputation model, and also allowing for uncertainty in estimation of the imputation model itself. The total variation in these imputed values thus accounts for the uncertainty.

Schafer[16] used a Markov chain Monte-Carlo procedure called 'data augmentation'[24] to implement proper multiple imputation methods. Let $\hat{\theta}$ be the estimator of the interest parameters, and let j be the parameters of the joint distribution of the data. Data augmentation allows us to draw from the 'posterior' distribution of $p(\hat{\theta}|\text{observed})$, and calculate standard errors or confidence intervals from these draws. We do not outline the data augmentation algorithm in full, other than to say that it is a probabilistic equivalent of the EM algorithm in Section 7.6.1; the reader is referred to Schafer[16,21] or Schafer and Graham[5] for good descriptions. Currently, algorithms for proper multiple imputation are available in *SAS*, *S-Plus* and *Stata* where the data are multivariate normal, multinomial (i.e. categorical) and the variables are mixed multivariate–categorical (i.e. follow a general location model).

7.6.4 Weighting, estimating equations and double robustness

Survey researchers have for a long time made adjustments for missing data using weights. These are constructed as being the inverse of the proportion responding in a stratum, with the weights declared in a weighted analysis of the complete data cases as probability weights (and not frequency weights), and with standard errors calculated using various methods, most commonly from the robust or sandwich parameter covariance matrix.[25,26] In practice, the missing data weights are commonly calculated from the predicted probability of response from a logistic model in which all available predictors of non-response are included (noting that the predictors must be available for responders and non-responders alike). This approach is very simple and flexible to use, effective in large samples, but only makes use of complete data cases. More recently, Robins and colleagues[27] have extended this approach within an estimating equations framework, improving the efficiency while remaining semi-parametric. Flexible and accessible routines for this approach are not yet readily available, but are likely to become widely used during the next decade.

This weighted estimating equation approach for dealing with missing data can be combined with a covariate adjustment/stratified-MAR approach for tackling the same problem. This delivers a property Robins refers to as double-robustness in which we can get unbiased estimates of effects provided that either the adjustment via the weights/estimating equations or that via the covariates is correct—we do not need both to be correct.[28]

7.6.5 Comparing proper methods

7.6.5.1 Modelling assumptions

As we shall show, the choice between using likelihood methods or multiple imputation is essentially down to the modelling assumptions the analyst is prepared to make. Up until this point, we have focused on only missing data assumptions (MCAR, MAR, etc.). However, all imputation methods make assumptions about the distribution of the missing values given the observed values. If these assumptions are incorrect, then estimates of the analyst's model parameters will be biased. For example, mean imputation assumes that the distribution of any given missing value is independent of the other variables in the data set. Regression imputation is more realistic because it allows the mean of the missing value distribution to depend linearly on the values of the observed data. Hot-deck imputation makes no parametric assumptions, other than that the distribution of the missing values given the observed values for an incomplete case is equal to the equivalent distribution amongst the complete cases. Thus mean imputation always performs poorly because its modelling assumptions are unrealistic. The modelling assumptions in regression and hot-deck imputation are more realistic, but both methods are more difficult to implement for complex missing value patterns.

7.6.5.2 Advantages and disadvantages of likelihood methods

The choice of likelihood method depends first on the analysis model $p(\text{data}|\theta) = p(Y|E,X;\theta)$, which could be, say, a linear regression or a Cox model; or $p(\text{data}|\theta) = p(\text{endogenous}|\text{exogenous};\theta)$ for structural equation models. When the covariates (or exogenous variables) are fully observed, estimation of θ can be performed using maximum likelihood (or alternatively least-squares) without having to make any more modelling assumptions than those usually made in the absence of missing data. This is because it is usually only the conditional distribution of the outcome given the covariates that is of interest (or the conditional distribution of endogenous given exogenous variables for structural equation models). However, when the covariates are incompletely observed, this is no longer the case and the likelihood method must incorporate modelling assumptions about covariate distribution.

For example, consider using the FIML method in SEM when confounder X is an exogenous variable that is incompletely observed. The modelling assumption commonly made is that the data are from a multivariate normal distribution. If X is highly non-normal, then it may be possible to transform it to have a symmetrical distribution, but this is not always possible; transformations are not an option for variables with nominal or ordinal categorical outcomes. Enders[29] conducted a simulation study to assess the sensitivity of FIML to modelling assumptions. For estimates of the regression parameters, it was found to be relatively robust to departures from the underlying multivariate normal assumption. For estimated standard errors, however, the method was not robust, and severe bias resulted.

In cases where the missing variables are categorical, an alternative approach to FIML is required. The general location model is suitable for data sets containing a mixture of normal and categorical variables; Little and Schluchter[30] developed an EM algorithm for the general location model. However, the parameters of the general location model do not always correspond to θ, and the calculation of estimated standard errors is not straightforward without statistical programming (the simplest method being to follow Oakes[31]). EM algorithms for Cox models with missing covariates are still being developed (e.g. Herring and Ibrahim[32]); the theory behind the EM algorithm is more complex for Cox models because complete data estimation is based on semi-parametric partial likelihood and not fully parametric likelihood.

7.6.5.3 Advantages and disadvantages of multiple imputation

Multiple imputation is more general than likelihood-based methods because it makes a distinction between the analysis model $p(Y|E,X;\theta)$, and a model for the complete multivariate data set, $p(Y,E,X|\varphi)$. Modelling assumptions about the distribution of the missing data given the observed data are implemented through the choice of $p(Y,E,X|\varphi)$. Schafer[16] developed proper multiple imputation methods based on $p(Y,E,X|\varphi)$ being multivariate normal (*Norm*), multinomial (*Cat*) and the general location model (*Mixed*); the first of these is implemented in *SAS* as well as *S-Plus*. If these choices are sufficient for your particular data set, then all is well.

In Section 7.2, we separated the study and analysis patterns, and thus far have considered only the analysis pattern. In this situation, as noted by Collins *et al.*,[33] multiple imputation based on a multivariate normal model is practically equivalent to the FIML method used in SEM. FIML has the advantage of not requiring multiple data sets, whereas studies have found multiple imputation to perform slightly better for standard error estimation and in small departures from the modelling assumptions,[29,44] although another study by Olinksy *et al.*[35] favoured FIML.

The real advantage of multiple imputation comes when the data do not follow a multivariate normal distribution. Compared with likelihood methods for non-normal multivariate distributions, such as the EM algorithm for the general location model, there are no problems obtaining estimates of θ when the analysis model parameters do not correspond to those of the general location model, and standard error estimates are easily calculated through the multiple imputation procedure. The first advantage comes from being able to specify separate analyst's and imputation models; but this can also be a source of potential bias if the imputation model is inconsistent with the analysis model, and the imputations are 'uncongenial'.[36] However, this is a minor problem in practice; provided that the imputation model is at least as complex as the analyst's model (in terms of interactions between variables), then bias due to uncongenial imputations will be small.[37] However, if the imputation model is simpler than the analysis model, then the bias could be substantial. For example, if the analysis model is a mixed effects/multilevel regression model with random terms at the household or area level, the analyst should be aware that imputation using the multiple imputation methods discussed thus far will be biased. Similarly, if missing repeated longitudinal measures are imputed without allowing for higher order associations between the measures, then biased estimates will result.

More recent work has involved combining different multiple imputation methods for data sets where the multivariate imputation models outlined above may be insufficient. Multiple imputation of repeated measures, as used in longitudinal and growth curve modelling, has been carried out by Longford *et al.*[38] and Di Stavola *et al.*,[39] based on estimates of the missing values under a suitable imputation model for repeated measures; Molenberghs *et al.*[40] develop a multiple imputation routine for Cox models with missing covariates. A generalization of this *ad hoc* approach to multiple imputation was developed by van Buuren *et al.*,[41] called 'multiple imputation by chained equations' (MICE) (http://www.multiple-imputation.com and the Stata utility). Using this approach, different imputation models can be chosen for different variables, depending on the distribution, and combined to produce a full set of imputations. The flexibility of this method for application to complex data sets makes it a promising approach. However, in theory, problems could arise if the choice of different imputation models does not correspond to a well-defined imputation model for the set of variables, and further theoretical work is required before MICE can be taken as the gold standard. Some simulation work by Faris *et al.*[14] found it to perform best out of a selection of multiple imputation methods. Another promising development is the non-parametric imputation approach developed by Paddock,[42] which makes no modelling assumptions and is applicable for non-monotone missing value patterns.

To demonstrate the last advantage of multiple imputation, recall that in Section 7.2 we made a distinction between the missing value pattern in the study data, and that in the variables used in a particular analysis. It may be true that variables measured in the study which are not included in the analysis are strongly associated with the non-response mechanism. Using likelihood methods, these variables would be included in the analysis model, thus complicating the likelihood method with further nuisance parameters. However, provided that a suitable imputation model is chosen, multiple imputations could be generated that take advantage of the extra information, and the same analysis model could be fitted to each. Collins *et al.*[33] call this an 'inclusive' strategy.

Van Buuren *et al.*[41] neatly summarized the main points necessary to avoid introducing bias into the estimates when following an inclusive strategy.

1. Include (at least) all variables in the analysis model in the imputation model.

2. Ideally include other variables (a) believed to be strongly associated with the non-response mechanism, and (b) strongly associated with the incomplete variables (for efficiency; see Section 7.5.3).

3. If possible, remove variables with high rates of non-response.

Step 1 ensures the results will be unbiased; steps 2 and 3 ensure that the imputation model will be as efficient as possible (i.e. have the smallest possible standard errors). Efficiency is important because a highly inefficient imputation model offsets the gain in information from the incomplete cases.

Ibrahim *et al.*[19] compare maximum-likelihood, full Bayesian, multiple imputation and weighted estimating equations, while Carpenter *et al.*[28] present a comparison of double robust and imputation methods.

7.7 Discussion

What can we conclude about the methods discussed in this chapter? First, it should be recognized that motivating the choice of missing data method should not be based on the maxim that filling in something is better than filling in nothing! There are important statistical arguments underpinning the way in which non-response adjustments are made and missing values are imputed, and it is important that these arguments are valid. For example, we have already cited work showing that filling in 'bad' values using mean imputation can be worse than complete cases analysis.[15]

It is reasonable to use complete cases analysis provided that the stratified-MCAR assumption is made plausible by the presence of a rich set of fully observed variables in the analysis, and the number of complete cases is sufficient. However, in life course epidemiology, missing value patterns are often too complex to give a sufficient number of complete cases. Similarly, the stratified-MCAR assumption may not be plausible. For example, Demissie et al.[43] considered Cox model analysis of a genetic exposure on the probability of getting cardiovascular disease when the exposure was incompletely observed. They found complete cases analyses to give severely biased results with MAR non-response mechanisms that are not stratified-MCAR.

When a complete cases analysis cannot be justified, intuitively appealing simple methods such as regression and hot-deck imputation become quite complicated. Regression imputation requires adjustments to both the parameter estimates (if a covariate in the analyst's model is incompletely observed) and the standard error estimates. Hot-deck imputation only requires adjustments of standard errors estimates, but such adjustments when continuous variables are incompletely observed are complicated and have yet to be implemented in standard software.

When faced with a complex missing value pattern, strategies such as dropping variables with a high proportion of missing values have been proposed. If the missing value pattern is non-monotone, this could simplify the missing value pattern and permit the use of, say, regression imputation for a monotone pattern. Alternatively, a proxy study variable with a high response rate could be substituted for the intended variable. However, in practice, proxy variables are also likely to be associated with the factors causing missing data, and so valid substitutions may not exist. In longitudinal studies with incomplete repeated measures, an oft-used strategy is 'last value carried forward'. This is another imputation method in which the imputation model is poor because any time trend in the outcomes will be distorted by imputation.

Some mention should be made of likelihood methods for Cox models, which are termed semi-parametric. Schafer and Graham[5] take the opinion that, if it is clear that the data are MCAR or MAR, then multiple imputation rather than likelihood methods are a better option, given the difficulties in implementing semi-parametric approaches. However, the situation where the data are MNAR cannot always be discounted, for regression and structural equation models as well as Cox models, and likelihood methods have been widely developed for non-ignorable non-response. An example of non-ignorable non-response specific to Cox models occurs when the follow-up time is related to the censoring indicator, so-called 'informative censoring' (see Chapter 9). Non-ignorable non-response is also likely in situations where the number of fully observed variables is small, or only weakly related to the outcome variable, in which case the stratified-MCAR or general-MAR assumptions are implausible. If the analyst is uncertain about whether the data are MCAR, MAR or MNAR, it is recommended to present a number of estimates obtained under different assumptions about the non-response mechanism. The exception to this rule is when auxiliary data are available; Faris et al.[14] call this 'data enhancement', and merge their sample with an administrative database to handle the missng data problem.

To conclude, the last few years have seen the theory and implementation of proper methods within the likelihood, Bayesian, multiple imputation and semi-parametric weighting frameworks move on considerably. Non-response adjustments can now be provided in a wide range of scenarios, without the limitations of simple methods elaborated on here. It is now possible to obtain non-response adjustments for complex multivariate, MAR data, with any missing value pattern, for a wide range of analytical models. The availability of such advanced methods in software packages such as *Stata* has also improved considerably, with the MICE method of van Buuren *et al.*[41] now implemented. Software for multiple imputation was reviewed by Horton and Lipsitz,[44] and lists of software can be found on the web (e.g. http://www.herc.research.med.va.gov/FAQ_I9.htm). As such, it is becoming more and more difficult to justify using simple methods. Proper methods are naturally extended to allow for NMAR data.

Further reading

Allison PD (2001). *Missing data*. Sage, Thousand Oaks, CA.

Brick J, Kalton G (1996). Handling missing data in survey research. *Statistical Methods in Medical Research* 5, 215–238.

Greenland S, Finkle WD (1995). A critical look at methods for handling missing covariates in epidemiologic regression analysis. *American Journal of Epidemiology* 142, 1255–1268.

Groves RM, Couper MP (1998). *Nonresponse in household interview surveys*. Wiley, New York.

Little RJA, Rubin DB (1989). The analysis of social science data with missing values. *Sociological Methods and Research* 18, 292–326.

References

1. Groves RM, Dilman DA, Eltinge JL, Little RJA, ed. (2002). *Survey nonresponse*. Section I. Wiley, Chichester.

2. Wadsworth MEJ, Butterworth SL, Hardy RJ, Kuh DJ, Richards M, Langenberg C, *et al.* (2003). The life course prospective design: an example of the benefits and problems associated with study longevity. *Social Science and Medicine* 57, 2193–2205.

3. Allison PD (2001). *Missing data*. Sage, Thousand Oaks, CA.

4. Little RJA, Rubin DB (2002). *Statistical analysis with missing data*, 2nd edn. Wiley, Hoboken.

5. Schafer JL, Graham JW (2002). Missing data: our view of the state of the art. *Psychological Methods* 7, 147–177.

6. Curran PJ (2003). Have multilevel models been structural equation models all along? *Multivariate Behavioral Research* 38, 529–569.

7. Groves RM, Couper MP (1998). *Nonresponse in household interview surveys*. Wiley, New York.

8. Robins JM, Gill RD (1997). Non-response models for the analysis of non-monotone ignorable missing data. *Statistics in Medicine* 16, 39–56.

9. Rubin DB (1976). Inference and missing data. *Biometrika* 63, 581–592.

10. Little RJA (1992). Regression with missing X's: a review. *Journal of the American Statistical Association* 87, 1227–1237.

11. Reilly MJ (1993). Data analysis using hot deck multiple imputation. *Statistician* 42, 307–313.

12. Reilly MJ, Pepe MS (1997). The relationship between hot-deck multiple imputation and weighted likelihood. *Statistics in Medicine* 16, 5–19.

13. Greenland S, Finkle WD (1995). A critical look at methods for handling missing covariates in epidemiologic regression analysis. *American Journal of Epidemiology* 142, 1255–1268.

14. Faris PD, Ghali WA, Brant R, Norris CM, Galbraith PD, Knudtson ML (2002). Multiple imputation for dealing with missing data in observational healthcare outcome systems. *Journal of Clinical Epidemiology* 55, 184–191.

15. Crawford SL, Tennstedt SL, Mckinlay JB (1995). A comparison of analytic methods for non-random missingness of outcomes data. *Journal of Clinical Epidemiology* 48, 209–219.

16. Schafer JL (1997). *Analysis of incomplete multivariate data*. Chapman and Hall, London.

17. Arbukle JL, Wothke W (1999). *AMOS 4.0 User's Guide*. SmallWaters, Chicago.

18. Dempster AP, Laird NM, Rubin DB (1977). Maximum likelihood estimation from incomplete data via the EM algorithm. *Journal of the Royal Statistical Society B* 39, 1–38.

19. Ibrahim JG, Chen MH, Lipsitz SR, Herring AH (2005). Missing-data methods for generalized linear models: a comparative review. *Journal of the American Statistical Association* 100, 332–346.

20. Schafer JL, Olsen MK (1998). Multiple imputation for multivariate missing-data problems: a data analyst's perspective. *Multivariate Behavioral Research* 33, 545–571.

21. Schafer JL (1999). Multiple imputation: a primer. *Statistical Methods in Medical Research* 8, 3–15.

22. Patrician PA (2002). Multiple imputation for missing data. *Research in Nursing and Health* 25, 76–84.

23. Rubin DB (1987). *Multiple imputation for nonresponse in surveys*. Wiley, New York.

24. Tanner MA (1996). *Tools for statistical inference*, 3rd edn. Springer, New York.

25. Horvitz DG, Thompson DJ (1952). A generalization of sampling without replacement from a finite universe. *Journal of the American Statistical Association* 47, 663–685.

26. Binder DA (1983). On the variances of asymptotically normal estimators from complex surveys. *International Statistical Review* 51, 279–292.

27. Robins JM, Rotnitzky A, Zhao LP (1995). Analysis of semi-parametric regression models for repeated outcomes in the presence of missing data. *Journal of the American Statistical Association* 90, 106–121.

28. Carpenter JR, Kenward MG, Vansteelandt S (2006). A comparison of multiple imputation and doubly robust estimation for analyses with missing data. *Journal of the Royal Statistical Society A* 169, 571–584.

29. Enders CK (2001). The impact of nonnormality on full information maximum-likelihood estimation for structural equation models with missing data. *Psychological Methods* 6, 352–370.

30. Little RJA, Schluchter MD (1985). Maximum likelihood estimation for mixed continuous and continuous categorical data with missing values. *Biometrika* 72, 497–512.

31. Oakes D (1999). Direct calculation of the information matrix via the EM algorithm. *Journal of the Royal Statistical Society B* 61, 479–482.

32. Herring AH, Ibrahim JG (2001). Likelihood-based methods for missing covariates in the Cox proportional hazards model. *Journal of the American Statistical Association* 96, 292–302.

33. Collins LM, Schafer JL, Kam CM (2001). A comparison of restrictive and inclusive missing data strategies. *Psychological Methods* 6, 330–351.

34. Wiggins RD, Sacker A (2002). Strategies for handling missing data in SEM: a user's perspective. In: Marcoulides GA, Moustaki I, ed. *Latent variable and latent structure models*. Lawrence Erlbaum, Mahwah, NJ, pp. 105–120.

35. Olinsky A, Chen S, Harlow L (2003). The comparative efficiency of imputation for missing data in structural equation modeling. *European Journal of Operational Research* 151, 53–79.

36. Meng XL (1994). Multiple-imputation inferences with uncongenial sources of input (with discussion). *Statistical Science* 10, 538–573.

37. Schafer JL (2003). Multiple imputation in multivariate problems when the imputation and analysis models differ. *Statistic Neerlandica* 57, 19–35.

38. Longford NT, Ely M, Hardy R, Wadsworth MEJ (2000). Handling missing data in diaries of alcohol consumption. *Journal of the Royal Statistical Society A* 163, 381–402.

39. Di Stavola BR, Silva ID, McCormack V, Hardy R, Kuh DJ, Wadsworth MEJ (2004). Childhood growth and breast cancer. *American Journal of Epidemiology* 159, 671–682.

40. Molenberghs G, Williams PL, Lipsitz SR (2002). Prediction of survival and opportunistic infections in HIV-infected patients: a comparison of multiple imputation methods of incomplete CD4 counts. *Statistics in Medicine* 21, 1387–1408.

41. Van Buuren S, Boshuizen HC, Knook DL (1999). Multiple imputation of missing blood pressure covariates in survival analysis. *Statistics in Medicine* 18, 681–694.

42. Paddock SM (2002). Bayesian nonparametric multiple imputation of partially observed data with ignorable nonresponse. *Biometrika* 89, 529–538.

43. Demissie S, LaValley MP, Horton NJ, Glynn RJ, Cupples LA (2003). Bias due to missing exposure data using complete-case analysis in the proportional hazards regression model. *Statistics in Medicine* 22, 545–557.

44. Horton NJ, Lipsitz SR (2001). Multiple imputation in practice: comparison of software packages for regression models with missing variables. *American Statistician* 55, 244–254.

Chapter 8

An overview of models and methods for life course analysis

Andrew Pickles and Bianca De Stavola

Abstract

We begin by considering the range of different aspects of the disease process that life course analysis must address. Given the essential longitudinal nature of much life course analysis, we illustrate the population average and subject-specific modelling frameworks for longitudinal and multivariate data. The bulk of the chapter then focuses upon the tools, both conceptual and statistical, for tackling the problem of causal analysis. This includes both traditional and more recently proposed methods, such as marginal structural models and instrumental variable methods, and approaches being adopted from other disciplines, such as structural equation modelling. We attempt to highlight both their specific strengths and their commonality. Two major concerns close the chapter, one relating to the implications for epidemiology of individual differences or non-uniform causal effects, and the second concerning the need to preserve objectivity within analysis.

8.1 Introduction

Undertaking research within a life course perspective poses numerous methodological problems. Important among these is how one can represent putative life course mechanisms within a statistical model: essentially problems of theoretical operationalization. A second related set of these problems concerns the complications and flawed inference that can arise when models are fitted using suboptimal data. In much epidemiological research, the methodological interest is almost exclusively directed to problems of this second kind. Without dismissing the need for appropriate data, we believe understanding the range and features of the statistical models that are relevant to a life course perspective should be our first task. Thus, we first discuss some of the conceptual models that are most frequently encountered in life course research. We then review how these can be formally studied using appropriate statistical frameworks. Since life course considerations emphasize the need to consider outcome profiles, Section 8.3 introduces the population-average and subject-specific approaches to multivariate and longitudinal analysis. Section 8.4 addresses the various problems and the methods that may help overcome them in the task of going beyond associational analysis to be able to make causal assertions and elucidate mechanisms. We include consideration of methods for measured, time-varying and unobserved confounders, chain-effect models that give insight into synergy, structural equation modelling to help account for measurement error, and multilevel modelling to consider ecological effects. Section 8.5 raises issues in relation to possible individual differences of effects. Section 8.6 concludes, raising two problems that have yet to be given sufficient consideration, individual variability in causal effects and the need to maintain greater objectivity throughout epidemiological analysis.

8.2 Conceptual models for disease mechanisms

8.2.1 General model

The possible alternative mechanisms that we might wish to represent are many and varied (see Chapter 1 and Kuh and Ben-Shlomo[1]). They are perhaps best characterized when contrasted with a non-life course model. This would regard current health as related only to contemporaneous individual exposures, e.g. X and Z (Fig. 8.1). The complexities that arise even in this simple framework need to be appreciated before more complex models are considered. To discuss them, we use Clayton's decomposition into a disease submodel (model I), and two further submodels, one for the exposure measurement (model II) and one for the exposure distribution (model III) (Fig. 8.2; Clayton[2]). Model I is equivalent to that described in Fig. 8.1 but replaces X with a 'latent' variable or 'true' exposure which is measured only with error by X. Model II relates the observed variable X to its latent self, accounting for possible additional bias arising from Z. Model III specifies the distribution or variation of the latent (true) exposure, which again can be influenced by Z. Thus with observational data, even when cross-sectional, just accounting for the likely presence of measurement error leads to substantial modelling complexity.

When a time dimension is added to this framework, more complex specifications become necessary, not only for the disease model (because several exposures that refer to different time points in the life course are involved), but also for the exposure submodel. Indeed, characterizing the relevant exposures becomes a major problem in its own right, and one in which the problems posed by measurement error become much more pernicious. Epidemiologists have some insight into the impact of measurement error under the

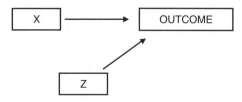

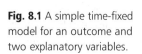

Fig. 8.1 A simple time-fixed model for an outcome and two explanatory variables.

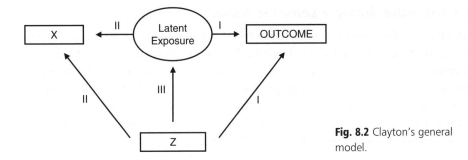

Fig. 8.2 Clayton's general model.

standard (time-fixed) model.[3,4] As we will argue, for the more complex life course (i.e. 'longitudinal') settings, this insight requires greater development, much of which can only be gained by the use of explicit statistical measurement models.

To be able to discuss these issues formally, we briefly review the disease models most relevant in life course studies. Then we consider the (statistical) causal models that one could adopt in order to deal with multiple exposures and confounders, and to include the relevant measurement and exposure submodels.

8.2.2 Cumulative exposure

There are numerous examples where contemporaneous risk is thought to be related to cumulative exposure over an extended period, such as the cumulative impact of social class on coronary heart disease,[5] poisons such as lead that are poorly eliminated from some tissues and thus accumulate, and some physiological capacities that are built up over an extended period. Peak bone mass is a good example here, dietary and exercise exposure throughout childhood and early adulthood contributing to the accumulation of a bone resource that may protect from skeletal fragility due to bone loss in late adulthood. In these cases, direct measurement, e.g. lead content of teeth and peak bone mass, directly provide a measure of the exposure incidence level integrated over some extended period of time, namely a cumulative exposure. In other cases, cumulative exposure, as the integration of point exposure level $x(t)$ over the period $T1$ to $T2$ of interest, $\int_{T1}^{T2} x(t)dt$, may need to be performed more explicitly. Usually, we have only a set of point exposure measures rather than the complete continuous exposure record. Solutions to this problem are often approached very informally. For example, Davey-Smith et al., in a study of mortality differentials,[6,7] consider cumulative exposure to social disadvantage from a simple count of father's occupation, own first occupation and current occupations that were manual occupations. Others have used a similar approach to study the impact of social disadvantage on mental and physical health.[8-9] This summary exposure could be mathematically represented by $\sum_{t=1}^{3} x(t)\Delta(t)$ for a binary indicator $x(t)$ which takes value 1 for exposure status at time t (e.g. manual occupation), 0 otherwise, where all periods of exposure $\Delta(t)$ are assumed to be of equal length. More generally, the problem corresponds to estimating cumulative exposure via an appropriate area under the curve (AUC).[10]

8.2.3 **Exposure during a sensitive period**

Under the cumulative exposure model described above, if exposure has been accumulated, it is only the total exposure and not the particular periods of exposure that is informative. However, it is clear that for some diseases, there can be sensitive periods during which exposure to the risk factor sets in place pre-conditions for disease. For example, Leon and Davey-Smith[11] contrast the importance of deprivation in childhood for adult stomach cancer, whereas it is adult deprivation that is relevant for many other adult cancers and diseases, such as coronary heart disease (CHD). Another example of a sensitive period model is the fetal origin hypothesis. This suggests that adverse circumstances *in utero* and early life lead to biological programming favouring adverse adult health. Thus a sensitive period is a time in an individual's life where exposure to certain factors can be crucial for his/her physical or psychological development that in turn can then influence later health. Meaney and colleagues[12] have shown that maternal licking of rat pups during the first days of life determines methylation of sections of DNA and subsequent altered expression of a gene, probably permanently, that is important in stress response. Formally this model can be specified in terms of several period-specific variables z_k holding the value taken by the exposure of interest during the kth period, $(t_{k-1} - t_k)$. Correlations among them, however, may make the results difficult to interpret (See Chapter 6).[13]

8.2.4 **Critical pathways of exposure**

A third model, often invoked in the study of social mobility, considers the impact of individual exposure trajectories as they develop throughout life. For example, a given total accumulated exposure, say to deprived socio-economic conditions, may have been achieved early or late in life. If early exposure is critical for the outcome of interest, then pathways that are characterized by early accumulation will have greater influence. If more than one life period is critical, pathways with greater exposure during those periods will be associated with the outcome. However, data limitations may make it impossible to distinguish sensitive period and cumulative exposure components empirically, as discussed by Hallqvist *et al.*[14] and Singh-Manoux *et al.*[15]

8.2.5 **Atypical trajectories**

The course of some chronic or episodic conditions may involve a change in presentation. In developmental psychopathology, the term heterotypic continuity is sometimes used for this process. An example of the more common homotypic continuity is where early oppositional behaviour occurs as a precursor of conduct disorder, which itself is considered to precede adult antisocial personality disorder (i.e. continuity within the same domain of behavioural disruption). However, Rowe *et al.*[16] suggest that in girls, early oppositional behaviour in fact precedes depression and not conduct disorder, contrary to expectations – an example of heterotypic continuity.

8.2.6 **Contextual effects**

A major theme within social medicine has been that variations in the wider social environment contribute to individual health over and above that of the personal characteristics

Table 8.1 Engel's data from 1848 on mortality ratios from Chorlton, Manchester

Class of street	Class of house		
	Best	**Middle**	**Worst**
Best	1/51	1/45	1/36
Middle	1/55	1/38	1/36
Worst	–	1/35	1/25

of that individual. Table 8.1 shows Engels' data from Chorlton, Manchester in 1848 (from Bartley *et al.*[17]) that recorded deaths in households cross-tabulated by the quality of their house and the quality of their street. These data clearly suggested that neighbourhood housing quality contributed to the risk of mortality over and above an individual's own housing conditions.

More generally, many authors have argued for the potential importance of social capital,[18] and Kuh and Ben-Shlomo[1] discuss the integration of eco-social factors into life course models. Measurement of these wider social characteristics have been fraught with problems, discussed in Chapter 3, but their geographical localization can be exploited to model their putative impact as a random effect, as discussed in the 'Multilevel models' section below.

8.2.7 Delayed effects

In some cases, exposure accumulated over a long period of time may act on health during some later point in life. In some instances, specific contemporaneous conditions may be required for that cumulative exposure to become active. In some individuals, exposure to childhood sexual abuse does not result in immediate psychiatric disorder, but may do so later when that individual is challenged by the need to form adult sexual relationships.[19] Rapid weight loss, resulting in rapid release of toxins previously stored in body fat, provides another example. Effects can thus arise due to an interaction between exposures accumulated over time and a current exposure or challenge.

8.2.8 Variable-based, individual-based and multivariate profile analysis

Operationalizing and distinguishing these and other mechanisms (we elaborate multistage mechanisms later) is a huge challenge. Study design of course plays a crucial role in order to ensure that the decisive contrasts and effects can be estimated and a strong interpretation placed upon these. However, in this chapter, we focus on analysis. In many life course questions, we conceive of our outcome as a profile of measures over some extended period or over several facets of health or behaviour. This concern is the principal distinctive feature of the 'individual-based' perspective whose proponents contrast it with 'variable-based' perspective where typically multiple variables are used to explain a single outcome measure. Some proponents have gone further and classified statistical methods as individual or variable based, a contrast that we do not consider that fruitful, since most methods can be elaborated to reflect better the interests of either of the two perspectives.[20]

Nonetheless, analysis of multiple outcome profiles is a key element of life course epidemiology in order to distinguish among the various mechanisms just introduced, and we start with a simple illustration of the analysis of such a multivariate outcome. A major emphasis is on the specification of a design matrix, the set of covariates and dummy variables that are manipulated to allow the estimation of different hypothetical effects. We also use this example to illustrate the two principal approaches to longitudinal data, namely the population-average (PA) and subject-specific (SS) methods. We then focus on a range of methods that can be used in our attempts to distinguish causal effects from mere associations. We conclude with a consideration of multilevel and random effects.

8.3 Multivariate association analysis

8.3.1 Subject-specific and population-average approaches

The usual method for exploring risk mechanisms of these various kinds is to fit models that structure the association among predictors and a set of outcomes measured over time. Such structured models are almost invariably some kind of generalized linear model, often logistic regression. When applied to repeated measures from the same individual, there is a need to take into account the residual correlation that will remain even after the effects of predictor variables are accounted for. There are two principal ways in which this can be done. The first approach, referred to variously as the marginal, population-average (PA) or generalized estimating equation (GEE) approach, essentially treats this correlation as nuisance.[21] The second approach, variously known as the subject-specific (SS), conditional or random effects approach, introduces subject-specific individual effects, often interpretable as persistent propensities or vulnerabilities that influence individuals but which may not yet be directly observable or measurable. Unfortunately, except in the case of standard linear models for a continuous response and for log-linear Poisson models for rates, these two approaches yield different estimates of effects of the predictors. In most cases, the population average estimate is smaller in size than the subject-specific estimate, though correspondingly smaller standard errors typically result in the z-statistics and P-values being very similar. This difference is not statistical 'artefact', but relates to the fact that the two approaches estimate different measures of association. Some argument persists about the relative appropriateness of the two effect estimates, the PA estimate being preferred by many within the public health field, the SS often being preferred by among those doing more basic science research. In practice, unless the researcher is specifically interested in putative subject-specific vulnerabilities, the mechanisms associated with them and how their development over time might be structured, then the PA approach is often the easier to implement and interpret. However, from the results of an SS model, it is possible to calculate approximate estimates of the results that would have been obtained from a corresponding PA model—whereas doing the reverse is more difficult. It is important, particularly for any meta-analysis/overview purposes, to know which kinds of effect are being reported.

In either approach, the data to be analysed usually require one outcome per record, with multiple records per subject when there are several outcomes to be analysed. It is necessary to manipulate the data carefully and construct and combine sets of dummy variables and predictors such that each outcome is predicted by the appropriate set of predictors. This is most easily illustrated by an example.

8.3.1.1 Quality of health during adulthood among those with learning difficulties

We examine self-rated quality of life when aged 33 and 43 years for participants of the National Child Development Study, a UK nationally representative birth cohort of boys and girls born in March 1958.[22] The outcome is ordinal with four categories (excellent, good, fair and poor), and the exposure of interest is learning difficulties in childhood (identified by IQ <70, measured prospectively when the participants were 11 years old). We examine whether the effect of the exposure persists after controlling for time-fixed confounders (sex and birth weight), and contemporaneous social circumstance (measured by social class, unemployment status and social adversity measured at age 33 and 43, respectively). We also assess whether quality of life has worsened or improved between age 33 and 43 years.

The data file consists of two records per subject, one for age 33 and one for age 43, unless data are missing in which case fewer records are available. To take account of the missing mechanism when adopting the PA approach, inverse probability weights were calculated based on a differential response associated with a variety of childhood measures. In contrast, SS models often exploit the properties of maximum likelihood to allow missing data to be assumed to be missing at random. Further discussion of missing data can be found in Chapter 7.

With one outcome per record, and any attrition weight specific to that record, the remaining variables need to include a subject identifier and the time-fixed predictors (with values merely repeated across age 33 and age 43 records), time-specific predictors (single variables but with different values on each record corresponding to each occasion of measurement) and a dummy variable indicating whether the record is for age 33 or 43 years. Once the data set is constructed, whether a variable is time varying or not is often not explicit in the model formulation. The age dummy variable, when specified in the model as a main effect, identifies the change over occasions in the reported health outcome, an effect that is assumed to be common to the whole cohort. Coefficients for interactions of the dummy age variable with any of the other predictor variables identify age-specific differences in the effects associated with these variables. Representation of more complex mechanisms often requires modest further data manipulation, for example within-subject cumulative totals for variables thought to have their effect through a lifetime dose, although care is necessary to avoid missing data undermining the validity of such simple summation.

We used an ordinal logistic regression model for the ordinal health outcome that, like ordinary binary logistic regression, gives effect estimates on the odds ratio scale.[23] The odds ratio associated with a given exposure refers to the relative odds of being in a given or higher level of the health outcome relatively to being at any lower levels, with the assumption that the odds ratio is the same for any grouping of the adjacent outcome categories. PA odds ratios (ORs) were estimated in *Stata* using the population-average svyologit procedure,[24] and the SS ORs using the *Stata* gllamm procedure.[25] The results are shown in Table 8.2.

The unadjusted PA OR for learning difficulties in childhood was 3.09 and the SS OR was 4.72. Note that the PA OR can be approximately derived from the SS OR by dividing the SS log-odds parameter by the square-root of the ratio of the scale variance of the logistic distribution ($\pi^2/3$, where π is 3.14) to the total error variance of the SS model, i.e. the sum of the scale variance of the logistic distribution and the variance of the random effect. This gives $\exp[\ln(4.72) \times ((\pi^2/3)/((\pi^2/3)+4.39))^{0.5}] = 2.76$, in this case rather smaller than the PA estimate of 3.09.

Table 8.2 shows that controlling for potential confounders (gender and birth weight) and for potential mediators (contemporaneous social and economic disadvantage), the learning disability effect estimates are somewhat reduced, although they nonetheless remain significant in both the PA and the SS model. The effects of age on quality of life remain practically unchanged, in both cases indicating a worsening of self-rated quality of life from age 33 to age 43.

The addition of an interaction between age and learning disability was not found to be significant in the PA model (Wald z-test $P = 0.8$). The result was supported by the similarity of the estimated effects of disability on quality of life at age 33 [OR = 1.82, 95 per cent confidence interval (CI) 1.07–3.09] and 43 (OR = 2.00, 95 per cent CI 1.15–3.47). The poorer outcome for learning-disabled individuals thus shows no sign of improvement even long after the ostensibly most 'learning-demanding' school age years.[22]

Table 8.2 Unadjusted and adjusted odds ratio (OR) of self-rated quality of life for the learning difficulties in childhood and age at measurement estimated by the population-average and subject-specific models

Variable	Population-average model*			Subject-specific model†		
	OR	95 per cent CI	P-value	OR	95 per cent CI	P-value
Unadjusted						
Learning difficulties	3.09	2.06–4.65	<0.001	4.72	3.00–7.41	<0.001
Age 43 years	1.29	1.23–1.35	<0.001	1.51	1.41–1.62	<0.001
Adjusted‡						
Learning difficulties	1.92	1.21–1.35	0.004	2.54	1.59–4.05	<0.001
Age 43 years	1.27	1.20–1.35	<0.001	1.46	1.35–1.59	<0.001

CI = confidence interval.

*Missing data treated by inverse probability weights.

†Missing data treated as missing at random.

‡Adjusted for gender, birth weight and contemporaneous unemployment status, social class and social adversity index.

8.4 **Statistical analysis of causal relationships**

8.4.1 **Epidemiology and causal analysis**

In the previous sections, we have described alternative causal mechanisms that may underlie the onset of the disease or the level of some chronic condition of interest. Each of these mechanisms comprises temporal and causal structures that often involve more than one point exposure and numerous potential confounding variables. We have assumed that they are investigated with prospective life course data so that at least some of the presumed relationships are justifiable. Nonetheless, the assessment of such complex relationships requires assumptions that are difficult or impossible to verify from available data. Careful qualification in the inferring of causation is thus essential.

The history of the estimated causal association between hormone replacement therapy and coronary heart disease (HRT–CHD) described by Davey-Smith[26] is instructive. Meta-analysis of the best observational studies (internally controlled and angiographic studies) inferred a relative *reduction* of 50 per cent in CHD mortality with ever use of HRT[27] and helped promote widespread use of HRT. In contrast, randomized trials of women with and without established CHD found that HRT *increased* CHD mortality rates by 30 per cent.[28,29] Was this discrepancy due to *residual confounding*, i.e. uncontrolled correlated risk factors? Checking that effects are specific to the expected outcome and do not extend to implausible outcomes provides one informal test for residual confounding. Petitti *et al.*[30] showed that in one observational study HRT was also associated with violent death, a biologically implausible association and thus suggestive of the presence of residual confounding effects. With the benefit of knowing the randomized controlled trial (RCT) findings, re-analysis of some observational studies has identified residual confounding. For example, Lawlor *et al.*[5] re-analysed one study and found that the incorporation of multiple controls for socio-economic position at several points in the life course resulted in positive risk estimates for HRT similar to those found in RCTs. Other explanations have focused on the differences in follow-up period of the two designs.[31]

Statistical causal modelling should be able to contribute to the solution to problems such as these and lead to unbiased estimates of causal effects. In their overview of causal models, Greenland and Brumback[32] identify four distinct and largely complementary approaches: (1) graphical causal models;[33,34] (2) potential outcome (counterfactual) models;[35] (3) sufficient component cause models[36]; and (4) structural equation models.[37,38] We cannot provide a complete overview of each here, but instead we point to particular aspects that seem to have special relevance to life course research, beginning with the more conceptual.

8.4.2 **Graphical models**

Figure 8.3 shows a simple graphical model in which Z is an intermediate variable, with values partly determined by the observed variable X and partly by the unobserved variable U. Both X and U influence Y directly and indirectly through Z. Unlike the path diagrams of structural equation modelling (SEM) (see below), graphical models are non-parametric and thus in

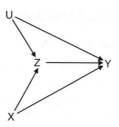

Fig. 8.3 Confounding of the causal relationship of X to Y occurs if Z is fixed because of the resulting confounding effect of unmeasured U.

themselves are not used for estimation. Their primary use is to identify the conditions under which independence and conditional independence between variables in the graph apply. Such identification can guide the choice of analysis (or experimental design) needed to estimate effects along one path which are uncontaminated by the effects of another.

Consider the direct path from X to Y. We might think that examining the relationship between X and Y in a sample selected to be homogeneous for Z would give an uncontaminated estimate of the X to Y effect because the variation in Z would have been eliminated. However, graphical theory tells that such an approach would be flawed, because selection on the basis of Z induces correlation between X and unmeasured U where none existed before, with the result that the simple relationship of X and Y in the sample selected for a specific value of Z is confounded by uncontrolled variation in U.[39] We should therefore be wary of examining relationships between, say, birth weight, and some late adult outcome, for samples that have been highly selected on some adolescent or early adult basis e.g. being a college student.

A related approach is that of Cox and Wermuth.[34] They too use graphical representations to define the dependence relationships among the variables of interest. Their approach is based on the theory of directed acyclic graphs (DAGs),[40] i.e. graphs where—when following the arrows that start from one variable—you cannot return to the same variable. In other words, DAGs are constructed making sure that no variable ever comes to explain itself. As in the case of Robins and Greenland's causal graphs, these graphs are used to formulate hypotheses but also to derive properties that lead to certain expected conditional independences among the variables, and these can be compared with the observed partial correlations. If the variables in a DAG can be arranged in boxes so that those in a particular box depend only on variables in boxes to their right (called univariate recursive regression graphs), simple univariate analyses can be applied to analyse the data (Fig. 8.4). Thus the partial regression coefficients obtained from sequentially regressing Y on Z, X and W, and Z on X and W would give empirical evidence for the assumed causal model.

Developments of this approach to include unmeasured variables are discussed in Wermuth and Cox.[41]

Fig. 8.4 Univariate recursive regression graph for Y, Z, X and W where all variables are observed.

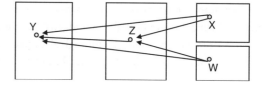

8.4.3 **Sufficient-component cause models, synergy and chains of effect**

8.4.3.1 Necessary and sufficient causes.

In certain settings, a variety of conditions have to be met before, during or even after a causal event happens for its effects to occur. In many studies, interest is focused only on one of the causal exposures in this chain, so that simplifying assumptions are made regarding the values taken by the others. These assumptions are not always appropriate, even if the study is defined in ways that meet them. Thus, with multiple causal exposures, a more developed conceptual framework (and terminology) is necessary. Rothman[36,42] proposed the idea of component causes, where each cause is *necessary* or *sufficient*. If the occurrence of just one of them is enough for the effects to be observed, this cause is sufficient. If several causes are present and yet no effect is observed unless one particular other cause is also present, then this latter is a necessary cause.

8.4.3.2 Sufficient-component causes and the additive model

The simple decomposition of necessary and sufficient causes has important implications regarding what we might expect to observe within our data. Figure 8.5(i) shows three causes A, B and C influencing a single outcome Y. These causes are each sufficient—only one needs to be present for the outcome to occur. Thus each leads to Y via a separate pathway.

Typically, one of them, say A, represents a composite path inclusive of all the other ways in which Y could occur in the absence of paths B and C. This allows us to focus on elucidating the causal mechanism relating to B and C without it being necessary (we hope) to explain every other possible way in which the outcome could have come about. Thus, we focus on the effects of B and/or C in elevating the rate of the outcome over and above some background rate that would be occurring as a result of the ever present generic path A.

Consider a hypothetical case in which B is exposure to smoking, C is poor exercise and the outcome Y is subsequent CHD. The causal model suggests that, in the absence of B and C, outcomes can only occur through the path defined by A, and that over some period of

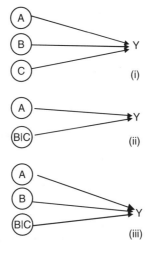

Fig. 8.5 Alternative pathways leading to an outcome Y: (i) independent paths from cause A, B and C; (ii) total synergy between cause B and C; (iii) partial synergy between cause B and C.

observation, the outcome might be observed according to rate a. For those also exposed to B, outcome will occur at rate a, through path A, and rate b, through path B. Similarly for those also exposed to C, the rates will be a and c. Both B and C are sufficient, i.e. exposure to either risk factor raises the subsequent rate of CHD. For people exposed to both B and C, in addition to the background cause A, some will succumb through path A, some through path B and some through path C. If the prevalences of B and C are small and uncorrelated, then comparatively few people will be exposed to both risk factors and still fewer will progress jointly down the B and C causal paths. This means that the expected rate of CHD for people exposed to both smoking and physical exercise is the sum of the rates arising through each possible path (including the background path), i.e. $a + b + c$.

Figure 8.5(ii) shows a rather different setting in which both B and C are necessary for the second pathway leading to Y, while the first still captures all other background causes. Since the rate is not increased if either B or C is absent, B and C are necessary but not sufficient causes, and people exposed to only one of them have base rate a. When they occur together, they form a sufficient cause and thus correspond to a pathway. In this case, there is total synergy between B and C, each risk factor potentiating the effect of the other with joint rate d.

Figure 8.5(iii) shows the case where B is sufficient for the second pathway, but is necessary but not sufficient for the third. C is also necessary but not sufficient for the third pathway. Here the presence of C only partially potentiates the risk posed by B. Partial synergy of this kind implies that B is a component of more than one sufficient cause, i.e. more than one pathway.

As discussed before, the expected outcome rate when all three causes are present under the model depicted in Fig. 8.5(i) is the sum of the cause-specific rates $a + b + c$. Different rates are expected under the other two models so that comparison of observed and expected rates can be used to test whether there is synergy between causes, using the first model as the benchmark (Table 8.3). An empirical test of whether there is synergy between B and C will therefore examine how well the three models fit the observed data.

This simple classification and thought experiment delivers some straightforward expectations and criteria for describing aspects of processes. It is therefore rather surprising to realize that it is almost entirely inconsistent with the way that we have been trained

Table 8.3 Outcome rates in the presence of different causes expected under the models shown in Fig. 8.5*

Exposure	Expected rates according to:		
	Model (i)	Model (ii)	Model (iii)
A	a	a	a
AB	$a + b$	a	$a + b$
AC	$a + c$	a	a
ABC	$a + b + c$	$a + d$	$a + b + d$

*Since A is the background rate and therefore always present, combinations without A are not shown.

and the way most of us actually analyse our research studies! The argument above suggests that our null expectation should be that the combined effect on an outcome of specific component causes will be additive in their individual rates. However, for perfectly sound statistical (and some good epidemiological) reasons, we have been taught that we should not combine effects additively on the rate scale but should do this on log scale, to which the logistic scale closely approximates when the base outcome rate is low. Table 8.4 shows the expected rates under a model that is additive on the log scale, i.e. equivalent to those from a Poisson regression (or logistic regression with low base rates) with additive effects for two specific risk factors B and C for a study where the outcome rate is low.

What we see is that the rate expected when B is present is b times the base rate. More critically, the expected rate when both B and C are present is not additive in their individual effects but multiplicative. In contrast to the Rothman additive model (i), if the base rate was 1 per 100 person-years (1/100py), and each component cause contributed a further 1/100py rate, then the rate expected when either B or C was present would be 2/100py, and when both risk factors B and C were present 3/100py. Under the main effects log-rate model, the corresponding rates would be 1/100py, 2/100py and 2/100py when either B or C are present, and 4/100py when both are present.

There are several implications. First, as Rothman and many others would understand it, substantial positive synergy is implied by a log-rate model that contains only main effects (cf. expected rate of 4/100py when B and C are present versus 3/100py under an additive model). Hence synergy is not at all synonymous with the need for a significant interaction term. Secondly, although the theory might tend to emphasize the possibility of positive potentiation of one risk factor by another, in practice we may be more likely to find we need negative interactions in log-rate regression analyses as a means of bringing the model closer to the often more plausible additive component cause model. Thirdly, it should be emphasized that the foregoing is not a criticism of log-rate or logistic regression, form of analysis that remain most elegant tools. The discussion above, however, does explain previous academic arguments as to whether synergistic effects are—or are not—present. The consensus among epidemiologists[43] is that synergy does not require or equate to an interaction within a log-rate regression. Most importantly, this does undermine the perhaps simple-minded, but ever so appealing, interpretation that the inclusion of a risk factor as a main effect within a log-rate regression represents the inclusion of a

Table 8.4 Outcome rates in the presence of different causes expected under the model shown in Fig. 8.5(i) when effects are additive on the log scales*

Exposure	Expected rates	
A	$\exp(\alpha)$	= base rate = a
AB	$\exp(\alpha + \beta) = \exp(\alpha)\cdot\exp(\beta)$	= ab
AC	$\exp(\alpha + \gamma) = \exp(\alpha)\cdot\exp(\gamma)$	= ac
ABC	$\exp(\alpha +\beta + \gamma) = \exp(\alpha)\cdot\exp(\beta)\cdot\exp(\gamma)$	= abc

*Since A is the background path and therefore always present, combinations without A are not shown.

separate pathway. It might be an approximation to it, but in fact it is more likely to be an elaboration of an alternative pathway model, to which we now turn.

8.4.3.3 Stages, chains and the multiplicative model

For many diseases, notably cancer, multiple stages of development have been considered. Defining these stages provides an opportunity for identifying temporal changes in aetiology: one set of factors may influence progress to an intermediate outcome, while another set may be important in the progression from intermediate to final outcome. Developing the single-stage models of the previous section, we now consider scenarios for a two-stage process with intermediate outcome *Y1* and final outcome of interest *Y2*.

In Figure 8.6(i), background factors A1 and A2 alone act to generate both intermediate and final outcomes. In Fig. 8.6(ii)–(iv), within each stage the presence of the additional risk factors, each representing a sufficient component cause with respect to their immediate outcome, acts as before in an additive fashion. However, at the second stage (and any postulated later stages), the background and risk factors cannot act on everybody; they can act only on those that have experienced the intermediate outcome. Achieving the intermediate outcome is a prerequisite either to being exposed to the second stage risk factors or to them having any effect. The result is that, unlike when combining effects within a stage, combining effects across stages is multiplicative—the larger the stage one effect the larger will be the number at risk to the second stage risk factors. With background factors alone influencing the two outcomes [as in Fig. 8.5(i)], the rate for outcome *Y2* is $a_1 a_2$, where a_1 is the base rate for *Y1* and a_2 the base rate for *Y2*. When another pathway is present for *Y1* [as in Fig. 8.6(ii)], the rate for *Y2* is $(a_1 + b_1) a2$, and when another is present for *Y2* [as in Fig. 8.6(iii)], it is $a_1 (a_2 + b_2)$. With additional pathways arising for both outcomes, the rate becomes $(a_1 + b_1)(a_2 + b_2)$. With background rates of 1/100py and additive within-stage component cause effects of 1/100py, the expected rates corresponding to Fig. 8.6 would become $(1/100 \times 1/100)py = 1/10,000py$ for model (i), 2/10 000py for models (ii) and (iii), and 4/10,000py for model (iv).

Fig. 8.6 Alternative pathways leading to an intermediate outcome *Y1* and a final outcome *Y2*: (i) only background factors acting on both outcomes; (ii) with an additional sufficient cause acting on *Y1* only; (iii) with an additional sufficient cause acting on *Y2* only; (iv) with an additional sufficient cause acting on *Y1* and another acting on *Y2*.

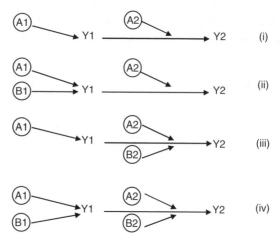

How the effects of risk and protective factors combine to increase or decrease the rate of the final outcome *Y2* will therefore depend upon which stages they impact upon, additive effects being expected if the factors operate on the same stage or multiplicative effects if they act on different stages. A main effects log-rate model is therefore rather more consistent with the idea of risk factors acting on different stages on a single but extended pathway, than it is with multiple distinct paths.

Synergy has often been conceptualized as some form of 'chemistry of the moment'—the immediate coincidence of risk factors being necessary for it to occur. In contrast, postulating an intermediate outcome (or outcomes), together with risk factors influencing rates both to and from it, provides all that is necessary for multiplicative and thus synergistic effects. Moreover, this synergy is one in which the exposure to each of these 'synergistic' risk factors could be separated by years. We would argue that this is much the more likely way in which synergy occurs rather than through 'chemistry of the moment'. A final elaboration of the argument is that the finding of partial synergy might suggest that one risk factor may operate on more than one intermediate outcome while the other operates on only one.

Multistage models also have implications for timing.[44] Where the relevant intermediate outcomes are not observed, the effect of changes in early risk factors on the final outcome may not be observed for some considerable time. A risk factor could be removed, but if it acts on an early stage then new cases could still continue to appear for years. Interventions on risk factors acting at later stages are likely to show their effects more immediately.

Chains of effects are conceptually appealing,[1] lending themselves to notions of developmental pathways and 'turning points'.[45] However, it is easy to leave an exaggerated impression as to the strength of risk effects that are transmitted over several links, though the effects of measurement error in the variables defining each link may work in the opposite direction, misclassification suggesting the links to be weaker than they may, in fact, be.[45]

8.4.4 Potential outcome models

8.4.4.1 Potential outcomes and counterfactuals

The traditional approach to the analysis of observational data, where by necessity exposures are not randomly assigned, is via some form of covariate adjustment (by either stratification or regression modelling). There are, however, numerous circumstances where this is not a satisfactory approach. We describe some alternative approaches to simple covariate adjustment, all of which draw upon the notion of *counterfactuals or potential outcomes*, a conceptual device that assists in the analysis of the effects of some potentially manipulable exposure by considering the comparison of an individual's outcome following their actual exposure history with potential outcomes that would have occurred had the exposure history been different. It should be noted that some warn that this conceptual device is both unnecessary and sometimes misleading.[46]

8.4.4.2 Counterfactuals and marginal structural means (MSM) modelling for measured confounders

Consider the diagram in Fig. 8.5. This is a small modification of that in Fig. 8.3 because now Z leads to X (and not vice versa), and U influences X as well as Z. Here X is the exposure of interest, Y is the outcome of interest, Z is all other measured risk factors and U is all unmeasured risk factors, both of which influence the value taken by the exposure as well as the outcome. Consider the case of a binary exposure. For a given subject, the causal effect of X is $\psi = E[Y_{x=1} - Y_{x=0}]$, where $Y_{x=1}$ and $Y_{x=0}$ are the values of Y when X is 1 and 0, respectively. However, we do not get to measure both of these quantities on the same sample of individuals: we can observe the outcome for the level of the X exposure that each individual actually experienced. We do *not* observe the counterfactual, the outcome for each individual had they experienced the other level of the X exposure. However, if we could define $\Pr(Y_{x=1} = 1)$ and $\Pr(Y_{x=0} = 1)$, then the causal risk difference $\Pr(Y_{x=1} = 1) - \Pr(Y_{x=0} = 1)$ or the causal OR $\Pr(Y_{x=1} = 1) \times \Pr(Y_{x=0} = 0)/\Pr(Y_{x=1} = 0) \times \Pr(Y_{x=0} = 1)$ could be calculated. Were X unconfounded, then estimates of the causal effects could be obtained from the crude effects, i.e. the observed probabilities. However, in observational studies, the absence of any confounding is implausible and therefore these crude estimates are not useful. Three related methods have been suggested to deal with confounding arising in this setting (Fig. 8.7).

8.4.4.3 Propensity scores for measured confounders

Consider the case where, in the population, the effect of X on the outcome Y may be confounded only by measured confounders Z. Exposure assignment is said to be strongly ignorable if the exposure X and the response Y are conditionally independent given the covariates Z. Rosenbaum and Rubin[47] proposed the propensity score approach for estimating the causal effect of X in this circumstance. For a binary exposure of interest X, the propensity score $e(Z_i)$ for a subject i is the conditional probability of exposure given the vector of observed confounders Z, i.e. $e(Z_i) = \Pr(X_i = 1 | Z_i = z_i)$. Such a propensity score is usually estimated by logistic regression, with X treated as the response variable and the confounders Z as the predictors. It can be shown that the estimate of the effect of X from an analysis that is also stratified by the propensity score gives unbiased estimates of the exposure effect under a wider range of conditions than an analysis that covaries for all the components of z. For example, if the covariates have greater variability, or different patterns of correlation in one exposure group than another, then direct covariate adjustment could increase the bias or even overcorrect.

The stratification or matching on propensity score results in exposed individuals being compared only with those unexposed individuals who had similar chances of being exposed. An alternative approach of including the propensity score as an additional covariate requires additional linearity assumptions to be met for valid causal inference.

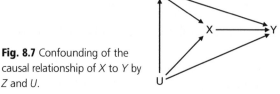

Fig. 8.7 Confounding of the causal relationship of X to Y by Z and U.

The matching and stratification approaches also tend to make explicit considerations (by defining a region of common support) of which subjects should be excluded from analysis because their propensity score is so close to 0 or to 1, either because matchable individuals of opposite exposure status are too rare or because for such individuals the exposure cannot reasonably be considered as manipulable.

8.4.4.4 Marginal structural means and time-dependent confounding

The propensity score approach is similar to the marginal structural means (MSM) approach proposed by Robins.[48] This uses a weighted analysis by directly comparing means marginalized over the confounders Z to yield unbiased estimates of the causal parameters. Each subject i is assigned a weight w_i equal to the inverse of the propensity score for their observed exposure, i.e.

$$w_i = 1/\Pr[X_i = x_i | Z_i = z_i]$$

If all individuals in this population are weighted using these values w_i, then in this overall weighted population the variables X and Z are no longer confounded. The analysis thus consists of fitting the usual models for the effects of X on Y, e.g. linear or logistic regression, but with subjects weighted by weights $\{w_i\}$. This must be done within a procedure that recognizes these weights as probability weights and requires that the procedure calculates the standard error, and thus P-values and confidence intervals, using the sandwich or robust estimator[49] or some other technique (such as bootstrap). In a longitudinal study, we will commonly be concerned with a time-dependent exposure, $X_0, X_1,...,X_K$, where we might wish to estimate the effect of a cumulative exposure. With no confounding, the association model

$$\text{logit}\left(\Pr\left[Y = 1 \mid X_0 = x_0, X_1 = x_1,..., X_k = x_k\right]\right) = \beta_0 + \beta_1\left(\sum_{k=0}^{k} x_k\right)$$

could be used to estimate the parameters of interest. With exposures confounded with $Z_0, Z_1,...,Z_K$, then we can again use weights for the probability of exposure, but now the weights are no longer defined as the conditional probability of a binary exposure, but instead as the conditional probability that a subject experienced their particular exposure *history*, i.e. a multinomial probability.

With complex confounder and exposure history, these weights can have excessive variability, giving rise to inefficient estimates of causal effects in the eventual weighted logistic analysis of cumulative exposure on outcome Y. To overcome this, stabilized weights are suggested. In the simple case of a single period of exposure, this involves replacing weight $w_i = 1/\Pr[X = x_i | Z = z_i]$ by stabilized weight $sw_i = \Pr[X = x_i]/\Pr[X = x_i | Z = z_i]$. In the multiperiod case, this simple formulation has the single exposure values and confounder vector replaced by their respective histories over the $(K + 1)$ periods. Diggle *et al.*[21] present a clear binary data example.

In the single period case, the practical advantage of the MSM approach over more routine covariate adjustment is not obvious. However, in the multiperiod time-dependent case, the advantage of the MSM approach is clearer. Both approaches attempt adjustment for Z_k, where Z_k is a confounder for later exposure. However, adopting the simpler covariate adjustment approach erroneously controls for the effect that earlier values of the exposure have on Z_k, i.e. the value of the confounder during period k. Thus it would also wrongly partial out causal effects that should be attributed to the exposure. An example of this approach is the study of the effect of antiretroviral therapy (the exposure) and CD4 counts (the confounder) on the risk of acquired immunodeficiency syndrome (AIDS).[50]

8.4.4.5 Explicit counterfactual models and G-estimation for measured confounders

For a continuous outcome and binary exposure of interest X we could construct an explicit counterfactual model along the following lines:

$$\text{Outcome if unexposed} = Y^* = \text{observed outcome} + \delta X$$

Where δ is a hypothetical value of the effect of exposure to X. If individuals were randomly assigned to exposure, then we could estimate the effect of exposure to X by finding the value of δ which makes our outcomes Y^* independent of X, i.e. the value of δ that gives Y^* a zero coefficient in the logistic regression in which Y^* predicted X. Exactly the same procedure can be followed in the presence of confounders, except that these are now also included in the logistic regression for X.

With a time-varying exposure, the process is modified to allow for the model of the counterfactual outcome Y^* to include the effects of partial and cumulative exposure to X, and for the logistic regression for X to include multiple records for each subject, with each record relating to a different exposure period. An elaboration and an example of this approach for survival data is illustrated in Chapter 9. A further elaboration of this approach replaces the observed exposure in the equation above by a variable that is related to exposure but not to potential confounders,[51] a modification that is strongly related to the instrumental variable approach that we now describe, and which is capable of accounting for both measured, and remarkably, unmeasured confounders.

8.4.4.6 Double robust estimators

It is possible to use a combination of methods for adjusting for confounders, such as using covariate adjustment and the weighting method described in Section 8.4.4.4. Such a combination offers the property of double-robustness, where unbiased estimates may be obtained provided either the covariate adjustment for confounders is correct or the weighting adjustment, or both. This gives the analyst two chances of correctly accounting for observed confounders.[52]

8.4.5 Instrumental variables and accounting for measured and unmeasured confounders

8.4.5.1 Instrumental variables and the exclusion restriction

The approaches described above require full information on all the confounders, since these are needed to define the propensity score and inverse probability weights or, in the case of G-estimation, to assess the independence of counterfactual outcome and exposure

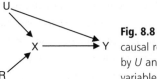

Fig. 8.8 Confounding of the causal relationship of X to Y by U and the instrumental variable R.

conditional on confounders. What if we do not have all this information? One way to deal with unmeasured confounding involves having data on a variable R that precedes and is related to exposure but is not directly related to the outcome or the unmeasured confounders (Fig. 8.8). Remarkably, what having such a variable allows is for the unbiased estimation of the effect of X on Y even when its effects are correlated with the error term. The 'exclusion restriction', that R is independent of Y given X and U, is key to being able to identify the effect of X on Y. A variable with these properties, if it exists, is said to be an instrument for the unbiased estimate of the causal effect of the exposure. Because the relationship between R and Y is completely via X and is unbiased, the causal effect of X on Y, β^{IV}, can be derived. For example, in the no covariate case, if all relationships are linear, then the instrumental variable (IV) estimator is the ratio of the coefficient in the regression of Y on R, β_{YR}, to the coefficient in the regression of X on R, β_{XR}. Typically this results merely in the magnitude of the estimated effect being increased over the naïve estimate. However, when calculated in the presence of measured covariates, this simple relationship no longer applies and the IV estimate can even be of opposite sign to the naïve estimate. In simple cases, β^{IV} can still be estimated by various versions of the two-stage approach just described,[53] or a model representing the complete causal diagram can be estimated by maximum likelihood. Instrumental variables have long been a feature of structural equation modelling,[54] but their very particular role has often been lost within many complex applications. In Section 8.4.6 we discuss SEM and a generalization of SEM, generalized linear latent and mixed modelling, that makes it better suited to the types of variables encountered in epidemiology. Skrondal and Rabe-Hesketh[55] illustrate such an approach to estimate an IV model for the effect of physician advice (binary) on a count of alcoholic drinks outcome (overdispersed Poisson), where the naïve positive association is reversed to suggest such advice as being protective.

8.4.5.2 Natural experiments and instrumental variables (IVs)

The IV approach is clearly powerful, but finding suitable instrumental variables R, and convincing other researchers of the appropriateness of the exclusion restriction, is rarely possible in entirely observational studies. Many social experiments make use of this approach in so-called encouragement designs in which a random subgroup (randomization being the IV) are encouraged to participate in some programme, the encouragement being designed to be sufficient to increase the proportion participating but not sufficient in itself to influence the outcome materially. Such a design and method of analysis is clearly suited to the evaluation of educational programmes that may be cast within a developmental framework (see Chapter 5). The other major source of IVs is from natural experiments.

Drastic lottery-based 'treatments' such as Vietnam military service used in classic analyses to evaluate the benefits of post-secondary school education[56] are both unusually convincing as an IV and rare. Nonetheless, at any one time, many differences exist across jurisdictional boundaries and areas defined following major point source accidental exposure. Geography and migration[57] can also provide suitable contrasts. Rutter et al.[58] provide a range of examples of natural experiments that have proved valuable in estimating environmental effects in development of psychopathology, many of which could be analysed using IV methods.

Recently this approach is finding novel application in Mendelian randomization studies where (presumed) functional genes are used as instruments for phenotypes thought to cause certain diseases. We illustrate this exciting possibility, but refer readers to Didelez and Sheehan[59] and Hernan and Robins[60] who highlight some of the limitations of the method.

Serum IGFBP-3 and mammographic features In breast cancer research, there is increasing interest in identifying functional genes linked to the production of growth hormones, as their levels are thought to be causally related to physiological features of the breast, such as lucent tissue, which are recognized risk factors for breast cancer.[61] The epidemiological evidence for the link between hormonal levels and mammographic features is however confounded by several other breast cancer risk factors, such as reproductive behaviour.

One growth hormone of current interest is insulin-like growth factor I (IgF-I) which is regulated by a protein called insulin-like growth factor-binding protein 3 (IGFBP-3). A putative functional gene for this protein, IGFBP3g, has been identified with genotypes AA, AC and CC. Mammographic features and both serum IGFBP-3 levels and IGFBP3g genotype are available for a stratified sample of 213 pre-menopausal women who participated in a prospective study carried out on the Channel island of Guernsey.[62] Of interest in this context is the relationship between IGFBP-3 and lucent area of the breast. A brief description of the data is given in Table 8.5.

Ignoring women with missing genotype, we use (natural) log transformations for both total area of lucent tissue and serum IGFBP-3 before fitting a linear regression model.

Table 8.5 Distribution of total area of lucent tissue and IGFBP-3 serum level by the putative genotype

Genotype	n	Total area of lucent tissue (cm²)		Serum IGFBP-3 (ng/ml)	
		Median	IQR	Median	IQR
AA	33	63.86	52.24	5188.5	1450.5
AC	66	53.41	38.53	4695.0	1214.0
CC	41	45.64	31.26	4681.0	1343.0
NK	33	45.57	39.86	4547.0	1469.0

n = number of women; IQR = interquartile range; NK = not known.

Table 8.6 Regression coefficients for the effect of 1 SD increase in ln(IGFBP-3) on ln(total lucent area)

	β	SE	95 per cent CI
Naïve estimate	0.09	0.05	(0.01–0.19)
Adjusted*	0.13	0.05	(0.03–0.22)
IV estimate from naïve model	0.53	0.27	(0.01–1.05)
IV estimate from adjusted* model	0.53	0.26	(0.02–1.03)

SE = standard error; CI = confidence interval IV = instrumental variable.

*Adjusted for age, parity, duration of breastfeeding and oral contraceptive use.

The naïve estimate of the effect of 1 standard deviation (SD) increase in ln(IGFBP-3) on ln(lucent area) is 0.094 (95 per cent CI 0.01–0.19; Table 8.6). This estimate may, however, be confounded by unmeasured (or unaccounted) factors that are correlated with the protein and also—directly or indirectly—influence total area of lucent tissue. A causal effect of IGFB-3 on total lucent area could nevertheless be estimated using an IV approach under the strong assumption that the putative gene IGFBP3g is related to total lucent area *exclusively* via serum IGFBP-3 (as in Fig. 8.8). This is known in IV methodology as the *exclusion* restriction. If this is correct, the results indicate that the causal effect may be, in fact, five times larger than originally estimated (0.53, 95 per cent CI 0.01–1.05). Before believing this finding, we should seek to confirm the applicability of the exclusion restriction, that conditional upon serum IGFBP-3 there is no association of IGFBP3g with lucent tissue area (a test commonly with rather low power). We could also test that it is not associated with known confounders and attempt to identify the source of some of the unaccounted negative confounding identified by the IV approach, by refitting the naïve regression model, but this time controlling for some known confounders for which information was actually available: age, parity, duration of breastfeeding and use of oral contraceptives. Adjusting for these factors slightly increases the naïve estimate to 0.13 (95 per cent CI 0.03–0.22). Interestingly applying the IV approach again while controlling for these same variables led to the same—but slightly more precise—estimate of the causal effect of ln(IGFBP-3).

8.4.6 Structural equation models (SEMs)

8.4.6.1 Path analysis

Path analysis, first systematically developed by Sewell Wright,[63] exploits linearity assumptions to allow the covariance between two variables on a path diagram to be decomposed into contributions arising from each legitimate path that connects them, with simple rules for determining the legitimate paths.[64,65] Implicit in these diagrams is the fact that the variables are modelled via a set of simultaneous equations. These would now be commonly estimated in software for structural equation modelling (e.g. Mplus[66]).

If, to the traditional diagram, a residual variance is added to each variable in the form of a double-headed arrow running both from and to that variable, then a rule for defining legitimate paths becomes: trace backwards from an intermediate variable or final out-come, change direction at a two-headed arrow, then trace forwards. These rules allow us to identify how the value of a later variable can be influenced by an earlier variable either by a direct path or by an indirect path via another variable. Multiplication of the (standard-ized) coefficients along each path gives the expected covariance (equivalent to standardized effect) for that path, and these may be summed to give the total, i.e. direct and indirect, expected covariances (or total standardized effects). Goodness-of-fit tests can also be computed by comparing observed and expected covariance matrices.

8.4.6.2 Triangulation and mediation

Path models can provide considerable insight into the mechanism by which variation in one variable gives rise to variation in some later variable, especially when variables that may play a critical intermediate role are included in the model. In this setting, the decomposition of total effects into direct and indirect components has become very useful. In particular, when it can be shown that there are no effects of the first variable on the last variable once the effects of the intervening variables have been accounted for, i.e. when effects are said to be mediated by intermediate variables with no residual direct effects, the interpre-tation is that the intervening variable lies on the causal pathway. Illustrated in Fig. 8.9, this argument corresponds to the removal of the direct path from the causal exposure X to outcome Y, leaving just the single pathway via Z. If the probability of Y occurring, given that the value of Z does not depend on X, i.e. $Pr(Y|Z,X) = Pr(Y|Z)$, then X has no direct effect on Y, with its effects being only indirect through Z.

Baron and Kenny[67] and Judd and Kenny[68] describe four steps in investigating such mediation in the context of SEM path models: (1) show that X is correlated with Y; (2) show that X is correlated with Z; (3) show that Z is correlated with Y; and (4) show that the effect (partial correlation) of X on Y controlling for Z is zero. In the regression framework, we would be comparing the regression of Y on X (model 1) and the regres-sion of Y on X and Z (model 2). The estimated coefficients identify component pathways (see previous section), while background effects due to possibly numerous other compo-nent causes are included within the error terms of the regressions. As commonly used, a significant coefficient for X in model 1, but a non-significant coefficient in model 2, is taken as evidence of mediation. Various more rigorous tests are available that assess the sig-nificance of the indirect effect from X to Y, i.e. of the product of the effects of X on Z and of Z on Y. Nonetheless, without further evidence, such a result could arise from Z being a

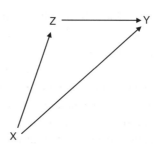

Fig. 8.9 Effects of X on Y partially mediated by Z.

confounder rather than a mediator, i.e. the association between X and Z in fact being merely correlational. Indeed, very little of this work on mediation takes any account of possible unmeasured confounders. Further, in many applications, the available data do not have the power to test all these correlations reliably.

This model has been used to study the direct effect of X on Y, treating Z as an *a priori* confounder or potential effect modifier. In certain settings, this has been contentious, for example in studies where the fetal origin hypothesis was investigated by regressing adult levels of systolic blood pressure (SBP) on birth weight controlling for adult body weight or body mass index (BMI; weight in kg/height in m^2).[69-72]

8.4.6.3 Measurement error

The major advantage of the SEM approach is its ability, when applied to studies with suitable measurement designs, to tackle the problem of measurement error. When some of the exposure variables are approximate measures for factors that were not measured precisely, latent variables can be introduced, as in Clayton's model.[2] In Fig. 8.10, three variables, X_1, X_2 and X_3, act as proxy (or 'manifest') measures for the unmeasured variable U, where U is thought to influence a final outcome Y (the SEM convention is to use squares for observed, i.e. manifest, variables, and circles for latent variables). Here the specification of the relationship between observed Xs and unobserved U defines the *measurement* submodel, while that between U and Y defines the *disease* or—more generally—*structural* submodel. Because U is not directly observed and does not usually have a quantifiable metric, its influence on the manifest variables can only be measured in terms of an arbitrary metric. One convention is to use the first of the proxy variables as reference and thus adopt its metric, e.g. that of X_1, so that the effect of the latent variable on Y becomes expressed in terms of X_1 units. Alternatively, the variance of the latent construct is fixed to be 1 and its effect on Y estimated in terms of 1 SD change in the latent variable.

In this simple example, the impact of accounting for measurement error in the exposure will be to increase the magnitude of the estimate of the effect of that exposure on the outcome, yielding the so-called 'disattenuated' effect. In more complex settings where several exposures are measured with error, such error can have far more pernicious effects. We illustrate these in the next example.

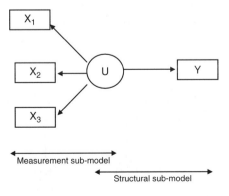

Fig. 8.10 Example of a path diagram for one distal outcome (Y) and a latent variable (U) measured by three proxy variables (X_1, X_2, X_3).

Table 8.7 Summary statistics for the repeated measures of childhood ability measured by Osborne and Suddick[73]

Age at measurement (years)	6	7	9	11
Mean	18.03	25.82	35.26	46.59
Standard deviation	6.37	7.32	7.80	10.39
Correlation matrix				
Age (years) 7		0.809		
9		0.806	0.850	
11		0.765	0.831	0.867

Measurement errors in children's ability scores Ability scores were collected in children aged 6, 7, 9 and 11 years to measure continuity in general ability.[73] Summary statistics for these data are shown in Table 8.7. As described in Dunn *et al.*,[74] a plausible starting model is the first-order autoregressive model shown in Fig. 8.11 where ability at one age, having taken into account ability at the previous measurements, is not associated with any earlier measure.

A feature of such a model is that an early measure may influence a later measure, but only through an intermediate measure. The model consists of three regressions (*Y1* on *Y2, Y2* on *Y3,* and *Y3* on *Y4*). In addition to estimating the standardized regression coefficients (0.809, 0.850 and 0.867, respectively), as one would do in standard regression modelling, we can assess the model's goodness-of-fit by comparing observed and expected covariances. This shows the autoregressive model to have a very poor fit [chi-square statistic of 61.82 with 3 degrees of freedom (df; the degrees of freedom are found from the difference between the 10 observed summary statistics and the seven estimated parameters which are the variances for *Y1, E2, E3* and *E4* and the three regression coefficients b1, b2 and b3)]. This poor fit immediately tells us that something is very wrong. For many researchers, the instinct is to conclude that additional relationships must exist, for example from *Y1* to *Y3* and *Y2* to *Y4*.

Those additional relationships correspond to 'sleeper effects', i.e. components of a given measure have no effect on the immediately following measure but yet can influence the subsequent one. There are circumstances where such effects are plausible (e.g. where the tests vary in content and those more far apart are more similar, say being more mathematical); however, in general, they are rightly considered implausible.

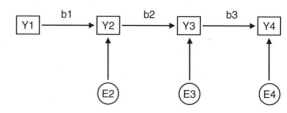

Fig. 8.11 A continuity model for the general ability data of Osborne and Suddick.[73]

One way to improve the model fit without adding these sleeper effects is to take the issue of measurement error seriously. In the classical measurement error model, the observed measurement is additively related to a 'true variable' F and a measurement error E of constant variance, i.e.

$$Y = F + E$$

The 'true variable' F is an example of a latent variable or factor, and in this simple case one that involves no regression coefficient (and is also therefore a simple random effect). Usually replicate measurements are necessary in order to identify and estimate the measurement error separately from the true variable. However, an SEM of the four measurements can be fitted with constraints, enabling the variance for F and E to be identified with only single measurements per occasion (Fig. 8.12). Imposing constraints such that the measurement error variance remains the same over the four occasions achieves identification of the model and involves only one more parameter than the previous model (three regression coefficients between the factors and variances for the factor $F1$, the disturbances $D2$, $D3$ and $D4$, and the single common measurement error variance for the Es). Allowing for measurement error results in a huge improvement in model fit (chi-square = 1.43 with 2 df). Clearly this model has no need of additional sleeper effects—it already fits so well. How has this come about?

In the model corresponding to Fig. 8.11, measurement error in the Ys attenuates the coefficients estimated in each regression of one Y on the previous one, i.e. smaller than they would have been in the absence of measurement error. This underestimation results in the predicted association among the most temporally distant variables $Y1$ and $Y4$—which is given by the product of the standardized regression coefficients b1, b2 and b3—being underestimated even more (a 10 per cent underestimation in each coefficient resulting in a $1 - 0.9 \times 0.9 \times 0.9 = 27$ per cent underestimation of their product). Allowing for measurement error corrects each regression coefficient and removes this gross underestimation of the model-predicted long-term association.

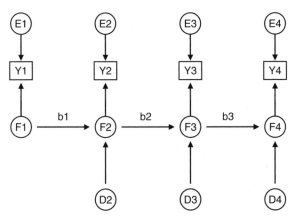

Fig. 8.12 Latent variable continuity model for the general ability data of Osborne and Suddick.[73] Observed variables Y, measurement error variables E, latent variables F and disturbances (variation in the factors not associated with the previous factor) D.

There are numerous implications from this very modest example. The first is that, in general, although measurement error in a covariate *X1* may result in systematic underestimation of its relationship with some response, it can also give rise to overestimation of the effects of some other covariate, *X2*, with which *X1* is correlated. Take the often repeated finding that current health is associated not only with contemporaneous risk factors, but also independently with the same risk factors measured in childhood (e.g. Krieger *et al.*[9]). Is this because the risk has its effect through an accumulation of risk exposure or is it an artefact of measurement error in the contemporaneous measurements and that these contemporaneous measures tend to be correlated with childhood measures? This latter possibility is rarely explored.

These data can be used to illustrate a further important point, namely that achieving a good model fit is not evidence for the correctness of the model, merely that it is one contender. A natural alternative model for data of this kind is a model in which each child is considered as having a trajectory over time (i.e. a growth curve) defined by an initial ability, represented by a latent intercept factor—or random effect—*F1*, and a latent rate of improvement, represented by a slope factor—or random coefficient *F2* (Fig. 8.13). The intercept factor 'loads', i.e. regresses, on all four measurements with a common regression coefficient λ. The growth (or slope) factor loads on all but the first, with either distinct factor loadings on each path (b1, b2 and b3) or with constraints such that the loadings vary in proportion with the time since the initial measurement (equivalent to allowing for the linear effects of time to be random). In almost all growth situations, values at the initial starting point are correlated with subsequent growth, requiring the two latent factors or random effects to be correlated. Again we can impose restrictions such that the measurement error variances (*E1–E4*) are constant. This model has one fewer parameter than the model of Fig. 8.12 but in fact fits these data better, giving a chi-square goodness-of-fit of 0.92 with 3 df.

Which of the two well fitting models should we choose? In this case, the choice is likely to rest upon theoretical considerations because we lack the data to discriminate effectively.

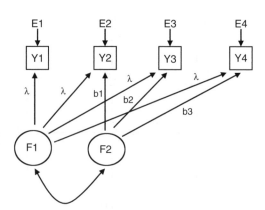

Fig. 8.13 Growth curve model for the general ability data of Osbourne and Suddick intercept and slope factors or random effects.

The last model has the fewer parameters and in addition has the advantage of cleanly partitioning initial cross-sectional variation from subsequent change. This has appeal, especially were the model extended to allow for the effects of exposures to be associated with both the intercept and slope factors.

8.4.6.4 SEM with continuous and discrete variables and interactions

These kinds of model can also be applied in the more common circumstance of epidemiology in which we have a mixture of continuous and discrete variables. Rabe-Hesketh et al.[75] show how the effects of occupation on CHD can be divided into direct and indirect effects through dietary differences in occupations. Here again measurement error in diet would be expected to attenuate the apparent importance of such indirect effects. Their application using a generalized linear latent and mixed model framework—a general modelling framework that includes SEMs (implemented within the *Stata* program gllamm) which uses non-parametric maximum likelihood—show how normality of the latent variable ('true' dietary intake) is not required.

One of the major limitations of SEM path models is their inability to represent interactions. In fact this is not a strict limitation, since multiple group methods, models that allow random coefficients (see next section), e.g. gllamm,[55] and a number of other approaches enable these to be considered.[76] Nonetheless, few substantive applications have pursued them.

8.4.7 Multilevel or hierarchical models

8.4.7.1 Clustered data and ecological effects

Hierarchical (or multilevel) models are used when individuals, or any other units of analysis, are correlated, for example because they are grouped in clusters. Common examples are where students are grouped within schools and children within families. Although developed independently within different statistical traditions (e.g. Goldstein[77] and Laird and Ware[78]), they can be described from within an SEM framework.

Their main feature is the modelling of the correlations within each cluster. This can be achieved by assuming that, for example, students in the same school share the same effect of the exposure variable of interest (e.g. the regression parameter in a linear regression model), but in general this effect varies across clusters. So the exposure effect can be seen as an unobservable ('latent') variable that varies at the level of the cluster, not of the individual, hence the term 'multilevel' used to describe these models. For a given distribution of this variable, its mean and variance can be estimated and used to describe the average effect across the clusters as well as its variability (spread).

An interesting application of this model concerns individual health outcomes, e.g. survival 1 year after diagnosis of a certain cancer, that are clustered within geographical areas. The approach allows the health outcomes to be decomposed into two elements, one associated with the individuals, and one associated with their local area. Typically they are assumed to be additive and uncorrelated, so that for individual i in area j, the outcome Y_{ij} is given by $Y_{ij} = \mu_{ij} + \delta_{ij}$. This decomposition results in two variances, $\Phi^2(\mu)$ and $\Phi^2(\delta)$, the individual and area level variation. Both of these sources of variation may be systematically related to measured characteristics of the individual, X_{ij}, and their area, Z_j, respectively, by $\mu_{ij} = \beta_x X_{ij} + u_{ij}$ and $\delta_j = \beta_z Z_j + d_j$; essentially regressions that help 'explain' variation at the individual and geographical levels, with each allowing for unexplained variation through the random errors u_{ij} and d_j that are assumed uncorrelated. The variables included in X and Z can be the same but measured at different levels. For example, one of the variables in X might be a manual occupation indicator for the individual, while one of the variables included in Z is the proportion in manual occupation in the area. The variances $\Phi^2(u)$ and $\Phi^2(d)$ now describe the residual or unexplained individual and area variations in health. The size of the area level variance has been seen to be of particular social and policy interest because, while we seem willing to accept individual variation in health as somehow inevitable (and anyway these are hard to distinguish from random measurement error in the individual's health outcome), systematic differences between communities should not be accepted. In standard (one-level) regression analysis, we are familiar with how including significant covariates reduces the size of the residual error variance. In the multilevel context, including individual covariates X_{ij} can reduce not only the size of the variance associated with residual individual differences, $\Phi^2(u)$, but also the size of the residual area differences, $\Phi^2(d)$. This is due to the fact that area-level variation not only reflects contextual effects, i.e. the effects of living in a particular area, but also compositional effects, i.e. the systematic differences in the make-up of local populations. There is thus an interest in the size of the area-level residual variation after having taken account of the compositional differences between areas as reflected in major individual-level predictors.

However, the multilevel model can also provide two distinct estimates for the effects of measured covariates; in our example β_x describes the variation associated with the manual occupation composition of the population in each area, while β_z describes how the geographical differences in health outcomes are associated with the proportion of manual workers. Note that, in parallel to what happens in standard one-level analysis, adding an exposure variable at the individual level can modify the estimated effect of a second exposure at either or both individual and area levels. Thus the results obtained from this type of model must be interpreted with care.

The assumptions described above are, however, very simple indeed. One further multilevel model elaboration allows for a much richer range of area-level effects to be explored. It is possible that the effects of some individual covariates are amplified in some contexts or areas more than others. For example, the effects of manual occupation may vary from area to area depending upon the nature of the work carried out by the major local employers of manual workers or upon their healthcare systems. In other words, the effect of the exposure is moderated by area. If information on the modifying factors is available, interaction terms between individual- and area-level predictors can be included in the model. Where these moderating area characteristics are unknown or unmeasured, then this requires the β_x coefficient to vary from area to area, i.e. to be random at the area level, leading to the individual component of the model to be specified by $\mu_{ij} = \beta_{x(j)} X_{ij} + u_{ij}$, with $\beta_{x(j)}$ distributed with mean β and variance $\Phi^2(\beta_x)$.

8.4.7.2 Modelling growth trajectories and their relationship to later disease

An interesting example where there is widespread interest in identifying whether time-changing exposures act cumulatively over time or instead specifically during 'critical' time periods is found in the literature on the relationship between childhood growth and onset of several chronic diseases.[79–82] Despite the increasing interest in this area, empirical investigations of how body changes in infancy, childhood and adolescence influence the occurrence of later disease suffer from limitations due to the quality of the available data. Indeed recorded childhood growth data for people at risk of adult diseases are difficult to obtain: when available, they may be based on recall or—even if recorded prospectively—they may be incomplete (because of either attrition or temporary losses to follow-up) or not available at the ages of greatest interest (e.g. peak height velocity or adiposity rebound[83]). Their precision may also vary over time, as the data collection process may be affected by changes in units and instruments (e.g. metric instead of imperial measurements).

Even in the absence of these problems, investigations of how childhood growth may influence the onset of a later disease remain challenging. Indeed these involve highly correlated variables—the repeated anthropometric variables—which depend on earlier factors, such as parental characteristics, also directly influence some of the adult risk factors. In trying to disentangle the effects of childhood variables on later disease, alternative biological models have been proposed: the critical period model and the critical size model. Discriminating between these models requires not only detailed childhood data but also appropriate analytical modelling. We illustrate some of the issues with an example from a study of childhood growth and breast cancer risk.

Childhood growth and breast cancer risk Prospective data on childhood growth, onset of menarche and adult life risk factors for breast cancer were available for 2187 female participants in the British 1946 national birth cohort[84–86] and introduced in Chapter 1. Childhood measurements of height and BMI were available for ages 2, 4, 6, 7, 11 and 14/15 years. Adult height (as a marker of the total height achieved by the end of the adolescent growth spurt) was self-reported at age 26 and measured at 36 and 43 years of age. A total of 59 women were diagnosed with breast cancer by 31 December 1999 (details in De Stavola et al.[82]).

The mean heights at different ages (up to adulthood) for breast cancer cases are consistently higher than those for the non-cases; the reverse is seen for the BMI mean values in childhood (Fig. 8.14). This is confirmed by the OR for breast cancer incidence estimated separately for each height and BMI value (Table 8.8).

To identify whether critical periods of growth or critical sizes reached by a certain age could be driving these relationships, yearly rates of change ('*velocities*') between consecutive anthropometric measurements were calculated (using in the denominator the exact differences in age at measurement) and their corresponding ORs for breast cancer incidence estimated separately (Table 8.9). They identify the periods between age 4 and 7 years and between age 11 and 15 as those when height gains have the greatest association with breast cancer risk. The joint analyses of all these components of growth are shown

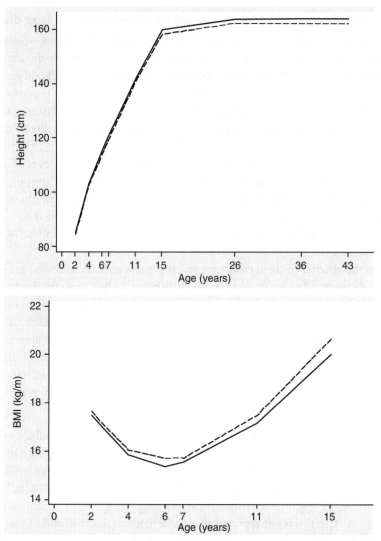

Fig. 8.14 Mean age-specific height and body mass index (BMI, kg/m²) by breast cancer status — cases, - - - non-cases; NHSD, 1946–1999.

in Table 8.10. Because of the reduced sample size, these analyses were initially based on the subsets of women for whom the relevant anthropometric measurements were available.

To overcome the limitations of these complete records analyses, a multiple imputation (MI) procedure (see Schafer[87] and Chapter 7) was also used to allow the inclusion of all 2187 eligible subjects in every analysis, assuming that missing data had occurred at random (MAR).[88] Since MAR is a less restrictive assumption than that of missing completely at random (MCAR) implicit in complete records analyses, the MI results are to be preferred. They show that in the model with the height intercept at age 2 plus all the consecutive height velocities (a decomposition of the model with just adult height), the height velocity

Table 8.8 Estimates of univariable breast cancer odds ratios (ORs) for 1 SD increase in anthropometric measures at different ages; results obtained on 2187 women followed-up to age 53 years

Variable	N*	D*	OR[†]	95 per cent CI
Childhood height (cm) measured at:				
2 years	1782	53	1.16	0.88–1.54
4 years	1944	56	1.12	0.86–1.46
7 years	1925	53	1.30	0.99–1.71
11 years	1862	51	1.16	0.88–1.53
15 years	1689	44	1.33	0.97–1.80
Adulthood height (cm) measured at:				
26 years[‡]	1758	50	1.28	0.96–1.69
36 years	1610	47	1.37	1.02–1.84
43 years	1567	40	1.36	0.99–1.86
BMI (kg/m^2) measured at:				
2 years	1705	50	0.93	0.69–1.25
4 years	1903	55	0.88	0.67–1.16
7 years	1853	52	0.89	0.66–1.19
11 years	1836	51	0.87	0.64–1.18
15 years	1664	43	0.79	0.56–1.11

CI = confidence interval.

*N and D are the total number of women and number of breast cancer cases included in the analysis, respectively.

[†]Odds ratios estimated by logistic regression using varying numbers of women and cases, depending on the data available on each variable.

[‡]Self-reported measure.

From MRC NHSD, 1946–1999.

from 4 to 7 years had the largest and most significant estimated effect (OR = 1.41, 95 per cent CI 1.08–1.85, P = 0.01; Table 8.10). In the model with all the BMI components up to age 15, only the 2–4 years velocity seems to be significantly protective (OR = 0.74, 95 per cent CI 0.57–0.97, P = 0.02). When all the height and BMI components were included in the same model, the effect of BMI velocity at ages 2–4 was strengthened in size and significance, with all the other effects left substantially unchanged (Table 8.10).

Thus the observation that breast cancer cases were taller and had slimmer body size throughout childhood, i.e. an observation of size at all childhood ages being important, has been dissected to show that fast height gains between 4 and 7 years and steep decreases in BMI between 2 and 4 years were the strongest positive predictors for breast cancer risk (P = 0.006 and P = 0.001, respectively). Height gains between 11 and 15 years were also, albeit marginally (P = 0.08), positively associated with increased breast cancer risk. Since in the final model with all growth components neither the coefficient for the height nor that for the BMI at age 2 years was significant, these results seem to support a critical

Table 8.9 Estimates of univariable breast cancer odds ratios (ORs) for 1 SD increase in anthropometric velocities at different ages, results obtained on 2187 women followed up to age 53 years

Variable	N*	D*	OR[†]	95 per cent CI
Height velocity (cm/year) at:				
2–4 years	1659	51	0.97	0.74–1.29
4–7 years	1744	53	1.33	1.02–1.74
7–11 years	1760	49	0.97	0.73–1.29
11–15 years	1600	43	1.16	0.85–1.57
15–adulthood[‡]	1283	37	0.89	0.63–1.25
BMI velocity (kg/m^2)/year at:				
2–4 years	1562	47	0.99	0.74–1.33
4–7 years	1651	51	1.03	0.78–1.36
7–11 years	1673	48	1.05	0.80–1.40
11–15 years	1559	42	0.89	0.65–1.21

CI = confidence interval.

*N and D are the total number of women and number of breast cancer cases included in the analysis, respectively.

[†]Odds ratios estimated by logistic regression using varying numbers of women and cases, depending on the data available on each variable.

[‡]Adult height measured at age 36.

From MRC NHSD, 1946–1999.

period of growth model rather that a critical size model. The results are, however, based on a small number of breast cancer cases and on MAR assumptions underlying the MI procedure.[88]

8.5 Individual differences in effect

One issue that has come to the fore in evaluation research has been the assumption of a common or uniform causal effect, i.e. whether the impact is the same for all individuals. Epidemiologists have tended to assume that even if the effect may be different from person to person, then our methods of analysis must be providing some estimate of the average effect. However, different study designs will deliver different subsets of the individuals exposed to some risk factor of interest, and if there is variation in effect then the average estimates from those different subsets may vary. In other words, we need to account for selection not just with respect to confounding but also with respect to the selection of individuals who are more or less sensitive to the risk factor in question. Thus those most exposed to infections are often the least able to ward off infection and, among marriages, those most damaging to children may have the higher rates of divorce. Alternatively, we must restrict our interpretation of our estimates of effect as being 'local' to the particular study design—making generalization more difficult.[89,90]

Table 8.10 Joint estimates of the effects of height and BMI changes obtained using the observed data or the multiple imputations procedure; MRC 1946 birth cohort: odds ratios (ORs) for 1 SD increase in anthropometric measures at different ages

Variable	Units	All height components up to adulthood				All BMI components up to age 15				All height and BMI components			
		Observed data		Observed and imputed data		Observed data		Observed and imputed data		Observed data		Observed and imputed data	
		(N* = 904, D* = 33)		(N = 2187, D = 59)		(N = 1062, D = 34)		(N = 2187, D = 59)		(N = 803, D = 30)		(N = 2187, D =59)	
		OR	95 per cent CI	OR	95 per cent CI	OR	95 per cent CI	OR	95 per cent CI	OR	95 per cent CI	OR	95 per cent CI
Height													
Intercept at 2 years	cm	1.08	0.71–1.66	1.18	0.87–1.61	–	–	–	–	1.17	0.71–1.92	1.21	0.87–1.69
Velocity 2–4 years	cm/year	1.02	0.67–1.56	1.14	0.86–1.51	–	–	–	–	0.77	0.45–1.30	1.04	0.75–1.43
Velocity 4–7 years	cm/year	1.53	1.04–2.24	1.41	1.08–1.85	–	–	–	–	1.59	1.02–2.47	1.54	1.13–2.09
Velocity 7–11 years	cm/year	1.44	0.92–2.25	1.17	0.82–1.67	–	–	–	–	1.44	0.89–2.31	1.17	0.81–1.69
Velocity 11–15ys	cm/year	1.23	0.78–1.93	1.32	1.01–1.73	–	–	–	–	1.13	0.69–1.85	1.29	0.97–1.71
Velocity 15–adulthood	cm/year	1.05	0.70–1.58	0.96	0.73–1.27	–	–	–	–	1.06	0.68–1.66	0.94	0.70–1.25
BMI													
Intercept at 2 years	kg/m^2	–	–	–	–	0.63	0.32–1.23	0.80	0.48–1.33	0.63	0.30–1.31	0.76	0.46–1.27
Velocity 2–4 years	k/m^2/year	–	–	–	–	0.70	0.36–1.36	0.74	0.57–0.97	0.45	0.21–0.97	0.63	0.48–0.83
Velocity 4–7 years	k/m^2/year	–	–	–	–	0.78	0.50–1.23	0.92	0.70–1.20	0.92	0.54–1.54	1.00	0.77–1.31
Velocity 7–11 years	k/m^2/year	–	–	–	–	1.10	0.77–1.57	0.97	0.74–1.29	1.06	0.69–1.63	0.93	0.70–1.23
Velocity 11–15 years	k/m^2/year	–	–	–	–	0.83	0.57–1.21	0.95	0.73–1.24	0.74	0.48–1.13	0.95	0.72–1.24

CI = confidence interval.

*N and D are the total number of women and number of breast cancer cases included in the analysis, respectively.

For example, an analysis associating change in exposure to change in outcome assesses effects local to the subpopulation for whom exposure changes. Whether an effect estimate from such an analysis applies to those for whom exposure did not change needs to be considered in just the same way that findings from a trial based on selected patients can generalize to the whole population of patients. Kurth *et al.*[91] have highlighted the extent of variability in estimates for the effect of a stroke treatment using the methods of Section 8.4.4, in particular the effect of excluding the 'unusual' patients, those patients that were of a type that were rarely given the treatment (and thus had propensity scores of <5 per cent). These were patients for whom the treatment probably should not have been given.

Do we find such a correlation between risk of exposure and magnitude of effect in epidemiology? In psychiatry, education and health-related behaviour, such a correlation is probably common. Children from homes with greater educational resource and support tend to have inherited genes from parents that may predispose them to benefit from education. Similarly, the obese may be exposed to the least exercise, but may be the group who would benefit most from it. In physical medicine, while such circumstances may be less obvious, that may not be sufficient justification to assume that variations in exposure and effect are independent. Socially modulated exposures such as famine (or just poor diet) may be greatest for those whose socio-economic position and health capital make them most vulnerable. Exposure over an extended period of time, for example to an industrial irritant, also provides scope for a mechanism that induces a negative correlation between exposure and sensitivity to exposure, as those most sensitive are removed or remove themselves from exposure.

As a consequence, we believe greater attention must be paid to defining the group to whom any effect estimate is supposed to apply and, in particular, supposed to generalize. This also has implications for systematic reviews of epidemiological studies, where a naïve assumption that studies are estimating a single common target parameter may be quite false, and heterogeneity of effect must be expected.

8.6 Discussion

This chapter has concerned itself for the most part with models and methods of analysis. These are important in their own right, but of equal importance is the recognition that these models and methods make demands on studies in terms of both design and data. It is therefore crucial that knowledge of analysis and the experience gained in analysing current studies be used to elaborate the design of future studies and future waves of data collection. It is through the future complementarity of design and analysis that we will gain most.

Each of the methodologies that we have described, several of them illustrated by an example, has distinct advantages and disadvantages. Currently no one method is universally superior or universally applicable. Recently, we have seen some convergence and generalization such that, for example, multilevel and SEM methods may now be seen as special cases of a more general framework. Similarly, propensity scores and marginal structural means modelling share much. In a number of other areas, however, the literature remains confusing, the similarities and differences among methods being much harder to identify. We have highlighted one area, that to do with effect heterogeneity, where the implications are that different methods of analysis and different study designs may be estimating different effects. We are yet to understand fully the implications for epidemiological research. In such circumstances, it may well be wise to undertake several analyses, and where different conclusions result to report findings with more caution while further investigating the reasons for inconsistency or pattern of effects.

Recent conflicting findings from RCTs and observational epidemiological studies have provoked a widespread concern as to the ability of epidemiology to deliver reliable findings, and life course research can claim no immunity from this concern. That life course methods may have a wider range of measured confounders is of some help, but probably of limited value without a clear structure for their use. Clearly more sophisticated methods of analysis may help, but only modestly so if the underlying observational design is flawed. However, RCTs differ from observational studies not just in terms of design. They also differ with respect to the practical steps taken to achieve objectivity, for example by the practice in RCTs of precise specification of the outcome measure and of the analysis that will be undertaken prior to obtaining the data—in other words blind to the data. In the longer run, we may find that an adaptation of such an approach may serve epidemiology better than the near untestable reliance on the ability of scientists and the research process to remain unbiased throughout. Recognition for the need for greater objectivity does not require any questioning of the integrity of individual scientists. The factors that influence research are simply too numerous and too pervasive to keep them all in check. However, several of the approaches we have described allow preparatory and extensive data analysis to be undertaken without the need for the outcome data, i.e. blind to the critical data. For example, this is true for the calculation of propensity scores where extensive exploration may be necessary for their specification but which can all be undertaken without knowledge of the outcomes. Once the propensity scores have been calculated, the final analysis of the outcome is often simple and could be easily specified in advance. Similar procedures to achieve objectivity may be achievable where instrumental variables are pre-specified. Thus, in the future, considerations of this kind may play as important a role in our choice of method and in our analysis strategy as the more familiar methodological considerations emphasized in the bulk of this chapter.

Further reading

Diggle PJ, Heagerty P, Liang K-Y, Zeger SL (2002). *Analysis of longitudinal data*, 2nd edn. Oxford University Press, Oxford.

Hernan M, Robins J (2006). Instruments for causal inference. An epidemiologist's dream? *Epidemiology* 17, 360–372.

Rosenbaum P R (2002). *Observational studies*, 2nd edn. Springer Verlag, New York.

Rothman KJ, Greenland S (2005). Causation and causal inference in epidemiology. *American Journal of Public Health* 95, S144–S150.

Skrondal A, Rabe-Hesketh S (2004). *Generalized latent variable modeling: multilevel, longitudinal and structural equation models*. Chapman and Hall/CRC, Boca Raton, FL.

References

1. Kuh D, Ben-Shlomo Y (2004). *A life course approach to chronic disease epidemiology*. Oxford University Press, Oxford.

2. Clayton DG (1992). Models for the analysis of cohort and case–control studies with inaccurately measured exposures. In: Dwyer JH, Feileib M, Lippert P, Hoffmeister H, ed. *Statistical models for longitudinal studies on health*. Oxford University Press, Oxford.

3. Carroll RJ, Ruppert D, Stefanski LA (1995). *Measurement error in non-linear models*. Chapman and Hall/CRC, London.

4. Carroll RJ (2000). Measurement error in epidemiological studies. In: Gail MH, Benichou J, ed. *Encyclopedia of epidemiologic methods*. John Wiley, Chichester.

5. Lawlor DA, Davey Smith G, Ebrahim S (2004). The association of socioeconomic position from across the life course with HRT use: an explanation for the discrepancy between observational and RCT evidence on HRT and CHD? *Amercan Journal of Public Health* 94, 2149–2154.

6. Davey Smith G, Hart G, Blane D, Gillis C, Hawthorne V (1997). Lifetime socioeconomic position and mortality: prospective observational study. *British Medical Journal* 314, 547–552.

7. Heslop P, Davey Smith G, Macleod J, Hart C (2001). The socioeconomic position of employed women, risk factors and mortality. *Social Sciences and Medicine* 53, 477–485.

8. Lynch JW, Kaplan GA, Shema SR (1997). Cumulative impact of sustained economic hardship on physical, cognitive, psychosocial, and social functioning. *New England Journal of Medicine* 337, 1889–1895.

9. Krieger N, Chen JT, Selby JV (2001). Class inequalities in women's health: combined impact of childhood and adult social class—a study of 630 US women. *Public Health* 115, 175–185.

10. Crowder MJ, Hand DJ (1990). *Analysis of repeated measures*. Chapman and Hall, London.

11. Leon D, Davey Smith G (2000). Infant mortality, stomach cancer, stroke, and coronary heart disease: ecological analysis. *British Medical Journal* 320, 1705–1706.

12. Fish EW, Shahrokh D, Bagot R, Caldij C, Bredy T, Szyf M, *et al.* (2004). Epigenetic programming of stress responses through variations in maternal care. *Annals of the New York Academy of Sciences* 1036, 167–180.

13. De Stavola BL, Nitsch D, dos Santos Silva I, McCormack V, Hardy R, Mann V, *et al.* (2006). Statistical issues in life course epidemiology. *American Journal of Epidemiology* 159, 671–682.

14. Hallqvist J, Lynch J, Bartley M, Lang T, Blane D (2004). Can we disentangle life course processes of accumulation, critical period and social mobility? An analysis of disadvantaged socio-economic positions and myocardial infarction in the Stockholm Heart Epidemiology Program. *Social Science and Medicine* 58, 1555–1562.

15. Singh-Manoux A, Ferrie JE, Chandola T, Marmot M (2004). Socioeconomic trajectories across the life course and health outcomes in mid life: evidence for the accumulation hypothesis? *International Journal of Epidemiology* 33, 1072–1079.

16. Rowe R, Maughan B, Pickles A, Costello EJ, Angold A (2002). The relationship between DSM-IV oppositional defiant disorder and conduct disorder: findings from the Great Smoky Mountains Study. *Journal of Child Psychology and Psychiatry* 43, 365–374.

17. Bartley M, Blane D, Davey Smith G (1999). Making sense of health inequality. In: Dorling D, Simpson S, ed. *Statistics in society: the arithmetic of politics*. Arnold, London.

18. Drukker M, Kaplan C, Schneiders J, Feron FJ, van Os J (2006). The wider social environment and changes in self-reported quality of life in the transition from late childhood to early adolescence: a cohort study. *BMC Public Health* 17, 6, 133.

19. Hill J, Pickles A, Rollinson L, Davis R, Byatt M (2004). Juvenile versus adult onset depression: multiple differences imply multiple pathways. *Psychological Medicine* 34, 1483–1493.

20. Pickles AR (1989). Statistical modelling of longitudinal data. In: Rutter M. ed. *The power of longitudinal data: studies of risk and protective factors for psychosocial disorder*. Cambridge University Press, Cambridge, pp. 62–76.

21. Diggle PJ, Heagerty P, Liang K-Y, Zeger SL (2002). *Analysis of longitudinal data*, 2nd edn. Oxford University Press, Oxford.

22. Collishaw S, Maughan B, Pickles A (2004). Age trends and chronicity of affective problems of adults with mild learning disability. *British Journal of Psychiatry* 185, 350–351.

23. Agresti A (2002). *Categorical data analysis*. Wiley, New York.

24. StataCorp (2005). *Stata statistical software: release 9*. StataCorp LP, College Station, TX.

25. Rabe-Hesketh S, Skrondal A, Pickles A (2002). Reliable estimation of generalized linear mixed models using adaptive quadrature. *Stata Journal* 2, 1–21.

26. Davey Smith G (2003). The HRT story: lessons for epidemiologists. *International Journal of Epidemiology* 32, 897.

27. Stampfer MJ, Colditz GA (1991). Estrogen replacement therapy and coronary heart disease: a quantitative assessment of the epidemiologic evidence. *Preventive Medicine* 20, 47–63.

28. Rossouw JE, Andesen GL, Prentice RL, La Croix Az, Kooperberg C, Stefanick KL, *et al.* (2002). Risks and benefits of estrogen plus progestin in healthy postmenopausal women: principal results from the Women's Health Initiative randomized controlled trial. *Journal of the American Medical Association* 288, 321–333.

29. Hulley S, Grady D, Bush T, Furberg C, Herington D, Riggs B, *et al.* (1998). Randomized trial of estrogen plus progestin for secondary prevention of coronary heart disease in post-menopausal women. Heart and Estrogen/progestin Replacement Study (HERS) research group. *Journal of the American Medical Association* 280, 605–613.

30. Petitti D, Perlman JA, Sidney S (1986). Postmenopausal estrogen use and heart disease. *New England Journal of Medicine* 315, 131–132.

31. Prentice R, Pettinger M, Anderson G (2005). Statistical issues in the women's health initiative. *Biometrics* 61, 899–911.

32. Greenland S, Brumback B (2002). An overview of relations among causal modelling methods. *International Journal of Epidemiology* 31, 1030–1037.

33. Robins JM (2001). Data, design, and background knowledge in etiologic inference. *Epidemiology* 10, 37–48.

34. Cox DR, Wermuth N (1996). *Multivariate dependencies*. Chapman and Hall, London.

35. Rosenbaum PR (2002). *Observational studies*, 2nd edn. Springer Verlag, New York.

36. Rothman KJ (1976). Causes. *American Journal of Epidemiology* 104, 587–592.

37. Bollen KA (1989). *Structural equations with latent variables*. Wiley, New York, NY.

38. Pearl J (2000). *Causality: models, reasoning and inference*. Cambridge University Press, Cambridge.

39. Robins JM, Greenland S (1992). Identifiability and exchangeability for direct and indirect effects. *Epidemiology* 3, 143–155.

40. Whittaker J (1990). *Graphical models in applied multivariate statistics*. Wiley, Chichester.

41. Wermuth N, Cox DR (2000). Statistical dependence and independence. In: Gail MH, Benichou J. ed. *Encyclopedia of epidemiological methods*. John Wiley, New York.

42. Rothman KJ, Greenland S (1998). *Modern Epidemiology*, 2nd edn. Lippincott-Raven, Philadelphia, PA.

43. Blot WJ, Day NE (1979). Synergism & interaction: are they equivalent. *American Journal of Epidemiology* 110, 99–100.

44. Pickles A (1993). Stages, precursors and causes in development. In: Hay DF, Angold A. *Precursors and causes in development and psychopathology*. Wiley, Chichester, pp. 23–50.

45. Pickles A, Rutter M (1991). Statistical and conceptual models of 'turning points' in developmental processes. In: Magnusson D, Bergman L, Rudinger G, Torestad B, ed. *Problems and methods in longitudinal research: stability and change.* Cambridge University Press, Cambridge, pp. 32–57.

46. Dawid AP (2000). Causal inference without counterfactuals (with discussion). *Journal of the American Statistical Association* 95, 407–448.

47. Rosenbaum PR, Rubin DB (1983). The central role of the propensity score in observational studies for causal effects. *Biometrika* 70, 41–55.

48. Robins JM, Hernan MA, Brumback B (2000). Marginal structural models and causal inference in epidemiology. *Epidemiology* 11, 550–560.

49. Huber P (1967). The behaviour of maximum likelihood estimates under non-standard conditions. In: *Proceedings of the fifth Berkely symposium on mathematical statistics and probability, vol. 1.* University of California Press, Berkeley, pp. 221–233.

50. Cole SR, Hernan MA, Robins JM, Anastos K, Chmiel J, Detels R, *et al.* (2003). Effect of highly active antiretroviral therapy on time to acquired immunodeficiency syndrome or death using marginal structural models. *American Journal of Epidemiology* 158, 687–694.

51. White IR (2005). Uses and limitations of randomization-based efficacy estimators. *Statistical Methods in Medical Research* 14, 327–347.

52. Neugebauer R, van der Laan M (2005). Why prefer double robust estimators in causal inference? *Journal of Statistical Planning and Inference* 129, 405–426.

53. Woolridge JM (2002). *Econometric analysis of cross-section and panel data.* MIT Press, Cambridge MA.

54. Goldberger AS (1972). Structural equation methods in the social sciences. *Econometrica* 40, 979–1001.

55. Skrondal A, Rabe-Hesketh S (2004). *Generalized latent variable modeling: multilevel, longitudinal and structural equation models.* Chapman and Hall/CRC, Boca Raton, FL.

56. Angrist J, Krueger A (1992). The effects of age at school entry on educational attainment: an application of instrumental variables with moments from two samples. *Journal of the American Statistical Association* 418, 328–336.

57. Elford J, Ben-Shlomo Y (2004). Geography and migration with special reference to cardiovascular disease. In: Kuh D, Ben-Shlomo Y. *A life course approach to chronic disease epidemiology,* 2nd edn. Oxford University Press, Oxford, pp. 144–164.

58. Rutter M, Pickles A, Eaves L, Murray R (2001). Testing hypotheses on environmental risk mechanisms. *Psychological Bulletin* 127, 291–324.

59. Didelez V, Sheehan N (2005). *Mendelian randomisation and instrumental variables: what can and what can't be done.* Research Report 05-02, Department of Health Sciences, University of Leicester.

60. Hernan M, Robins J (2006). Instruments for causal inference. An epidemiologist's dream? *Epidemiology* 17, 360–372.

61. Torres Mejia G, De Stavola B, Allen DS, Perez-Gavilan JJ, Ferreira JM, Fentiman IS, *et al.*(2005). Mammographic features and subsequent risk of breast cancer: a comparison of qualitative and quantitative evaluations in the Guernsey prospective studies. *Cancer Epidemiology Biomarkers and Prevention* 14, 1052–1059.

62. dos Santos Silva I, Johnson N, De Stavola BL, Torres Mejia G, Fletcher O, Allen DS, *et al.* (2006). The insulin-like growth factor (IGF) system and mammographic features in pre- and postmenopausal women. *Cancer Epidemiology Biomarkers and Prevention* 15, 449–455.

63. Wright S (1921). Correlation and causation. *Journal of Agricultural Research* 20, 557–585.

64. Heise DR (1975). *Causal analysis.* Wiley-Interscience, New York.

65. Wright S (1934). On the method of path coefficients. *Annals of Mathematical Statistics* 5, 161–215.

66. Muthen LK, Muthen BO (2004). *Mplus user's guide*. Muthen & Muthen, Los Angeles, CA.

67. Baron RM, Kenny DA (1986). The moderator–mediator variable distinction in social psychological research: conceptual, strategic and statistical considerations. *Journal of Personality and Social Psychology* 51, 1173–1182.

68. Judd CM, Kenny DA (1981). Process analysis: estimating mediation in treatment evaluations. *Evaluation Review* 5, 602–619.

69. Barker DJP (1998). *Mothers, babies and health in later life*. Churchill Livingstone, Edinburgh.

70. Leon DA, Lithell HO, Vågerö D, Koupilova I, Mohsen R, Berglund L, *et al.* (1998). Reduced fetal growth rate and increased risk of ischaemic heart disease mortality in 15 thousand Swedish men and women born 1915–29. *British Medical Journal* 317, 241–245.

71. Lucas A, Fewtrell MS, Cole TJ (1999). Fetal origins of adult disease—the hypothesis revisited. *British Medical Journal* 319, 245–249.

72. Tu YK, West R, Ellison GT, Gilthorpe MS (2005). Why evidence for the fetal origins of adult disease might be a statistical artifact: the 'reversal paradox' for the relation between birth weight and blood pressure in later life. *American Journal of Epidemiology* 161, 27–32.

73. Osbourne RT, Suddick DE (1972). A longitudinal investigation of the intellectual differentiation hypothesis. *Journal of Genetic Psychology* 110, 83–9.

74. Dunn G, Everitt B, Pickles A (1993). *Modelling covariances and latent variables using EQS*. Chapman and Hall, London.

75. Rabe-Hesketh S, Pickles A, Skrondal A (2003). Correcting for measurement error in logistic regression using non-parametric maximum likelihood estimation. *Statistics in Medicine* 3, 215–232.

76. Schumacker RE, Marcoulides GA (1998). *Interaction and nonlinear effects in structural equation modelling*. Lawrence Erlbaum, London.

77. Goldstein H (2003). *Multilevel statistical models*, 3rd edn. Edward Arnold, London.

78. Laird NM, Ware JH (1982). Random-effects models for longitudinal data. *Biometrics* 38, 963–974.

79. Cheung YB, Low L, Osmond C, Barker D, Karlberg J (2000). Fetal growth and early postnatal growth are related to blood pressure in adults. *Hypertension* 36, 795.

80. Eriksson J, Foirsen T, Tuomilehto J, Osmond C, Barker D (2001). Size at birth, childhood growth and obesity in adult life. *International Journal of Obesity* 25, 735.

81. Horta BL, Barros FC, Victora CG, Cole TJ (2003). Early and late growth and blood pressure in adolescence. *Journal of Epidemiology and Community Health* 57, 226.

82. De Stavola BL, dos Santos Silva I, McCormack V, Hardy RJ, Kuh DJ, Wadsworth ME (2004). Childhood growth and breast cancer. *American Journal of Epidemiology* 159, 671–82.

83. Roland-Cachera MF, Deheeger M, Bellisle F, Sempe M, Guillord-Battaille M, Patois E (1987). Adiposity rebound in children: a simple indicator for predicting obesity. *American Journal of Clinical Nutrition* 39, 129.

84. Wadsworth ME, Mann SL, Rodgers B, Kuh DJ, Hilder WS, Yusuf EJ (1992). Loss and representativeness in a 43 year follow up of a national birth cohort. *Journal of Epidemiology and Community Health* 46, 300–304.

85. Wadsworth MEJ, Butterworth SL, Hardy RJ, Kuh DH, Richards M, Langenberg C, *et al.* (2003). The life course prospective design: an example of benefits and problems associated with study longevity. *Social Science and Medicine* 57, 2193–2205.

86. Wadsworth MEJ, Butterworth SL, Montgomery SM, Ehlin A, Bartley MJ (2003). Health. In: Ferri E, Bynner J, Wadsworth MEJ, ed. *Changing Britain, changing lives: three generations at the turn of the century*. Institute of Education Press, London, pp. 207–236.

87. Schafer JL (1999). Multiple imputation: a primer. *Statistical Methods in Medical Research* 8, 3–16.

88. Little RJA, Rubin DB (1987). *Statistical analysis with missing data*. John Wiley, New York.

89. Angrist J, Imbens G, Rubin D (1996). Identification of causal effects using instrumental variables. *Journal of Economics* 71, 145–160.

90. Hirano K, Imbens G, Rubin D, Zhou X-H (2000). Assesing the effect of an influenza vaccine in an encouragement design. *Biostatistics* 1, 69–88.

91. Kurth T, Walker A, Glynn R, Chan KA, Gaziano JM, Berger K, *et al.* (2006). Results of multivariable logistic regression, propensity matching, propensity adjustment, and propensity-based weighting under conditions of nonuniform effect. *American Journal of Epidemiology* 163, 262–270.

Chapter 9

An overview of methods for studying events and their timing

Andrew Pickles and Bianca De Stavola

Abstract

This chapter explains the concepts of censoring and time scales, and introduces proportional hazards, accelerated failure time and proportional odds models. More complex models for competing events, for multiple events of the same and of different types and for multistate processes are then considered. Errors in the dating of events are discussed. For profiles of event occurrence over an extended period, we illustrate a typological analysis. Finally, the problem of time-varying confounding is described and ways in which it can be addressed using marginal structural models and G-estimation considered.

9.1 Introduction

There are events that are inevitable but it is still interesting to study them. Indeed, we all die, but there is huge variation in why and when we eventually do so. For example, in Western societies the diseases with later onset, such as Alzheimer's disease, are becoming increasingly common as mortality rates from other causes with earlier onset have declined. We may all experience for brief periods of time other conditions, such as respiratory problems or depression. What may be more important than their mere occurrence is the time until recovery and, following that, the time until any recurrence. We therefore need the ability to analyse the timing of events, the duration of episodes and, for recurrent events, the structure of event histories. Because of the original field of application, these methods often remain known as *survival analysis* even where the outcome of interest is not death. This chapter describes these tools and generalizations of them that may be particularly suited to questions posed within life course research.

The chapter begins with a brief introduction to the main features of survival data. Then the most widely used models are introduced. These include the proportional hazards models but also the lesser known accelerated failure time models and ordinal response models. Issues such as those arising when event times are not observed precisely, or are not observed because of possibly correlated competing events, are then discussed and more complex modelling approaches are reviewed. Recent methods developed for dealing with time-varying confounding factors and models for identifying patterns of events over the life course are then described.

9.2 **Basics**

9.2.1 **Data and censoring**

To analyse event rates, we need data on the timing of these events. If we could observe every study participant until they all suffer the event, the data would consist of individual event times. However, in most situations, events are observed only for some—but not all—study participants, so that different types of 'times' are recorded. Those of participants who experienced the events are true event times; for the others they are censored, i.e. they are times when the participants were last observed and were event free at that time.

Standard survival analysis methods deal with these missed event times by assuming that the reason why censoring occurred was not related to the (unseen) timing of the event of interest. This is not always true, however. For example, the event of interest may not be observed because it is preceded by another related event, e.g. cardiovascular death occurring before lung cancer diagnosis. When such events have similar causes, such as smoking, the censoring created by the earlier event is not independent of the process that would have led to the main event of interest. This presents an example of informative missingness, also discussed in Chapter 7, and limits the applicability of standard survival methods in ways that will be discussed later.

Another form of censoring arises when the event of interest changes in nature with the passage of time. For example, a woman may experience her first birth as a teenager, or as an adult. The teenage birth is often considered non-normative behaviour, often being linked to single motherhood, poor socio-economic circumstances and low education attainment. In contrast, the later birth is thought normative. Thus—although biologically similar (though they may have different long-term risks for breast cancer and some other health outcomes)—these two events may require separate consideration, for example by imposing an age limit when dealing with teenage events (i.e. artificially censoring the times for births to older women) or by jointly analysing normative and non-normative reproduction as separate but related events. Thus, besides the censoring that is inherent to the way data are collected, there is censoring that may be created by the analyst. Artificial censoring may also give raise to analytical difficulties if it is not independent of the process that underlies the event of interest.

9.2.2 **Time scale**

Survival data can be viewed differently according to the time scale in which they are sorted. Event and censoring times are recorded from a particular starting point, the recruitment into the study, until either the event occurs or the follow-up is interrupted. This information is usually collected in terms of dates (date of entry and either date of the event or date last seen). In many clinical applications, these dates are not interesting *per se* because it is the length of time between them, i.e. the total follow-up time, that matters. In many other applications, and especially in epidemiology, other time dimensions derived from those dates are more important. For example, the individual ages at which entry and exit occurred, or the amount of time elapsed since a landmark date (e.g. first employment in the nuclear industry), may have more relevance for the events being studied (e.g. radiation-induced cancer).

9.2.3 Proportional hazards (PH) survival models

The better known survival models are specified in terms of the rate (or hazard) function for the event of interest. Formally the rate is the instantaneous probability that the event of interest occurs at time t, given that it has not yet occurred. It is often denoted $\lambda(t)$ to stress that the rate may vary with time t, where t is the adopted time scale. Once the rate function is specified, we can work out the survival function, $S(t)$, which is the cumulative probability that the event of interest has not yet occurred by time t.

The simplest form that can be specified for the rate is that of a constant, $\lambda(t) = \lambda_0$. This implies that the instantaneous probability of the event is the same for every value of t. In particular it means that it does not depend on the length of time already spent in the study, or on the changing age of the participants. In most studies, this may not be a realistic assumption and more general models that allow the rate to vary with time may be more appropriate. A well known example of a parametric model with time-varying rates is the Weibull model. However, researchers have often preferred greater flexibility, and a less structured way to relax the constancy assumption is to break the follow-up times into shorter periods during which it is plausible to assume that the rates are constant. The rate then changes in steps, for example is constant at level λ_0 between entry (denoted as time t_0) and t_1, then constant but at a different level $\lambda_0 + \delta_1$ between time t_1 and t_2, etc. (Fig. 9.1, where $t_1 = 5$, $t_2 = 10$, etc.), i.e.:

$$\lambda(t) = \lambda_0 \, I(t_0 \leq t < t_1) + (\lambda_0 + \delta_1) \, I(t_1 \leq t < t_2) + (\lambda_0 + \delta_2) \, I(t_2 \leq t < t_3) + ... \quad (9.1)$$

where $I(t_i \leq t < t_{i+1})$ is an indicator that t is between t_i and t_{i+1}, and δ_i is the difference between the rates in (t_i, t_{i+1}) and those in (t_0, t_1).

Simple conditional independence assumptions result in it being possible to pool information across individuals and bands of time and estimate the rates in each band as the number of events divided by the total person-years of exposure, giving the person-years method,[1] a generalization of the Poisson model for rates.[2] This is also the model used by demographers to estimate life expectancies in different populations. In that context, it takes the name of *life table* method.[2]

As described so far, the rate in any interval has been assumed to be identical for all study participants. This can be relaxed by introducing explanatory variables, most commonly assuming a log-linear form for the rate. For example, considering for simplicity only one such variable and a time constant rate, the rate becomes

$$\lambda_0(x_1) = \exp(\beta_0 + \beta_1 \, x_1) = \lambda_0 \exp(\beta_1 \, x_1) \quad (9.2)$$

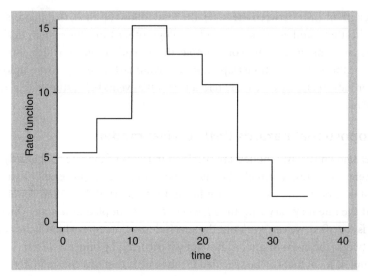

Fig. 9.1 A stepwise rate function defined over 5-year intervals.

where x_1 is a covariate observed at the start of the study and $\lambda_0 = \exp(\beta_0)$ is the baseline hazard. The exponential function in equation 9.2 is used to guarantee that the rate is positive, while the regression coefficient β_1 (which can take either positive or negative values) represents the effect on the (natural) log-transformed event rate of a unit increase in the value of x_1, with a positive coefficient implying a higher rate. The equivalent specification for the stepwise model is

$$\lambda(t; x_1) = [\lambda_0 \, I(t_0 \leq t < t_1) + (\lambda_0 + \delta_1) \, I(t_1 \leq t < t_2) + ...] \exp(\beta_1 x_1) \qquad (9.3)$$

A very well known generalization of this model leaves the step function unspecified as in

$$\lambda(t; x_1) = \lambda(t; 0) \exp(\beta_1 x_1) \qquad (9.4)$$

where $\lambda(t; 0)$ is the baseline rate (hazard) function for an individual with $x_1 = 0$. This construction implies that the event rates expected for two levels of x_1 remain in the same ratio [$\exp(\beta_1)$ if the difference in levels is 1] regardless of t, i.e. they remain proportional. This is the proportional hazards (PH) model proposed by D. R. Cox more than 30 years ago.[3] A way to assess this proportionality assumption is to calculate the observed cumulative event rate of subjects with different values of x_1 and plot them against t. When both axes are log-transformed, the observed cumulative rates (i.e. the negative of the log survival probabilities) should be parallel if the assumption is appropriate.

To obtain estimates of the covariates' effects, Cox's seminal paper introduced the concept of partial likelihood, in which it was not necessary to specify the baseline rate or how it might vary over time. The partial likelihood takes each event in turn, from the earliest to the latest, and compares the characteristics of the persons who actually experience the event at time t to the characteristics of all those who are still to experience the event (i.e. remain eligible for the event), in a similar way to how time-matched case–control studies are designed and analysed. Because of these time-matched comparisons, results are affected by the choice of analytical time scale: if it is time since entry into the study, event-affected individuals are compared with event-free individuals with follow-up times at least as long; if in contrast it is age, the comparison is with event-free individuals who are at least as old. The group to whom affected persons are to be compared thus changes with the choice of time scale.

9.2.4 Accelerated failure time (AFT) survival models

A completely different approach to the analysis of survival data focuses not on the rates but on the observed event times, and examines how risk factors shrink, or protective factors stretch, those times. Since times to events are always positive, the times are usually log-transformed (on the natural log scale) before being related to a set of explanatory variables and an error term η, as in

$$\log_e (t; x_1) = b_0 - b_1 x_1 + \eta \tag{9.5}$$

If η follows a normal distribution, the corresponding rate function first increases and then decreases with time; if instead it follows a Weibull distribution, the rate is monotonic, i.e. either always increases or always decreases with time. When observations are censored, we cannot directly observe $\log_e(t)$, and more complex calculations are required to determine the probability of the event not having occurred up to the time of censoring.

This specification in equation 9.5 implies a multiplicative effect of x_1 on the event time t, with a unit increase in x_1 leading to a multiplication of the expected event time by a factor equal to $\exp(-b_1)$. If b_1 is positive, a unit increase in x_1 reduces the expected event time and therefore accelerates the event rates, giving rise to the accelerated failure time (AFT) model, and explaining the negative sign in equation 9.5 for the regression coefficient of the explanatory variable.

Until recently there has been little interest in these models in epidemiology, despite their availability in many software packages. The main reason has been the extraordinarily elegant statistical properties of the Cox PH model of the previous section. Among all AFT models, only for the Weibull model are the rates corresponding to different values of the exposure proportional. Thus, in general, AFT models should be considered when there is evidence of non-proportional effects. However, unlike the Cox PH model, they all require the specification of the baseline rate via the distribution of η. This is much more parametric than the PH model and a significant disadvantage of the AFT approach. Recent years have seen the potential contribution of AFT models being re-considered since they lend themselves to a counterfactual approach to causal modelling (see Chapter 8).

9.2.5 Proportional odds (PO) survival models

Event times are not always recorded precisely. For example, when study participants are only assessed at regular times—say yearly—event dates may be known to occur only to a

1-year accuracy. For such interval-censored data, the PH and AFT models are not appropriate and instead a class of models for ordinal data are often used. This class includes the proportional odds (PO) model,[4] which specifies the odds of reporting the event between regular observation times as a function of a baseline odds, which may vary with time, and a set of explanatory variables. With one such variable, the odds are modelled as,

$$[1 - S(t; x_1)]/S(t; x_1) = \omega (t; 0) \exp(\alpha_1 x_1) \qquad (9.6)$$

where $S(t; x_1)$ is the cumulative probability of surviving up to time t with covariate value x_1, and $\omega (t; 0)$ represents the time-changing odds of failure when x_1 is equal to zero. The PO model is similar to applying logistic regression to a set of binary observations for the occurrence of an event in a sequence of discrete time intervals. In this model, unlike the PH model, the different baseline odds of the event in the different intervals are estimated. This approach is also used to deal with time-changing exposure variables, e.g. $x_2(t)$, that may have values updated at regular intervals.[5] All these classes of models (PH, AFT and PO) are now all easily fitted with standard software.

9.3 Modelling effects over the life course for a single event outcome

When used in their simplest forms, though they measure effect in different ways, all these models assume that the effect of a predictor is constant over time. Particularly with life course data, that may cover an extended period of time, this is often not plausible for two main reasons.

First, the values of one or more predictor variables may vary over time. To reflect their changing impact on overall survival, separate sections of the follow-up should be considered where their values are updated. All of the methods described above are surprisingly easily extended to this circumstance, though for the person-year methods the changes in covariate values and time interval bands (e.g. the bands shown in Fig. 9.1) must coincide. It should also be noted that these time-varying covariates should be exogenous, i.e. they should change for reasons that do not depend on the survival process being investigated. An example of endogeneity concerns the case where the covariate is an indicator of progression towards the event, a problem to which we shall return (also see time-varying confounding in Chapter 8).

Secondly, the predictors may vary in their impact even where their values remain fixed. Baseline predictors often appear to 'wear out', becoming less predictive the further from the baseline is the event risk being considered. Various reasons for this are possible; for example, the baseline measure might proxy for a contemporaneous measure and become increasingly inaccurate as a proxy with increasing time from baseline. Alternatively, a risk factor might influence only a subgroup of the population and, as time goes by, those remaining to experience the event are the subgroup invulnerable to this risk ('the healthy survivor effect'). Another possibility is that a predictor could become more (or less) important particularly where the nature of the event changes with time. For example, in the case of all-cause death rates in the teenage years, the important risk factors are those for accidental and violent deaths, while those important in older age are risk factors for coronary heart disease and cancer.

Testing and allowing for time variation in risk factors and in their effects is thus likely to be of special importance within life course analysis. We show an example of time-varying effects by examining time to first birth among the participants in the UK 1958 National Child Development Study cohort.[6] Table 9.1 shows the event data and the survival probabilities separately for male and female cohort members. We are interested in the factors that predict the rate of first parenthood up to age 33 years and explore the contribution of two exposures observed when the cohort members were aged

Table 9.1 Number of events and probability of surviving without parenthood by age intervals and sex in the 1958 National Child Development Study

Age intervals (years)	At risk at start of interval	Becoming parents	Lost to follow-up	Probability of surviving	(95 per cent CI)
Boys					
14–15	4201	3	0	0.999	(0.998–1.000)
16–17	4198	26	0	0.993	(0.990–0.995)
18–19	4172	103	0	0.969	(0.963–0.973)
20–21	4069	238	0	0.912	(0.903–0.920)
22–23	3831	416	0	0.813	(0.801–0.824)
24–25	3415	489	0	0.697	(0.682–0.710)
26–27	2926	467	0	0.585	(0.570–0.600)
28–29	2459	486	0	0.470	(0.455–0.485)
30–31	1973	347	0	0.287	(0.372–0.402)
32–33	1626	183	1443	0.309	(0.293–0.324)
Girls					
14–15	4355	4	0	0.999	(0.998–1.000)
16–17	4351	167	0	0.961	(0.955–0.966)
18–19	4184	324	0	0.886	(0.877–0.895)
20–21	3860	450	0	0.783	(0.771–0.795)
22–23	3410	556	0	0.655	(0.641–0.669)
24–25	2854	506	0	0.539	(0.524–0.554)
26–27	2348	488	0	0.427	(0.412–0.442)
28–29	1860	392	0	0.337	(0.323–0.351)
30–31	1468	291	0	0.270	(0.257–0.284)
32–33	1177	116	1061	0.222	(0.209–0.235)

CI = confidence interval.

11 years: disadvantaged social circumstances (on a continuous scale) and the teacher's report of antisocial behaviour (coded 1 for 'yes' and 0 for 'no').

Were we to fit a standard Cox PH model, this would assume that each predictor raises the hazard by a certain factor throughout the period of study data, here from age 14 to age 33 years. A plot of the log-log-transformed survival probability against logged time scale for each category, of say, antisocial behaviour, should give parallel straight lines were this true. Figure 9.2 shows this clearly not to be the case for this exposure and this is seen even after adjusting for the differences by sex (data not shown).

This suggests that we should allow for age-varying effects for the predictors. Table 9.2 shows the results obtained when fitting a Cox PH regression model with and without interaction terms between the time scale (i.e. age) and, respectively, sex, antisocial behaviour and childhood social class. The results are unequivocal in that for all three predictors, the interaction terms are highly significant. The age–product interaction terms were constructed centring age at 18 years so that the main effect of each risk factor corresponds to their effects at age 18 and are all significant and positive, while the interaction terms indicate that these effects decline or even reverse with increasing age. Analysis that imposed early censoring or the inclusion of interactions that would allow the effects of covariates on risk to change over time should thus be more routinely considered.

9.4 Survival analysis for more complex data

9.4.1 More complex models

The models described in the previous section can be generalized to deal with more complex analytical settings, such as competing risks, correlated events and sequences of events.

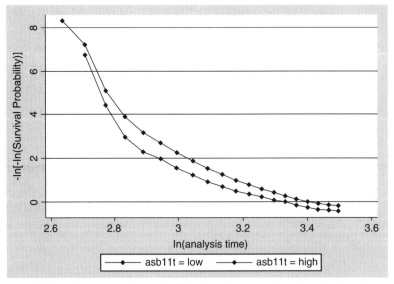

Fig. 9.2 Plot of minus log-log survival probability from first parenthood against log time by category of antisocial behaviour when aged 11 (asb11t).

Table 9.2 Cox proportional hazard model results for age at first birth until age 33 in the UK National Child Development Study

Risk factor	Categories/units	Model 1		Model 2	
		Rate ratio	(95 per cent CI)	Rate ratio	(95 per cent CI)
Sex	Male	1	1		
	Female	1.46	(1.39–1.54)	2.64	(2.37–2.93)
Interaction with time*		–	–	0.92	(0.91–0.93)
Antisocial behaviour	No	1	1		
	Yes	1.31	(1.21–1.42)	1.92	(1.66–2.23)
Interaction with time*		–	–	0.94	(0.92–0.96)
Childhood social class	Scale 1–7	1.22	(1.19–1.26)	1.64	(1.55–1.77)
Interaction with time*		–	–	0.96	(0.95–0.97)

CI = confidence interval.

*The time scale (age) was centred at 18 years.

There is often a choice of available approaches: selecting which one is the most appropriate depends on the final aims of a study. These are discussed after a brief review of the methods.

9.4.2 Competing risks

9.4.2.1 Types of competing risk

Competing risks (i.e. failures) arise when an individual is exposed to several events, with the occurrence of any of them preventing (because they terminate the follow-up) or modifying the occurrence of any other.[7] Since competing events are likely to share common causes, their event times are rarely independent. This happens, for example, in a study of lung cancer mortality when study participants also die from other smoking-related reasons. It also happens when loss to follow-up is not independent of the process being studied, e.g. when participants in a study of time to pregnancy refuse to continue participation because of marital break-up.

Different modelling considerations arise when the competing events exclude the occurrence of other events, or when they modify them. We will examine these two settings separately.

9.4.2.2 Terminating competing events

A common approach to model competing risks that prevent the occurrence of other events is to fit separate PH models for each competing cause, treating all other causes as a censoring event (the 'cause-specific Cox regression model'). A generalization of this approach leads to the joint estimation of all cause-specific hazard ratios after some simple data manipulation.[8] The difficulty, however, lies in the interpretation of the estimated hazard ratios as they represent effects in the absence of all the other causes, i.e. conditional on having first suffered any other event type. If the event times are not independent, this condition restricts the results to a selected subset of individuals and therefore are not easily generalizable.

An alternative approach which involves modelling the probability of experiencing the failure of interest as the first event by time t [the 'cumulative incidence' $CI(t)$] was suggested by Fine and Gray.[9,10] This is not conditional on the other events being absent because $CI(t)$ by definition depends on the rate of occurrence of all the risks (more specifically on surviving the other risks). The estimates obtained from this model measures the effect of the exposures on $CI_k(t)$, where k is the failure of interest, as opposed to their effects on λ_k, the event rate for failure k. The model can nevertheless be fitted using standard Cox PH software after some data manipulation that involves modifying the members of each risk set.[9,10] The effects estimated by the Fine and Gray model will be denoted 'competing risks' relative risks to distinguish them from the cause-specific ones described above. These two approaches are illustrated with an example.

Manual occupation and mortality due to myocardial infarction and stroke The Uppsala Birth Cohort Study (UBCoS) holds all live births recorded at the Uppsala Academic Hospital in Sweden during the period 1915–1929 (http://www.chess.su.se/ubcosmg/info/indexinfo.htm). Detailed information on the course of pregnancy and birth, and linkage to census and mortality registries, is available on 11 849 out of 14 193 live births. Of interest is the association between disadvantaged socio-economic position in adulthood, as measured by manual occupation at the time of the 1960 census, and mortality due to myocardial infarction (MI) and stroke. For simplicity, analyses are restricted to 6168 males. A total of 1374 (1064 due to MI, 222 to stroke and 88 to other causes) were recorded from the beginning of 1961 to the end of 2002. Table 9.3 summarizes the number of events by occupational status, and their corresponding rates.

MI deaths occur at much higher rates than the other causes of death, leading to the 'prevention' of the occurrence of other causes of mortality. The stroke-specific hazard ratios for manual occupation may therefore give downwardly biased estimates of its marginal effect if, for example, men in manual occupation have increased rates of both stroke and MI death but the latter are larger in absolute terms, with MI deaths occurring first. Modelling the cumulative incidence function, as in the Fine and Gray approach, leads instead to relative risk for the probability of experiencing stroke as the first event by time t, which would not be biased but give a measure of effect on a different scale (i.e. in terms of effects on the cumulative incidence).

Table 9.4 reports the results obtained from these two approaches. The estimated hazard ratios are not very different because MI is by far the more common cause of death. They do nevertheless have different meanings: the cause-specific ones are conditional on surviving the other causes, while the competing risk ones refer to the probability of each failure being the actual cause of death. These results agree with those of Tai *et al.*[11] who show that the bias of the cause-specific estimates is negligible when the mean failure time

Table 9.3 Mortality due to MI, stroke and other causes in male UBCoS male participants by occupation recorded at the 1960 census

Occupation in 1960	n	MI			Stroke			Other		
		Deaths	Rate*	95 per cent CI	Deaths	Rate*	95 per cent CI	Deaths	Rate*	95 per cent CI
Non-manual	3121	515	4.61	4.23–5.03	114	1.02	0.85–1.23	47	0.42	0.32–0.56
Manual	3047	549	5.17	4.76–5.62	108	1.02	0.84–1.23	41	0.39	0.28–0.53
All	6168	1064	4.89	4.60–5.19	222	1.02	0.89–1.16	88	0.40	0.33–0.50

MI = myocardial infarction; CI = confidence interval.
*Rate per 1000 person-years.

Table 9.4 Relative risks for the effect of manual occupation on fatal MI, stroke and other causes of death estimated using the cause-specific and competing risk methods;[9,10] male UBCoS participants

Occupation	Cause of death					
in 1960	MI		Stroke		Other	
	RR	95 per cent CI	RR	95 per cent CI	RR	95 per cent CI
Cause-specific analysis						
Non-manual	1	–	1	–	1	–
Manual	1.18	1.04–1.33	1.05	0.81–1.37	0.98	0.65–1.49
Competing risk analysis						
Non-manual	1	–	1	–	1	–
Manual	1.12	0.99–1.26	0.99	0.76–1.29	0.91	0.60–1.39

MI = myocardial infarction; RR = relative risk; CI = confidence interval.

of the main event is shorter, the correlation among the times to each competing risk is modest (i.e. ρ <0.3) or the magnitude of the effect is small.

9.4.2.3 Modifying competing events

When competing events modify instead of preventing the rates for other events, multivariate failure time models are appropriate. For example, different, but not mutually exclusive, types of disease progression could follow diagnosis of a chronic condition, as with diabetic patients who may suffer from retinopathy, leg ulceration, nephropathy, etc. One approach to model these parallel failure time data specifies only their marginal distributions by a Cox PH model, leaving their dependence structure completely unspecified.[12] The hazard ratios estimated from this model represent marginal effects of the exposures on each failure type. Alternative multivariate models assume that an unobserved variable underlies the correlations among the failure types.[13,14] The choice of distribution for this latent variable, however, may be too restrictive, with results not being robust to departures from the assumed distribution.[12] If the time sequence of these competing events is of interest instead, multistate models could be used (see later section).

9.4.2.4 Mixed competing events

When the competing events are a mixture of terminating and modifying events, e.g. when they involve both disease progression and death, various modelling choices are available. They could all be treated as terminating, and the univariable models discussed earlier could be used (as in CASCADE, 2002,[10] where the Fine and Gray model was used). Alternatively, multivariate models could be used. In the latter case, there is a choice of specifications of the follow-up time of terminating events: they can be censored when a modifying event occurs in order to study time to first event, or they can be left uncensored to model their marginal cause-specific hazards. Li and Lagakos[15] stress how the interpretation of either set of results requires care, as shown in the example below.

Birth weight and fatal and non-fatal myocardial infarction Consider again the males in the UBCoS study. This time we examine the effect of low birth weight (categorized as <3 kg versus ≥3 kg) on fatal and non-fatal MI, with deaths from other causes treated as an additional censoring factor. Depending on whether we study time to fatal MI, ignoring any intermediate non-fatal events (to obtain marginal cause-specific hazard ratios), or we censor the follow-up time when such intermediate events occur (to obtain hazard ratios for each failure type being the first event), different results are found (Table 9.5). There is some borderline evidence that low birth weight increases the marginal cause-specific hazard of fatal MI, but no evidence that it affects the hazard for fatal MI to be the first event.

9.4.3 Multiple events and shared frailty models

When the event of interest is recurrent, i.e. may occur more than once to the same individual, the term event history is often used. In event histories, the sequence of event times is likely to be correlated, either because certain individuals are more likely to experience the event, or because the occurrence of one such event increases the likelihood of another occurring. For example, certain children may be more likely to suffer from respiratory infections than others, and it could also be the case that each infection in turn lowers a child's ability to fight the next infection. Ignoring these correlations would lead to biased estimates of the precisions of all the model's parameters and can bias estimates in some circumstances. There are two possible approaches to deal with them: (1) some correction for these correlations is made to the estimated precisions; or (2) a more general model is assumed in which the correlations are considered as arising from individuals varying in their propensity for the events (i.e. in their so-called 'frailty'). The first approach uses robust methods such as GEE techniques (see Chapter 8). The second instead leads to generalization of the standard survival model (PH or AFT). If the rates for the first, second, … j[th] event

Table 9.5 Hazard ratios for the effect of low birth weight on fatal and non-fatal MI, and other causes of death estimated using different specifications of the Wei, Lin and Weissfeld model;[12] male UBCoS participants

Birth weight (kg)	Event type				
	Non-fatal MI			**Fatal MI**	
	HR	**95 per cent CI**		**HR**	**95 per cent CI**
Cause-specific analysis					
≥3	1	–		1	–
<3	1.19	1.0–1.41		1.15	0.97–1.36
First event analysis					
≥3	1	–		1	–
<3	1.19	1.0–1.41		1.01	0.79–1.28

MI = myocardial infarction; HR = hazard (rate) ratio; CI = confidence interval.

suffered by person i are denoted $\lambda_{i1}, \lambda_{i2}, \ldots \lambda_{ij}, \ldots$ the Cox regression PH model could be extended as in,

$$\lambda_{ij}\ (t;\ X_{1ij}) = \lambda(t;\ 0)\ \exp(\beta_0 + \beta_1\ X_{1ij} + v_i) \tag{9.7}$$

where v_i follows a pre-specified distribution and is constant for every individual but randomly varies between individuals.[16] The AFT model can be similarly extended. Both approaches are available in several well-known statistical packages.

9.4.4 Multivariate analysis of event and other response data

In Chapter 8, we illustrate the value of being able to analyse a profile of responses, whether they be different or repeated measures, or both. Event data could form one of these response variables. A particular example of interest is where the event outcome is relatively rare and so we wish to strengthen our findings by undertaking an analysis jointly with a surrogate variable, a variable whose variation may show evidence of effects that precede the event. Further interest arises where a risk factor is thought to have its impact on the event of interest through the surrogate variable (usually a biomarker), in other words the surrogate variable lies on the causal pathway and is a mediating variable.

We know of no life course example, but Skrondal and Rabe-Hesketh[17] provide an excellent illustration of this approach in a clinical context. In their example of prednisone treatment for liver cirrhosis, measures were taken of a biomarker that measured liver function (prothrombin). The data consist of biomarker data measured at various time points, together with a time of death or censoring for each subject. In their generalized mixed model approach, a growth curve (see Chapter 8) is fitted to the available biomarker data, which allows the estimation of a biomarker latent variable that serves to provide an estimate of the biomarker data for each subject at any time (not just those time points at which measures were taken). This latent biomarker score then contributes to the set of covariate values for each patient among each risk set being considered for death. Treatment is allowed to influence the biomarker, and both treatment and the biomarker can influence the death rate. Their conclusions were that while the treatment may have some modest beneficial direct effect on the death rate, it had a significant harmful effect on liver function, which in turn increased the death rate. When direct and indirect effects were summed, the results implied a non-significant harmful impact of treatment on death.

9.4.5 Multistate models

In survival analysis, the occurrence of an event may be considered to be a transition from one state (e.g. health) to another (e.g. death; Fig. 9.3). Generalizations of this setting could include an intermediate state, as shown in Fig. 9.4, or competing risks, as shown in

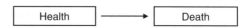

Fig. 9.3 A simple two-state model.

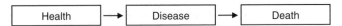

Fig. 9.4 A three-state model.

Fig. 9.5. More complex multistate models include transitions back to an earlier state, as in Fig. 9.6, for example.

The transition rates, i.e. the instantaneous probability of moving from one state to the next, are defined as the rates in the usual survival model, for example via a PH model. The estimation of multistate models that do not include back-transitions (i.e. as in Figs 9.3–9.5) can be carried out in stages, considering one pair of states at a time. Where back-transition is possible (as in Fig. 9.6), the fitting procedure is more complex. Although life course studies often involve investigations of pathways across discrete states, for example from manual to non-manual social class,[18] these models have seldom been used.

9.4.6 **Multivariate events**

A related development in event history analysis concerns the joint analysis of several parallel events, i.e. where one event does not censor the potential observation of the other event and where the events are not ordered on pathways as in multistate modelling. There are often two distinct concerns that motivate such analyses. The first concern is determining whether different kinds of events share or have distinct (measured) risk factors; the second concern is the potential mechanism for interdependency of these events. If only the first is of interest, then a marginal modelling approach, in which the interdependency is treated as a nuisance rather than of substantive interest, is often the most straight-forward.[12] For the second, multivariate survival models can be fitted once both the event time distributions and their correlation structure are specified.[19,20] Here results are likely to be sensitive to these choices and therefore subject-matter knowledge is essential.

In the past, correlation among disease occurrence that was observed within families, co-morbidity and the identification of shared risk factors have all given valuable insight into aetiological mechanisms. Statistical complexities have largely prevented this approach being exploited with respect to survival and event timing analysis, but progress has been made especially in the context where the dependency may have genetic origins.

Each of the univariate modelling methods described earlier can be generalized to deal with such data; Neale *et al.*[21] illustrate a generalization of an AFT model; Pickles and

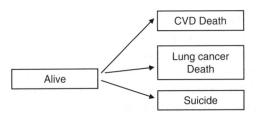

Fig. 9.5 A competing risks multistate model.

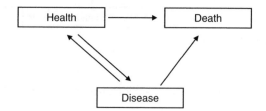

Fig. 9.6 A three-state model with recurrent disease.

Crouchley[22] and Yashin and Iachine[23] illustrate frailty modelling i.e. the extension of random effects modelling to PH survival models; and Pickles *et al.*[24] illustrate the fusion of covariance structure analysis with multivariate ordinal response modelling for censored data.

In principle, this approach could be used to examine the association between events quite distant in time across the life course, such as age at menarche and age at breast cancer occurrence.[25] As yet examples concern events that are more closely linked in time. Falcaro and Pickles[26] show how, among US adolescent twins, the association in the age of first tobacco smoking and alcohol consumption without parental permission are correlated, and that this correlation seems to arise, as a result not of shared environmental factors, but of shared genes. This is consistent with the view that, with essentially ubiquitous risks such as tobacco and alcohol availability, it is often the factors underlying risk-taking behaviour that determine variation in exposure within a particular population.

9.5 **Measurement errors in reporting event times**

Not all life course studies can be undertaken prospectively. Retrospective recall of events is notoriously slippery but, while there are a number of studies that show poor reliability and validity of poor retrospective measures, there are remarkably few studies of well-designed retrospective measurement. There are also circumstances where prospective measurement is problematic or impossible. Hence recall should not be discarded out of hand.[27] However, while there is an extensive literature on how study design and analysis can take account of errors of measurement for standard continuous and discrete data, there is very little guidance on errors in reported timing. Two common forms of error have been identified from survey studies of relatively frequent events. The first is a tendency for a systematic bias for events to be reported as occurring more recently than they did in fact occur. This has been called telescoping.[28] The second, which also generates as a side effect an additional apparent telescoping, is that random errors in timing increase the further ago the event occurred, i.e. heteroscedastic or non-constant variance measurement error. These measurement errors can be empirically investigated by comparing reports made at different times (including contemporaneous) but also by the use of current status data, meaning the information on the cross-sectional age of occurrence distribution available from the binary variable representing having experienced the event or not, a variable which is not itself subject to errors in reported timing.

Pickles *et al.*[29] proposed a model incorporating both these forms of error. Applied to data on maternal reports of the timing of breast development and menarche of their daughters, they showed that systematic telescoping predominated with the former, while heteroscedastic measurement error predominated with the latter. They attributed this difference to the nature of the events being reported, 'soft' events (often implicitly measured by some ill-defined threshold on a continuum) being especially prone to telescoping. However, telescoping is not universal. Rabe-Hesketh *et al.*[30] found evidence for secondary school boys to report ages of onset of smoking systematically earlier rather than later.

9.6 Time-varying confounders

9.6.1 What is a time-varying confounder?

The estimation of the effect of an exposure on an outcome of interest based on observational data always leads to the considerations of potential confounders, i.e. alternative explanations for the observed effects. Methods for assessing the presence of confounding in the exposure's estimated effect are available, e.g. stratification and multiple regression, although they depend on unverifiable assumptions on the relationships among exposure, confounders and outcome.[31] Further difficulties are encountered when the exposure varies with time. Mark and Robins[32] define a time-varying confounder Z as a variable whose current value predicts the outcome Y and whose past values predict the current value of the exposure of interest X. If past values of X also predict current values of Z, then standard survival analyses with time-updated exposures will give biased effect estimates whether the confounder is included or not. Chapter 8 gave the example where in HIV, CD4 count predicts outcome and influences subsequent treatment, and treatment influences both CD4 and outcome. Two alternative—but related—approaches have been suggested to deal with this. These are briefly sketched below.

9.6.2 Propensity score weighting (marginal structural models)

When we are concerned with a time-varying exposure $X(t)$, measured for example at times $t_0, t_1, \ldots, t_K$, and taking values $X_0, X_1, \ldots, X_K$, there are several ways in which its association with disease can be explored. For example, we may wish to estimate its cumulative effect. Considering for simplicity a logistic model for the outcome Y where cumulative X is the exposure of interest

$$\text{logit}\left[\Pr\left(Y \mid x_0, x_1, \quad , x_K\right)\right] = \beta_0 + \beta_1\left(\sum_{t=0}^{K} x_t\right) \tag{9.8}$$

$\exp(\beta_1)$ represents the odds ratio per unit increase in cumulative X. If X is binary, it represents the effect of one additional occurrence of observed $x = 1$.

If $Z(t)$ is a potential confounder—and Z is observed at times $t_0, t_1, \ldots, t_K$, where it takes values $Z_0, Z_1, \ldots, Z_K$, the routine approach would be to include the Zs as additional covariates. However, where the confounding variable has an effect on later values of X

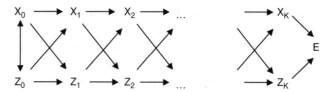

Fig. 9.7 Simplified diagram of correlated time-varying exposure X and confounder Z on an event outcome E.

(Fig. 9.7), then this approach may 'over-control' and the estimated cumulative effects of X will be biased. On the other hand, if $Z(t)$ is not controlled for, the estimated effect of $X(t)$ is also biased because it includes a component due to $Z(t)$.

We have seen in Chapter 8 that an alternative to the use of regression or stratification to control for confounders is to construct weights based on the propensity score, an approach derived from marginal structural models (MSMs; Robins *et al.*[33]). In that approach, the probability of being exposed or unexposed to X was related to the confounder Z, usually through a logistic model, and observations were weighted by the inverse of the predicted probabilities. With time-fixed variables, the weight is $w_i = 1/\mathrm{Pr}(X = x_i|Z = z_i)$. With time-varying variables, the denominator is the conditional probability that a subject experienced their particular exposure history $(X_0, X_1,...,X_K)$. This essentially corresponds to weighting the available observations so that in the weighted sample $X(t)$ is not correlated with $Z(t)$. However, with complex confounder and exposure history, these weights can have excessive variability, giving rise to inefficient estimates. To overcome this, stabilized weights have been suggested. In the simple case of a single period of exposure, this involves replacing $w_i = 1/\mathrm{Pr}(X = x_i|Z = z_i)$ by $sw_i = \mathrm{Pr}(X = x_i)/\mathrm{Pr}(X = x_i|Z = z_i)$. In the multiperiod case, the single exposure values and confounder vector are replaced by their histories over the preceding periods.

In the single period case, the practical advantage of the MSM approach over more routine covariate adjustment is not obvious. However, in the multiperiod time-dependent case, the advantage of the MSM approach is clear. Like stratification and covariate adjustment, MSM aims to control for Z_k because it is a confounder for later exposure values. However, unlike the other approaches, MSM does not control for the effects of Z_k that should be attributed to earlier values of the exposure because it is on its causal pathway.

9.6.3 G-estimation in survival analysis

An alternative approach to deal with time-dependent confounding is G-estimation. This is most easily described in the potential outcomes or counterfactual framework (see Chapter 8), in which subjects have two survival times, one when exposed and one when unexposed, only one of which is observed. If a subject is never exposed, the counterfactual survival time when continuously unexposed, U_i, is assumed to be equal to their observed failure time T_i multiplied by a factor, $\exp(\delta)$. With a time-varying exposure, we need to construct a binary indicator variable, $e(t)$, that distinguishes periods of exposures from those of non-exposure, where $e_i(t) = 1$ if subject i is exposed at time t, 0 otherwise. The adjustment factor to obtain the counterfactual survival time for an entirely unexposed history when subject i is exposed during certain periods identified by $e_i(t)$ is calculated as

$$U_{i\partial} = \int_0^{T_i} \exp\left[\delta e_i(t)\right] dt \qquad (9.9)$$

As usual, we may wish to adjust for the fact that exposure may be associated with J measured confounders $\{z_{ij}(t)\}$, for $j = 1, 2, \ldots, J$. G-estimation searches for the value of δ that gives no association between counterfactual survival time and observed exposure history, or more specifically a zero estimate for the parameter α in the following equation:

$$\text{Logit}\left[e_i(t)\right] = \alpha U_{i\partial} + \sum_j \beta_j z_{ij}(t) \qquad (9.10)$$

The process involves two steps. In step 1, a range of values of δ are considered, and for each value of δ the values of $\{U_{i\partial}\}$ are calculated from equation (9.9). Then in step 2, for each set of $\{U_{i\partial}\}$, the parameter α is estimated. The two values of δ that give the smallest (in magnitude) positive and negative values of α then provide the range of values for a new finer grained search for the δ that will give an estimate of α as close to zero as possible. A 95 per cent confidence interval (CI) for δ can be obtained as the values of δ that deliver logistic models with Wald statistics for $\alpha = 0$ with $P = 0.025$. Extensions beyond binary exposures appear possible, though conceptually clumsy.

We illustrate this approach with a simplified version of Sterne and Tilling's analysis of the effects of current smoking on occurrence of MI/death from coronary heart disease in the Caerphilly Prospective study (CaPS), taking into account the time-varying confounder of fibrinogen level, raised levels of which will be partly caused by previous smoking.[34] The data concern 1756 subjects followed for 14 years from baseline, with post-baseline examinations made on up to three occasions. In this time, there were 244 MI events and a large set of potential time-changing confounding variables, of which we use just age and elevated fibrinogen (fibrinogen above the 75th percentile).

A simple Weibull survival analysis suggested a highly significant effect of baseline smoking status that shortened time to MI, controlled for baseline fibrinogen and age [log-hazard ratio: -0.323 (95 per cent CI -0.545 to -0.099)] implying reduction by $100 \times [1 - \exp(-0.323)] = 100 \times (1 - 0.723) = 28$ per cent (Table 9.6). In contrast, an analysis using baseline, lagged and current values for smoking and the confounders gave results that suggested no significant role for smoking, particularly in the case of current smoking. The worry is that the effects of smoking on coronary heart disease have been attributed to fibrinogen, which is acting as a mediator for these effects and not just a confounder as usually understood.

Adopting the G-estimation approach, we search for the value of δ that, when used to generate counterfactual survival times, i.e. a survival time as if the person had always been a non-smoker, gives times that at each occasion of measurement are not associated with actual smoking, once the effect of age and fibrinogen are controlled for. Using the *Stata* procedure stgest,[35] the G-estimate of δ was found to be 0.294 (95 per cent CI

Table 9.6 Estimated log hazard ratios (HR) for smoking measured at different times controlled for different potential confounders

Smoking measured at:	Controlled for baseline confounders		Controlled for concurrent confounders		Controlling by G-estimation	
	log HR	95 per cent CI	log HR	95 per cent CI	log HR	95 per cent CI
Baseline	−0.323	−0.545, −0.099	−0.117	−0.497, 0.264	–	–
Lagged	–	–	−0.199	−0.632, 0.235	–	–
Current	–	–	−0.001	−0.335, 0.332	−0.294	−0.426, −0.073

CI = confidence interval.

0.073–0.426), implying smoking-unexposed counterfactual times of $\exp(\delta) = 1.342$, or 34 per cent longer, and that for the log hazards ratio for current smoking to be −0.294, implying a causal survival hazard ratio for current smoking of 0.745 (95 per cent CI 0.653–0.930). The G-estimation has provided a single estimate of the causal effect of smoking that has properly taken account the confounding due to fibrinogen. Clearly this revised analysis has strikingly different clinical and public health implications. More routine application of G-estimation is complicated by the need to address censoring properly (which has not been done here) and the fact that uninformative censoring can become informative on the counterfactual time scale.

9.7 Typologies of life course pathways

When events can frequently recur over time, it is often the pattern of rates over successive time periods that may be of primary interest. Possible examples include the pattern of onset and recurrence of epileptic seizures, ischaemic events or commission of crimes (e.g. Naglin and Tremblay[36]). As this type of data is usually collected at regular intervals, data may consist of sequences of binary indicators of whether the event had or had not been experienced between observation times. Thus extensions of the PO model are appropriate, where the correlation among the repeated observations on the same subjects is accounted for, for example, with models akin to growth curve models for repeated binary responses (see Chapter 8). However, such an approach sometimes tends to impose more structure on the patterns of variation in rate than available theory can justify. In these circumstances, discrete random effects and latent class methods provide a more flexible alternative. This may be best regarded as a form of model-based cluster analysis used to identify typologies of variation in rate over time.

We illustrate this approach using the data from the British 1946 national birth cohort on attainment and loss of bladder control as represented in six binary status measures obtained at ages 4, 6, 8, 9, 11 and 15 and published in Croudace et al.[37] Our analyses are based on the (corrected) published table and do not (though could) take account of the sample stratification weights. The objective is to identify distinct 'bladder control trajectories', or latent classes, and the factors that might be associated with them.

Let p_k be the probability of being in latent class k, with the sum of these probabilities over all, say K, classes summing to 1. Given that an individual belongs to class k, in an unstructured model the probability of a positive event ($y = 1$) being recorded for subject i at time t is given by

$$\text{logit}[\Pr(y_{it} = 1|k)] = e_{tk} \qquad (9.11)$$

The trajectory of class k is thus represented by a set of outcome rates (on a logistic scale), one for each occasion of measurement $\{e_{1k}, e_{2k}, e_{3k}, e_{4k}, e_{5k}, e_{6k}\}$, shared by all subjects that belong to the same class. In the original paper, this model was fitted using Mplus.[38] Here we estimate the same model using the *Stata* procedure gllamm (www.gllamm.org).[35] A sequence of models is fitted, each one having one more latent class than the preceding model, and the relative fit of the models are compared. In some cases, there is a maximum number of classes that can be fitted, say M. Models with more than this number of classes fit no better but merely split one or more of the M classes into two or more identical subclasses. The model with M classes is described as the non-parametric maximum likelihood estimator (NPMLE). Although there is some interest in finding this model, its existence can be incorrectly understood to imply that there does exist a discrete typology with M types. Both statistical theory and simulation show that the NPMLE exists even when the underlying population is drawn from a distribution of continuously varying trajectories. In other words, a typology based on a finite number of classes may simply be a good way of representing variation, discrete or continuous, in the population. The classes may provide a useful classification, but it cannot be interpreted that each and every individual conforms to just one of these types. The classes represent a good approximation given the available data. In practice, the objective is usually some compromise between parsimony, i.e. wanting a small number of classes, and fitting the data well enough. In addition, there may be theoretical interest in the possible existence of a particular kind of class. For example, in criminology, there has been particular interest in a class with persistent and early onset antisocial behaviour. In our case, while the four-class solution gave a marked improvement in fit compared with the three-class solution, the improvement offered by a five-class solution, while statistically significant, was gained at the expense of undesirable complexity. The four-trajectory class solution was chosen and is presented in Fig. 9.8. The original authors attached the labels 'normal' to class 3, 'persistent' to class 4, 'chronic' to class 2 and 'onset' to class 1.

These trajectory classes have been defined without reference to potential risk factors. However, the association of trajectory class membership with risk factors can be examined using posterior class membership probabilities or by extending the model to allow class probabilities to vary. In the former approach, we calculate the posterior probability $\Pr(k = c|y_{i1}, y_{i2}, y_{i3}, y_{i4}, y_{i5}, y_{i6})$ obtained using Bayes' theorem as the probability of the observed response history for class c, $\Pr(y_{i1}, y_{i2}, y_{i3}, y_{i4}, y_{i5}, y_{i6}| k = c)$, divided by the sum of such probabilities for all latent classes $k = 1, \ldots, K$. Tabulating the means of these probabilities by sex gave the results in Table 9.7, indicating the normal class to be more common in girls, with all abnormal classes, especially the chronic class 2, being less common.

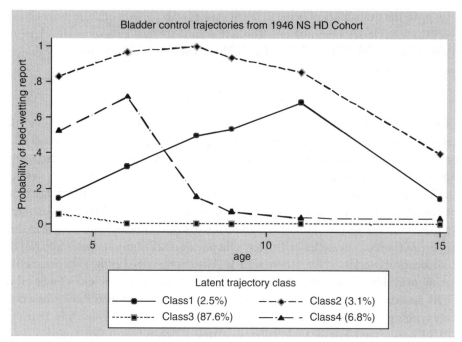

Fig. 9.8 Four bladder control trajectory classes from UK 1946 NSHD birth cohort (class 1 = onset, 2 = chronic, 3 = normal and 4 = persistent).

To implement the second approach, the model is extended to allow

$$\text{logit}[\Pr(y_{it} = 1|k] = a_0 + a_{1k} \times \text{sex}_i \tag{9.12}$$

giving $K - 1$ parameters to describe differences in rates by sex as in the standard model for effects on a directly observed multicategory outcome, namely the multinomial logit model. This extended model gives a 4 df likelihood ratio chi-square reduction of 22.72, indicating a significant improvement in model fit. With class 4 as the reference class, estimated log-odds coefficients for sex were 0.21 (SE 0.38) for class 1, −0.38 (SE 0.32) for class 2, and 0.50 (SE 0.21) for class 3. The tabulated posterior probabilities from this model were similar to those without sex as a covariate (Table 9.8).

The overall event probability at each age is obtained by summing the event probabilities of each trajectory class (see Fig. 9.8), weighting that sum by the size of that class.

Table 9.7 Distribution of boys and girls by bladder control trajectory classes: simple model without sex difference in prior probabilities (class 1 = onset, 2 = chronic, 3 = normal and 4 = persistent)

	Class 1	Class 2	Class 3	Class 4
Boys	2.8%	4.1%	85.5%	7.7%
Girls	2.1%	2.0%	90.0%	5.9%

Table 9.8 Distribution of boys and girls by bladder control trajectory classes: extended model with allowance for sex difference in prior probabilities (class 1 = onset, 2 = chronic, 3 = normal and 4 = persistent)

	Class 1	Class 2	Class 3	Class 4
Boys	2.8%	4.1%	85.5%	7.7%
Girls	2.2%	1.8%	91.1%	4.9%

Our analyses show that these weights will be different for boys and girls, and so give different overall rates by age. However, unlike the more traditional PH event models, there is nothing in these models that imposes a restriction that the difference in age-specific rates (or any function of them) between boys and girls should remain constant. Boys could be at higher risk at some points and at lower risk at others.

9.8 Discussion

As we have seen, survival and event history analysis has some distinctive problems, terminology, methods and uses. While a process of familiarization is necessary, there is clearly considerable scope for the application of these methods within a life course framework. In every case, such an application requires very careful consideration to allow the simplest appropriate analysis to be undertaken. We have emphasized that in spite of its distinctive features, users of event analysis need to continue to be alert to all the usual problems of confounding, sample selection, and so on. We emphasize this point because the complexities of life course research questions and data, the added complications arising from time-varying exposures and the expectation of time-varying effects, correlation among events, frailty and imperfect measurement—to name but some—all conspire to call for more and more modelling complexity, leading to levels of sophistication that are at the boundary of what we can currently do. Our advice is to first deal with each problem separately, for example by breaking the analyses into consecutive time windows, and to compare results obtained using different approaches, before attempting to bring all components together.

Further reading

Clayton D, Hills M (1993). *Statistical models for epidemiology.* Oxford University Press, Oxford.

Crowder JM (2001). *Classical competing risks.* CRC Press, London.

Hougaard P (2000). *Analysis of multivariate survival data.* Springer-Verlag, New York.

Machin D, Cheung Y-B, Parmar M (2006). *Survival analysis a practical approach.* Wiley, Chichester.

Mark SD, Robins JM (1993). Estimating the causal effect of smoking cessation in the presence of confounding factors using a rank preserving structural failure time model. *Statistics in Medicine* 12, 1605–1628.

Nagin DF, Tremblay RE (1999). Trajectories of boys' physical aggression, opposition, and hyperactivity on the path to physically violent and non-violent juvenile delinquency. *Child Development* 70, 1181–1196.

References

1. Breslow NE, Day N (1987). *Statistical methods in cancer research, Vol II—the design and analysis of cohort studies.* IARC, Lyon.

2. Clayton D, Hills M (1993). *Statistical models for epidemiology.* Oxford University Press: Oxford.

3. Cox DR (1972). Regression models and life tables. *Journal of the Royal Statistical Society B* 34, 187–203.

4. Bennett S (1983). Analysis of survival data by the proportional odds model. *Statistics in Medicine* 2, 273–277.

5. D'Agostino RB, Lee ML, Belanger AJ, Cupples LA, Anderson K, Kannel WB (1990). Relation of pooled logistic regression to time dependent Cox regression analysis: the Framingham Heart Study. *Statistics in Medicine* 9, 1501–1515.

6. Fogelman K (1983). *Growing up in Great Britain.* MacMillan, London.

7. Gooley TA, Leisenring W, Crowley J, Storer BE (1999). Estimation of failure probabilities in the presence of competing risks: new representations of old estimators. *Statistics in Medicine* 18, 695–706.

8. Lunn M, McNeil D (1995). Applying Cox regression to competing risks. *Biometrics* 51, 524–532.

9. Fine JP, Gray RJ (1999). A proportional hazards model for the subdistribution of a competing risk. *Journal of the American Statistical Association* 94, 496–509.

10. CASCADE Collaboration (2002). Changes over calendar time in the risk of specific first AIDS-defining events following HIV seroconversion, adjusting for competing risks. *International Journal of Epidemiology* 31, 951–958.

11. Tai B-C, De Stavola BL, de Gruttola V, Gebski V, Machin D. (2007). First event or marginal estimation of cause-specific hazards for analysing correlated multivariate failure time data? *Statistics in Medicine* in press.

12. Wei LJ, Lin DY, Weissfeld L (1989). Regression analysis of multivariate incomplete failure time data by modeling marginal distributions. *Journal of the American Statistical Association* 84, 1065–1073.

13. Clayton DG, Cuzick J (1985). Multivariate generalizations of the proportional hazards model. *Journal of the Royal Statistical Society B* 148, 82–117.

14. Hougaard P (1986). Life table methods for heterogeneous populations: distributions describing the heterogeneity. *Biometrika* 71, 75–83.

15. Li QH, Lagakos SW (1997). Use of the Wei–Lin–Weissfeld method for the analysis of a recurring and a terminating event. *Statistics in Medicine* 16, 925–940.

16. Keiding N, Andersen PK, Klein JP (1997). The role of frailty models and accelerated failure time models in describing heterogeneity due to omitted covariates. *Statistics in Medicine* 16, 215–224.

17. Skrondal A, Rabe-Hesketh S (2004). *Generalized latent variable modeling: multilevel, longitudinal and structural equation models.* Chapman and Hall/CRC, Boca Raton, FL.

18. Singh-Manoux A, Ferrie JE, Chandola T, Marmot M (2004). Socioeconomic trajectories across the life course and health outcomes in mid life: evidence for the accumulation hypothesis? *International Journal of Epidemiology* 33, 1072–1079.

19. Lawless JF (1987). Regression methods for Poisson process data. *Journal of the American Statistical Association* 82, 808–815.

20. Prentice RL, Williams BJ, Peterson AV (1981). On the regression analysis of multivariate failure time data. *Biometrika* 68, 373–379.

21. Neale MC, Eaves LJ, Hewitt JK, MacLean CJ, Meyer JM, Kendler KS (1989). Analyzing the relationship between age at onset and risk to relatives. *American Journal of Human Genetics* 45, 226–239.

22. Pickles A, Crouchley R (1994). Generalizations and applications of frailty models for survival and event data. *Statistical Methods in Medical Research* 3, 263–278.

23. Yashin IA, Iachine IA (1995). Genetic analysis of durations: correlated frailty model applied to survival of Danish twins. *Genetic Epidemiology* 12, 529–538.

24. Pickles A, Crouchley R, Simonoff E, Eaves L, Meyer J, Rutter M, *et al.* (1994). Survival models for developmental genetic data: age of onset of puberty and antisocial behavior in twins. *Genetic Epidemiology* 11, 155–170.

25. De Stavola BL, dos Santos Silva I, McCormack V, Hardy RJ, Kuh DJ, Wadsworth MEJ (2004). Childhood growth and breast cancer. *American Journal of Epidemiology* 159, 671–682.

26. Falcaro M, Pickles A (2007). A flexible model for multivariate interval-censored survival times with complex correlation structure. *Statistics in Medicine* 26, 663–680.

27. Hardt J, Rutter M (2004). Validity of adult retrospective reports of adverse childhood experiences: review of the evidence. *Journal of Child Psychology and Psychiatry* 45, 260–274.

28. Huttenlocher J, Hedges LV, Bradburn NM (1990). Reports of elapsed time: bounding and rounding processes in estimation. *Journal of Experimental Psychology—Learning, Memory and Cognition* 16, 196–213.

29. Pickles A, Pickering K, Taylor C (1996). Reconciling recalled dates of developmental milestones, events and transitions: a mixed GLM with random mean and variance functions. *Journal of the Royal Statistical Society A* 159, 225–234.

30. Rabe-Hesketh S, Yang S, Pickles A (2001). Multilevel models for censored and latent responses. *Statistical Methods in Medical Research* 10, 409–427.

31. Hernan MA, Hernandez-Diaz S, Werler MM, Mitcell AA. (2002). Causal knowledge as a prerequisite for confounding evaluation: an application to birth defects epidemiology. *American Journal of Epidemiology* 155, 176–184.

32. Mark SD, Robins JM (1993). Estimating the causal effect of smoking cessation in the presence of confounding factors using a rank preserving structural failure time model. *Statistics in Medicine* 12, 1605–1628.

33. Robins JM, Hernan MA, Brumback B (2000). Marginal structural models and causal inference in epidemiology. *Epidemiology* 11, 550–560.

34. Sterne JAC, Tilling K (2002). G-estimation of causal effects, allowing for time-varying confounding. *Stata Journal* 2, 164–182.

35. StataCorp (2005). *Stata statistical software: release 9*. StataCorp LP, College Station, TX.

36. Nagin DF, Tremblay RE (2001). Parental and early childhood predictors of persistent physical aggression in boys from kindergarden to high school. *Archives of General Psychiatry* 58, 389–394.

37. Croudace TJ, Jarvelin MR, Wadsworth ME, Jones PB (2003). Developmental typology of trajectories to nighttime bladder control: epidemiologic application of longitudinal latent class analysis. *American Journal of Epidemiology* 157, 834–842.

38. Muthen LK, Muthen BO (2003). *Mplus users guide*. Muthen & Muthen, Los Angeles, CA.

Afterword and conclusions

Andrew Pickles, Barbara Maughan and
Michael Wadsworth

The present state of life course epidemiology

Life course epidemiology remains in its infancy. Even the mapping of conceptual models
to data requirements is still to be completed, and many years of ingenious measurement,
imaginative design and analysis, research investment and effort are required before it is
likely to fulfil its promise.

The first volume in this series assembled an extensive overview of the form and potential contribution of life course epidemiology to the full range of disease areas.[1] Across
disease areas, life course epidemiology and the long-term historical perspective that it
fosters are transforming the way we approach many research questions and public health
policy challenges. The life course perspective has concentrated thinking about how to
measure long-term exposures, for example to poverty; has encouraged the development
of new ideas and models to account for the association of exposures with outcomes, such
as the hypothalamic–pituitary–adrenal (HPA) model; and has played an essential part in
the development of genetically informed research design. In public health, life course
thinking challenges established approaches to intervention and prevention, and new
studies are now required to test whether intervention earlier in the risk pathway is indeed
effective. As chronic diseases and states of mental and physical frailty associated with ageing become increasingly prevalent in many societies, the design of effective prevention
strategies in public health is pressing.

While there are tremendous opportunities for life course research, there remains, nevertheless, a wide range of challenges to be addressed. This volume has attempted to provide
an overview of both the opportunities and the challenges.

Life course, developmental processes and gene–environment interplay

Enormous strides are being made in understanding developmental processes, particularly with respect to biology. An issue highlighted in Chapters 3 and 5 is that currently the
integration of social environmental exposures into these developmental processes is
often quite limited. Chapter 5 highlights the need for transductional mechanisms that
link these exposures to a biological response or adaptation made by the individual, which
then may carry the longer term risk. Perhaps not surprisingly, this has proven comparatively easy to do for psycho-social health, and these same mechanisms may have a more
widespread impact on physical health. This would seem to be the case for early experience

influencing the development of the HPA system, which may then influence not just anxiety but many other aspects of health. Similarly, suboptimal early allergen or viral exposure appears to result in miscalibration of the immune system, which may then present a longer term vulnerability. In both examples, the organism could be regarded as 'learning' about or needing to 'learn' from the early environment, and this may be a model that applies more generally.

Awareness of the need to integrate genetic and environmental influences, while well advanced in some areas such as psychiatry, cancer and immunology, is much less complete elsewhere. In mainstream epidemiology, there remains both enthusiasm[2] but also considerable scepticism as to the likely importance of gene–environment interactions or, more particularly, our ability to find them.[3] One reason may be that the kinds of environmental factors considered are less obviously heterogeneous or modifiable. While a 'psychosocial' exposure such as parental divorce may typically be disadvantageous, it is also obvious that for some children it could be beneficial—most notably, perhaps, when it involves release from a discordant household or separation from an abusing parent. It is less clear if there are any circumstances or individuals for whom exposures such as smoking could deliver a health benefit. With cross-over effects or interactions that lead to a reversal of the direction of effect, for which main effects are non-significant, analysis for interactions are essential to identify the high risk genes. However, for risk factors such as smoking where reversal of direction interactions are implausible, then in the search for the contributing gene to a change in level (as opposed to direction) interaction, there is no or little gain in power to be had from incorporating into the analysis the interaction and, with several environmental measures, a considerable cost with respect to exacerbating the multiple testing problem. From this point of view, searching for interactions at this stage of the game is often seen as unnecessary, and those gene–environment interactions that have been identified are viewed as almost certainly false positives. The contrary point of view is that in terms of developmental and evolutionary theory, such interactions must be common; that there are overwhelmingly convincing proof of concept animal models; and that if we are interested in understanding the mechanisms, then it is the interaction that must be the scientific target. The disciplinary differences in perspective may be valid, but perhaps an appropriate generalist position is a sceptical allegiance to the pro-interactions school when backed by cogent prior theory and evidence as to its plausibility. However, we should acknowledge that interactions are not a universal expectation, that the risk of false positives is very high, and findings will require replication from large studies.[3]

Chronic methodological problems and solutions

Life course research is not immune from the loss of faith that has afflicted epidemiology more generally over its ability to deliver robust and valid findings. Even after some years, we are yet to understand fully why large and prestigious observational studies identified hormone replacement therapy as beneficial for breast cancer and heart disease while randomized trials found clear evidence of harm (discussed in Chapter 8). Some proposed answers, such as that the harmful risk is short term, or that there is a need to control for socio-economic confounding over the lifetime, may suggest that life course epidemiology, with its emphasis on long-term measurement and developmental change, may contain the means to resolve this conundrum and perhaps help re-establish the position of epidemiology more generally. While there may be an element of truth in this suggestion, it pre-supposes an ability to apply epidemiological methods to a standard that the research community has previously achieved only rarely. Rigour needs to be maintained from the stage of design, through sample selection and measurement, to analysis and reporting. While one could press for near perfection at every stage, this would, in fact, be both impractical and ineffi-cient. Instead, we need to assess the quality of the whole package. There are circumstances where we can trade the increased random measurement error of a cheaper but less reliable measure for a larger sample, provided our set of measures is complemented by methods of analysis that can deal with measurement error. This places still further emphasis on the importance of properly functioning interdisciplinary teams, to formulate studies with a sufficient grasp of the whole theory, design, measurement and analysis process to enable the right cost-effective and pragmatic decisions to be made.

We have also seen (in Chapters 2–5) the critical role of scientific imagination, most obvious in the identification of the natural experiments, interventions and instrumental variables that can transform our ability to deal with residual confounding. The need to bring ideas from experimental and observational approaches together goes beyond merely proposing intervention. Epidemiology generally still pays insufficient attention to the importance of objectivity within the experimental tradition. The Campbellian tradi-tion of quasi-experiments in the social sciences emphasized a range of experimental practices that improved validity and which could be adapted to the design of observa-tional studies.[4] Many of these relate to objectivity, an issue raised at the end of Chapter 8 as a criterion that should also be applied to analysis. Thus while greater effort should continue to be expended to ensure blindness in order to assist in bias reduction at the stage of data collection, so too greater effort should be made to pre-specify as far as pos-sible any plan for analysis, and to undertake as much exploratory analysis as possible without access to (and thus blind to) outcome data. Broadly interpreted, this requires a change in the culture of epidemiology, one in which if each step is not actually moni-tored by independent reviewers, then it is undertaken as far as possible as if it were.

Review, synthesis and collaboration

Mention of replication inevitably leads on to the more general question of assessing consis-tency of findings. To date, life course epidemiology remains very much at the stage of nar-rative reviews, with formalized meta-analysis of effects still rare. Perhaps the major reason is that we are still exploring mechanisms, and have too slight an evidence base to define a single target parameter confidently in order to justify quantitative review. However, we have elsewhere expressed concern as to the variability and conceptual lack of precision in the supposedly causal effect estimates that many studies provide. Further clarification and resolution of this issue is a pre-requisite for us to progress to more systematic synthesis.

Achieving this objective would also be much enhanced by efforts in harmonization of measurement (discussed in Chapter 4). However, given the constraints on participant measurement burden that all studies face, harmonization may come only at the expense of novelty and improvement—something that must also be avoided. Chapter 4 raised the use of calibration samples (inside or external to a main study), samples that receive multiple instruments, and thus enable mapping of one measure, or different versions of a measure, onto another. The combined data can be conceived as a missing data problem, and tackled using the methods of Chapter 7, such as multiple imputation,[5] or can be approached using instrumental variable methods introduced in Chapter 8. These methods are as much relevant to the pooling of studies to yield a common estimated effect as they are to the pooling of studies where the focus is on their difference, i.e. comparative studies.

The future

Chapter 4 highlighted the range of major large-scale health data resources that are or will shortly be available to the life course researcher. Social science-based life course studies are also increasing in size and number, and increasingly include biological measures.[6] It is tempting to think that with so much still to investigate and analyse, there is no need to design and initiate any new studies—in particular birth cohorts. How could we possibly need a new birth cohort when we now have them by the handful? Moreover, we know the years that must pass before they can deliver statistical power with respect to many health outcomes, and the much increased pace of scientific development must mean that measurement protocols quickly become old-fashioned and irrelevant to current science. This viewpoint must be taken seriously, but we consider there are strong counter-arguments. In many societies, social and health environments have been transformed over the last century; in others, such transformation has been achieved in just a few decades—something that presents both challenges but also experimental opportunities. With such external change, research questions necessarily change too. Whereas our current concerns are with childhood weight trajectories and outcomes such as diabetes, we will soon be able to explore the potential early risk factors and mechanisms for late-onset diseases such as Alzheimer's. This is likely to highlight areas of measurement, such as imaging, that are poorly covered by even the most recent of current studies. We can thus argue that we need new studies that start out with a range of novel measures to tackle these novel questions. By itself, however, this is unlikely to suffice. We must also recognize that much of our comparative wealth of current data arises not from the foresight of previous generations of scientific committees, but often from the obsessions of individual scientists, who persuaded and cajoled the sceptics into thinking that there were potential short-term benefits to be had from each data collection proposal, until each study had attained sufficient scientific momentum to advance. It is likely that novel measurement alone will not deliver an irresistible case. We will need to continue to be opportunistic, both with respect to funding opportunities and with respect to the possibilities that become available through building on administrative systems, traditionally strong in Nordic countries, but becoming more widespread as e-infrastructure spreads.

In addition, we may need to explore more imaginative designs than we have up to now. Of these, studies with data missing by design (discussed in Chapter 4 and 7) are currently among the most promising. Missing data by design is entirely different from the missing data that we usually encounter day to day, in that we know the factors that accounted for its missingness. As a consequence, we are able to apply adjustment methods at the analysis stage that we know, rather than merely hope, are correct. What does data missing by design offer? It can enable (1) expensive and detailed measurement, e.g. imaging, to be focused on the subset of individuals likely to be of most interest and to offer most power for estimating some key effect; (2) reduction in the measurement burden, since not all individuals need receive the whole measurement protocol; (3) reduction in cross-contamination (bias), where use of one measure may influence the result obtained from a subsequent measure; and (4) the use of adaptive measurement that reduces irrelevant assessment. The potential gains from combining these ideas are yet to be fully exploited in the design of life course studies.

A key advance in measurement that would transform the kinds of studies we might undertake would be the ability to measure, without excessive intrusion, tissue-specific gene suppression/expression. The animal models that have elaborated epigenetic mechanisms described in Chapters 1 and 5 immediately suggest the urgent need for such studies in early human development as soon as the technology allows. Moreover, the very limited data we have from identical twins indicate that genetic expression continues to diverge well into mature adulthood. Epigenetic phenomena may thus be contributing to disease processes not only through the impact in early development but also through continuing change throughout the life course; that raises the possibility of modifying and possibly reversing epigenetic status.

The essential task is to continue to develop fully interdisciplinary research and the development of a portfolio of studies with extensive biosocial measurement and varied design, so that the impact of interacting developmental, environmental and genetic effects on the risk of and resilience to illness and the processes of ageing can be precisely evaluated.

References

1. Kuh D, Ben Shlomo Y, ed. (2004). *A life course approach to chronic disease epidemiology*, 2nd edn. Oxford University Press, Oxford.
2. Todd JA (2006). Statistical false positives or true disease pathways. *Nature Genetics* 38, 731–733.
3. Shadish WR, Cook TD, Campbell DT (2001). *Experimental and quasi-experimental designs for generalized causal inference*. Houghton Mifflin, Boston.
4 Marchini J, Donnelly P, Cardon LR (2005). Genome-wide strategies for detecting multiple loci that influence complex diseases. *Nature Genetics* 37, 413–417.
5. Collishaw S, Maughan B, Goodman R, Pickles A (2004). Time trends in adolescent mental health. *Journal of Child Psychology and Psychiatry* 45, 1350–1362.
6. Finch CE, Vaupel JW, Kinsella K, ed. (2001). *Cells and surveys—should biological measures be included in social research?* National Academic Press, Washington, DC.

Index

Note: page numbers in bold refer to figures and tables